The Clinical Laboratory Assistant/ Phlebotomist

by Jacquelyn R. Marshall, BA, MT, MA

Clinical Allied Healthcare Series

Kay Cox-Stevens, RN, MA
Series Editor

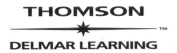

THOMSON

DELMAR LEARNING

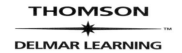

THOMSON
DELMAR LEARNING

The Clinical Laboratory Assistant/Phlebotomist
by Jacquelyn R. Marshall, BA, MT, MA

Series Editor and Executive Director:
Kay Cox-Stevens

Senior Editor and Project Coordinator:
Valerie Harris

Editors:
Karen Bijlsma and Cory Jones

Production Artists:
Kristen Farish, Valerie Harris, Karen Bijlsma, and Cory Jones

Illustrators:
Alan Borie, Samuel Benge, and Valerie Harris
Additional Graphics obtained from the LifeART™ Collections from Techpool Studios, Inc., Cleveland, OH.
Selected photographs courtesy Gazelle Technologies, Inc. and PhotoDisc, Inc. Used under license.

Cover Design:
Harris Graphics

Library of Congress Catalog Card Number
98-070063

ISBN 0-89262-434-5

NOTICE TO THE READER

Dedication

This book is dedicated to Deborah Frey, who, as a long-term clinical laboratory professional, has never compromised her devotion to providing the highest standard of patient service.

Contents

Acknowledgements

As a clinical laboratory technologist for over twenty years and a supervisor of clinical laboratory assistants/phlebotomists, I have a great deal of respect for the position of clinical laboratory assistant/phlebotomist. I began my clinical laboratory career in this position, realizing immediately the importance of treating the patients with respect and possessing the necessary skills to make blood drawing as painless and possible.

I would like to thank those clinical laboratory professionals that I have observed over the last twenty-three years who have dedicated their careers to serving the patient above all other considerations.

Kay Cox-Stevens, RN, MA and Series Editor, for conceiving this Clinical Allied Healthcare Series and for her insightful suggestions about this textbook.

Harold Haase, Publisher of Career Publishing, Inc. and his hardworking staff for having a vision of creating entry-level training programs for many areas of the healthcare profession.

The staff of Mt. Diablo Hospital Medical Center Clinical Laboratory in Concord, California for their cooperation and patience in allowing photographs to be taken while they were in the midst of one of their busiest times of the year. Special thanks go to Penny Beitler and Debbie Frey.

Glenda Willerford for her excellent photographic skills and her willingness to buy a new Nikon camera to provide well-focused pictures for this textbook.

Guy B. Mulder, DVM, MS, the Senior Veterinarian of University Laboratory Animal Resources at the University of California, Irvine for his careful review of Chapter Thirteen and his helpful suggestions for obtaining blood samples from animals.

Introduction

To work in the medical field is to make a real contribution to your fellow man. This is a career that will ask much of your mind and heart and give much in return. The satisfaction gained from calming a frightened child or brightening the day of a lonely patient will enrich you. The pride felt will be lasting when your observations and skills someday help to save a patient's life. This is a career where you can really make a difference!

Some of you have already made a decision to seek a career in some area of healthcare. Some of you are just exploring your options. Everything you learn will build a foundation of skills and knowledge, so learn well. Become competent in everything you are taught along the way and be your own task master. We all must be responsible for our own education. If at some point you discover you didn't learn a skill well enough, go back and practice until you do. Remember, some day a patient's life may depend on you and your mastery of what you are taught.

Today's healthcare industry places many demands on care givers. We must keep costs down, document everything we do, and have more knowledge and skills than ever before because of new technology. This textbook series was designed to help you build a sound foundation of knowledge and provide many opportunities for cross-training. The more you can learn, the better. Always remember, however, to practice the art, the science, and the SPIRIT of your new career. Good luck!

Kay Cox-Stevens, RN, MA
Series Editor

Contributors

About the Author
Jacquelyn Marshall, BA, MT, MA, has worked as a clinical laboratory assistant/ phlebotomist and clinical medical technologist for over twenty years. She began her medical career working as a clinical laboratory assistant for three years. During that period, she went back to college to become a clinical laboratory technologist. In one of her positions as a clinical laboratory technologist she served as supervisor of clinical laboratory assistants.

Mrs. Marshall has served as a science curriculum writer/consultant for the Center for Occupational Research and Development (CORD) in Austin Texas. She also has been a technical medical curriculum writer for the State of California, developing Model Curriculum Standards for Vocational Health Occupations throughout California. She also has taught a vocational clinical medical assistant/phlebotomist course for four years.

Mrs. Marshall currently is a free-lance medical writer and is author of seven textbooks, including *Fundamental Skills for the Clinical Laboratory Professional*. She also has developed several instructor's guides, and has edited and contributed to three medical series.

About the Series Editor
Kay Cox-Stevens, RN, MA conceived this textbook series, and recruited and coordinated the authors in the development of each of their texts. She is the author of *Being a Health Unit Coordinator,* and the editor of a Medical-Clerical Textbook Series for Brady. Before entering education, she worked in medical/surgical and critical care nursing and in the inservice department as a clinical instructor.

Formerly a Professional Development Contract Consultant for special projects and curriculum development for the California Department of Education, Professor Cox-Stevens has also served as chairperson of the California Health Careers Statewide Advisory Committee, and been a Master Trainer for Health Careers Teacher Training through California Polytechnic University of Pomona. She also is a founding member of the National Association of Health Unit Coordinators. Professor Cox-Stevens is currently Program Coordinator of the Medical Assistant Program at Saddleback College in Mission Viejo, California, and operates her consulting business, Achiever's Development Enterprises.

Editor's Note

I would like to take this opportunity to thank the authors of this series. Their dedication and sense of mission made it a joy to work on this challenging project.

I would also like to express my sincere gratitude to the staff of Career Publishing, Inc. and most particularly to Valerie Harris, Senior Editor, for her professional and talented assistance throughout. I also would like to express my appreciation to Harold Haase, Publisher, for his enthusiasm for this project and for his humanistic approach to education.

Kay Cox-Stevens, RN, MA
Series Editor

Chapter One
Introduction to the Career of Clinical Laboratory Assistant/Phlebotomist

Objectives

After completing this chapter, you should be able to do the following:

1. Define and correctly spell each of the key terms.

2. Describe several tasks a clinical laboratory assistant/phlebotomist might perform.

3. Explain the role of the clinical laboratory in a healthcare facility.

4. List locations of various types of clinical laboratories.

5. Identify several job titles associated with the clinical laboratory.

6. Identify at least five potential employers for the clinical laboratory assistant/phlebotomist.

7. Explain why cross-training is important in the healthcare environment.

8. Name four organizations that provide continuing education for the clinical laboratory assistant/phlebotomist.

Key Terms

- autopsy
- clinical laboratory manager
- clinical laboratory technologist
- cross-training
- inpatient

- outpatient
- pathologist
- phlebotomist
- sputum
- stool

Introduction

phlebotomist: Also known as the clinical laboratory assistant/phlebotomist; a clinical laboratory employee whose duties include obtaining blood specimens, requisitioning laboratory tests in the computer, transporting specimens, preparing specimens for testing, and performing testing in different areas of the clinical laboratory.

Today's **clinical laboratory assistant/phlebotomist** plays a vital role in the **clinical laboratory.** One of his or her most important duties is to obtain blood specimens from patients. The act of taking blood from a vein is called **phlebotomy**, and one who draws blood is called a **phlebotomist.** However, the clinical laboratory assistant/phlebotomist does not only draw blood. In many healthcare facilities, he or she may enter the patient's name into the laboratory computer, transport specimens, process specimens for testing, perform simple tests, and carry out many other tasks. Further, due to budget cuts in the healthcare environment because of financial pressures, the clinical laboratory assistant is now performing duties in some facilities that were formerly restricted to the clinical laboratory technologist (such as operating laboratory instruments and drawing arterial blood gases). Careful training is extremely important for the clinical laboratory assistant/phlebotomist, especially because of the increasing responsibilities given to this position.

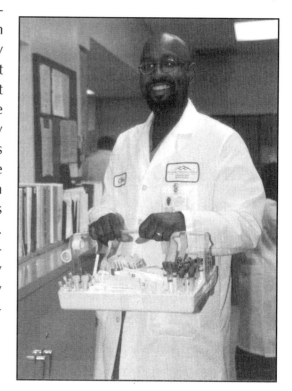

Figure 1-1: The clinical laboratory assistant/phlebotomist has a variety of duties.

The Clinical Laboratory

The clinical laboratory, often called the medical laboratory, is a separate section of a healthcare facility. The clinical laboratory is a place where blood, urine, **sputum, stool,** and tissues are analyzed in a precise, accurate, and timely manner.

sputum: mucous coughed up from the lung.

stool: feces.

The results of the analyses performed in the clinical laboratory give valuable information to physicians about a patient's medical condition. There are a number of conditions and diseases that can be rapidly diagnosed by the laboratory, including diabetes, heart attack, strep throat, and leukemia, to name a few. The laboratory can provide valuable information that can help the physician make a complicated diagnosis. Most physicians in a variety of specialties rely on the clinical laboratory for information relating to treatment as well. Laboratory tests monitor patient conditions during drug therapy, infection reduction, blood sugar adjustment, and heart attack damage.

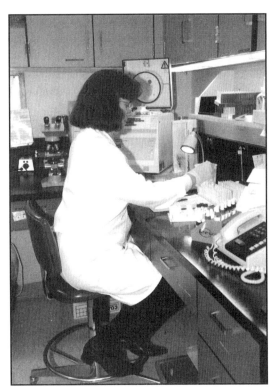

Clinical laboratories come in many sizes, from a corner of a doctor's office to a large multi-department facility in a medical center. The clinical laboratory can appear in many areas of our communities, providing an invaluable role in keeping the community healthy and productive. Laboratories can be found in such places as public health departments, health maintenance organizations (HMO's), physicians' offices, research facilities, veterinary clinics, insurance companies, armed forces health facilities, and every kind of hospital. In the healthcare facility, the clinical laboratory continually interacts with almost every other department, providing critical services for **inpatients** and **outpatients** served by the facility itself.

Figure 1-2: Small laboratories often may be found in physicians' office complexes.

inpatient: a patient who is admitted into a healthcare facility and receives treatment within the facility itself.

outpatient: a patient who receives treatment from a facility without being admitted into the hospital.

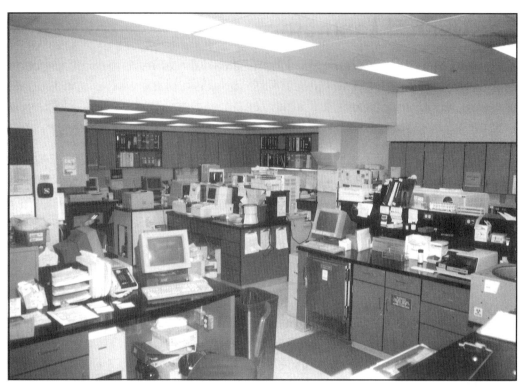

Figure 1-3: A large multi-department clinical laboratory is likely to be found in a medical center.

Thinking It Through ...

Sally is a very busy clinical laboratory assistant at Mercy General Hospital Clinical Laboratory. Today is a particularly hectic day. Sally has already been to several floors in the hospital this morning obtaining early morning blood specimens. She has been to the emergency room, once to draw blood from a man possibly having a heart attack and another time to obtain blood from a woman who was seriously injured in a car accident. She has been called up to the intensive care nursery to get blood from a newborn who has an infection and is about to hurry over to Diagnostic Imaging (X-ray) to obtain blood from a patient who is feeling very faint. And that's only in the first two hours of Sally's shift!

Figure 1-4 illustrates the clinical laboratory's relationship to other parts of a healthcare facility. The clinical laboratory is generally categorized as a part of the Diagnostic Services of a hospital.

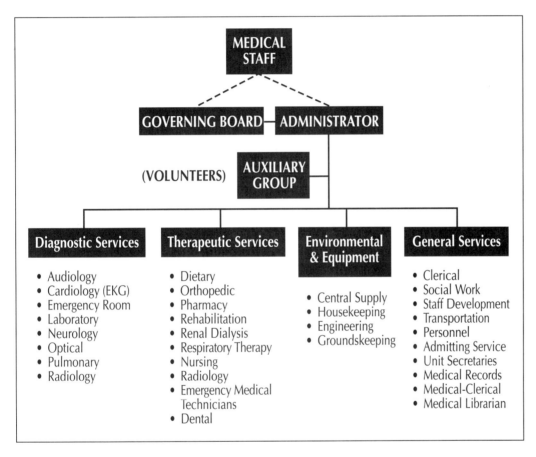

Figure 1-4: A Typical Hospital Organization Chart

Clinical Laboratory Personnel

As medical science has advanced over the past several centuries, the use of laboratory tests has increased to help the physician understand the human body. In the early 1900's, the first clinical laboratories were staffed by physicians who were developing the fundamentals of medical laboratory science. As more tests were developed, training programs began for non-physician personnel who were interested in working in such an environment. Today, the clinical laboratory employs a variety of personnel with several different job titles, many of which may vary from laboratory to laboratory as well as from state to state. The following table shows an organizational chart for a large clinical laboratory with commonly used job titles.

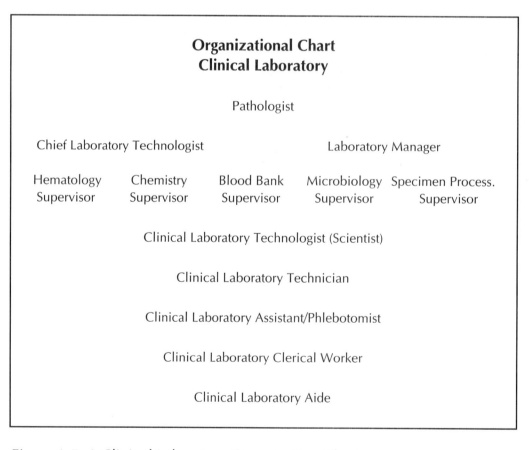

Figure 1-5: A Clinical Laboratory Organization Chart

Clinical Laboratory Aide

The **clinical laboratory aide** is an unskilled position, often not requiring any prior training (although there are short training courses available in some areas). This position can be full or part-time. Generally, it involves cleaning soiled laboratory glassware, restocking supplies, and doing general cleanup in the clinical laboratory.

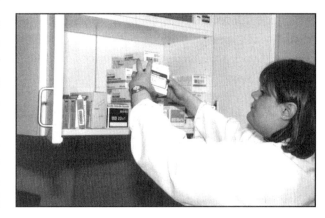

Figure 1-6: Restocking supplies is one of the main duties of the laboratory aide.

Clinical Laboratory Clerical Worker

A **clinical laboratory clerical worker** generally is required to have a high school diploma and some prior clerical training. Often this position will be filled by clerical staff in a healthcare facility who have worked elsewhere in the facility. Other job titles include laboratory secretary and medical laboratory secretary.

The clinical laboratory clerical worker interfaces continually with the laboratory computer system, performing such tasks as entering tests into the computer and retrieving results for physicians. The clerical worker also answers calls on a very busy telephone system and distributes reports to physicians, hospital floors and the medical records department of a healthcare facility. An employee in this position also files laboratory reports, enters laboratory tests to be drawn into the computer, takes messages, and performs many other clerical duties. This is a busy, responsible position.

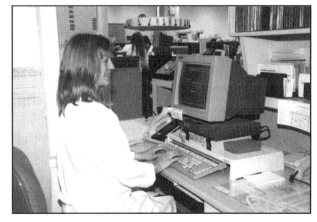

Figure 1-7: The laboratory clerical worker interfaces continually with the laboratory computer system.

Clinical Laboratory Assistant/Phlebotomist

The general requirements for the clinical laboratory assistant/phlebotomist position include a high school diploma and completion of an approved clinical laboratory assistant/phlebotomist program. There are many titles for this position, including venipuncture technician, laboratory assistant, phlebotomist, and clinical laboratory assistant.

Some hospitals have two job descriptions to fit this position: the laboratory assistant and the phlebotomist. But increasingly, these two positions are grouped together as one job with many responsibilities. Such responsibilities include the following:

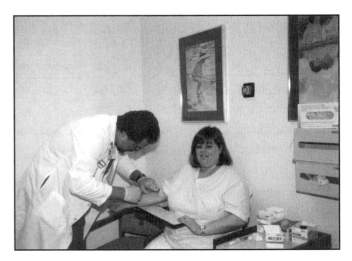

Figure 1-8: The clinical laboratory assistant/ phlebotomist has many responsibilities, including obtaining blood specimens.

- obtaining blood specimens
- requisitioning (requesting) laboratory tests on the computer
- transporting specimens
- preparing specimens for testing
- performing simple tests in different departments of the clinical laboratory

Clinical Laboratory Technician

The **clinical laboratory technician** has several titles, including medical laboratory technician (MLT) or laboratory technician. This position requires graduation from a two-year associate degree program at a college. The armed services also provides training for these positions. Graduates of this training have several semesters of practical and theoretical classes related to the clinical laboratory. Students have a great deal of "hands-on" training in their programs. Graduates are eligible for examination by the Board of Registry of the American Society of Clinical Pathologists and the National Certification Agency for Medical Laboratory Personnel. Clinical laboratory technicians can perform testing in the laboratory under the direction of a clinical laboratory technologist.

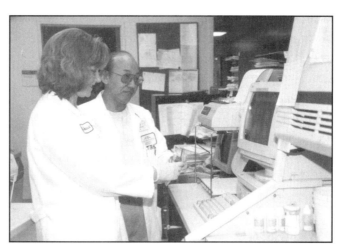

Figure 1-9: The clinical laboratory technician must be a graduate of a two-year associate degree program at a college.

Clinical Laboratory Technologist

The **clinical laboratory technologist,** also called a clinical laboratory scientist or a medical technologist, has a four year bachelor of science degree with one additional year or more of study in a medical technology program. Today, the clinical laboratory technologist is often employed as a supervisor of one of the departments in the clinical laboratory and is responsible for all the test results that are produced by that department. This person is able to perform all tests in the clinical laboratory.

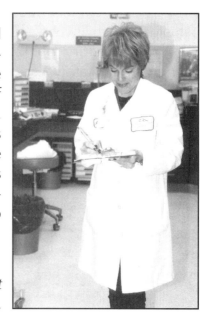

Figure 1-10: The clinical laboratory technologist often serves as department supervisor.

clinical laboratory technologist: a clinical laboratory professional often employed as a supervisor of one of the clinical laboratory departments; responsible for results produced during laboratory testing.

Laboratory Manager/Chief Laboratory Technologist

clinical laboratory manager: a professional with a business or management education who is responsible for business operations in the clinical laboratory.

In many large clinical laboratories, both a **clinical laboratory manager** and a **chief laboratory (medical) technologist** work in the laboratory. The laboratory manager may have a business or management education and is responsible for all business operations in the laboratory, including long-range planning and budgeting. The laboratory manager may also be in charge of all personnel considerations. Some states require that a laboratory manager be a clinical bioanalyst, a licensed position that requires graduate work. The chief laboratory technologist is often in charge of all laboratory testing procedures; however, some laboratories combine this position with that of the laboratory manager.

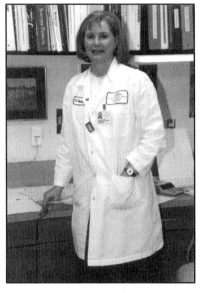

Figure 1-11: The laboratory manager often has an education in business or in management.

Pathologist

pathologist: a physician with a specialty in pathology (the study of disease); oversees laboratory operations and aids other physicians in the diagnosis and treatment of disease.

A **pathologist** is a physician trained in the cause and nature of disease. Generally, the pathologist has completed four years of college, four years of medical school, and five or more years of specific training. Several pathologists may work in the clinical laboratory. Clinical pathologists are involved in the day-to-day clinical laboratory operations, including interpreting laboratory tests, while anatomical pathologists concentrate on performing tissue testing, **autopsies,** and so on.

autopsy: an examination after death of organs and tissues of the body to determine a cause of death or pathological condition.

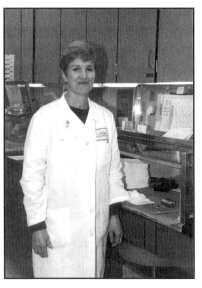

Figure 1-12: Pathologists are physicians trained in the cause and nature of disease.

Career Opportunities

The overall employment opportunities for the clinical laboratory are good. The rapidly-growing older population is increasing demand for laboratory services and will continue to do so in the future. New, more powerful diagnostic tests will encourage more testing and require personnel to run the tests. Due to budgetary cutbacks, laboratory assistants/phlebotomists will be given even more responsible tasks to perform than are presently required in the laboratory. This will increase their versatility and security in the healthcare field.

Some people feel more comfortable working in a small facility while others thrive on the busy pace of a large workplace. As a clinical laboratory assistant/ phlebotomist, you can choose among many different types of employment. Working in a large facility often has the advantage of better benefits, more choices in shifts, and opportunities for **cross-training**. Often in large healthcare facilities, if your job disappears in the clinical laboratory and you have more seniority than someone at your pay level (or there is an opening) in another department, the facility may want to cross-train you for another position outside the laboratory. The best advice in today's healthcare environment for the employee is BE FLEXIBLE AND LEARN AS MANY NEW SKILLS AS YOU CAN!

cross-training: the gaining of skills of other job descriptions in addition to one's own position.

However, if you do not want to work in a fast-paced environment, there are many opportunities open to the clinical laboratory assistant in smaller clinics, doctor's offices, and other facilities that see fewer patients and give you a more personal connection with them. Some employment opportunities for this position are listed below:

- healthcare facilities such as public, private, and military hospitals
- clinics
- doctor's offices/complexes
- insurance companies
- private laboratories
- research facilities
- universities

Career Ladder for the Clinical Laboratory Assistant/Phlebotomist

After you have gained valuable experience as a clinical laboratory assistant/ phlebotomist, you will have also observed many different positions in the healthcare setting that may require various amounts of additional training. Many laboratory assistants eventually become nurses, respiratory therapists, radiology technicians, and even doctors; or they may decide that they are happy with the job that they have. Whatever career path you choose to follow, it is always good to keep your eye open for training opportunities within the hospital, where you may be trained in-house for other positions. You may also discover that you might like to become supervisor someday and can take courses to learn to be a better leader/manager. So, if you work hard and have a good attitude, one of the greatest advantages of working in the healthcare environment is the variety of jobs that can become open to you.

Professional Organizations

From the beginning of your employment as a clinical laboratory assistant/ phlebotomist, you should see yourself as a responsible professional. As such, you should be aware of any organizations that exist to promote professionalism in the clinical laboratory. Always be aware of new advances in the field (there will be several each year).

Four national organizations that see the clinical laboratory assistant as a vital part of the healthcare team are listed below. All sponsor continuing education programs for the laboratory assistant. (See Chapter 27 for information about certification for the laboratory assistant/phlebotomist.)

- The American Society of Clinical Pathologists (ASCP)
- The American Society for Medical Technology (ASMT)
- The American Society of Phlebotomy Technicians (ASPT)
- The National Phlebotomy Association (NPA)

Chapter Summary

The clinical laboratory, often called the medical laboratory, is a department within a healthcare facility. The clinical laboratory is a place where blood, urine, sputum, stool, and tissues are analyzed in a precise, accurate, and timely manner. The clinical laboratory assistant/phlebotomist works with other personnel in the clinical laboratory, including the pathologist, laboratory manager, chief clinical laboratory technologist, clinical laboratory technologist, clinical laboratory technician, clinical laboratory clerk, and clinical laboratory aide.

The clinical laboratory assistant/phlebotomist should always be aware of new advances in the field. There can also be many opportunities in the clinical laboratory setting for cross-training.

Name _____

Date _____

Student Enrichment Activities

Complete the following exercises.

1. Name three conditions/diseases that can be diagnosed rapidly by clinical laboratory testing.
    A. _____
    B. _____
    C. _____

2. What are the educational requirements for the following positions in the clinical laboratory?
    A. pathologist _____

    _____

    B. clinical laboratory assistant/phlebotomist _____

    _____

    C. clinical laboratory technician _____

    _____

    D. clinical laboratory technologist _____

    _____

3. Name five employers who may hire a clinical laboratory assistant/phlebotomist.
    A. _____
    B. _____
    C. _____
    D. _____
    E. _____

4. What is the primary function of the clinical laboratory?

    _____

    _____

    _____

5. Why should clinical laboratory assistants/phlebotomists participate in
   continuing education?

   _____

   _____

   _____

   _____

   _____

   _____

6. Why is cross-training so important in today's healthcare environment?

   _____

   _____

   _____

   _____

   _____

Chapter Two
Departements in the Clinical Laboratory

Objectives

After completing this chapter, you should be able to
do the following:

1. Define and correctly spell each of the key terms.

2. Name the different departments in a typical
   clinical laboratory.

3. Discuss tasks that the clinical laboratory assistant might
   perform in various departments of the clinical laboratory.

4. Name several tests that are commonly run in each
   department of the clinical laboratory.

Key Terms

- activated partial thromboplastin time
- anemia
- antigen/antibody reactions
- blood bank
- clinical chemistry
- coagulation
- complete blood count
- cytology
- Gram stain
- hematology
- hemoglobin

- histology
- microbiology
- Pap smear
- pathogenic
- platelets
- prothrombin time
- red blood cells
- serology
- specimen processing
- turbidity
- urinalysis
- white blood cells

Introduction

Until recently, clinical laboratory assistants/phlebotomists usually did not have much interaction within the clinical laboratory itself. Most duties were focused on drawing blood and bringing specimens back to the laboratory. Today, clinical laboratory assistants play a very important role in many laboratories by working in the various departments of the laboratory.

Clinical Laboratory Departments

histology: the study of the microscopic structure of tissue.

cytology: the science that deals with the formation, structure, and function of cells.

Clinical laboratories vary in the way their departments are set up. Laboratories generally have two divisions: clinical analysis (where the tests are performed), and anatomical and surgical pathology (where tissue samples are studied).

The anatomical and surgical pathology division is concerned with the study of the microscopic structure of cells and tissues. Before the pathologist analyzes tissue from autopsies and surgeries, the tissue must be processed and stained. This process is performed in the **histology** department, under the direction of a histologist. Another department in this division is **cytology**, where body fluids and tissues are prepared by a pathologist or **cytologist** who then examines the tissues for signs of disease, such as cancer. The **Pap smear** is one of the most common examinations performed in cytology. Generally, the laboratory assistant/phlebotomist does not work in this section, but often may bring specimens to these areas.

The clinical laboratory assistant/phlebotomist will spend a great deal of time in the clinical analysis division. This section is divided into departments including hematology, clinical chemistry, microbiology, **blood bank** (immunohematology, immunology/serology, and specimen processing). Larger facilities may have an education section as well.

Hematology

The **hematology** department performs tests to identify diseases of the blood and blood-forming tissues. (See Figure 2-1.) Such elements include red and white blood cells as well as platelets. **Red blood cells** (erythrocytes) carry oxygen throughout the bloodstream, delivering oxygen to the cells of the body. This oxygen is bound to the pigment **hemoglobin** in the red blood cell. Physicians often measure the hemoglobin content in the blood to measure blood loss, to diagnose **anemia**, and to determine how much oxygen is getting to the tissues and cells.

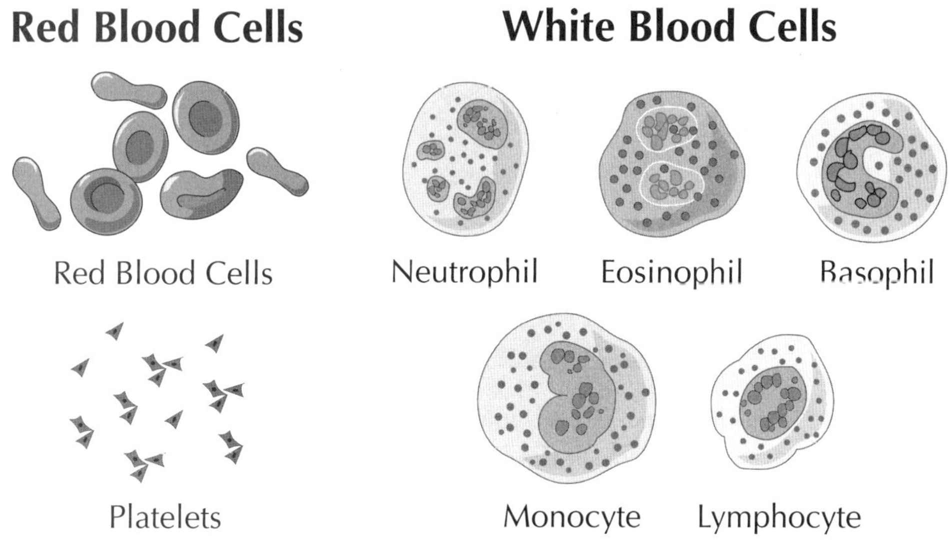

Pap smear:
the scraping and examination of cells from the body, especially the cervix and the vaginal walls; used in the detection of cancer; Papanicolaou test.

hematology:
the clinical laboratory department concerned with the qualitative and quantitative evaluation of the formed elements of the blood and bone marrow.

red blood cells:
also known as erythrocytes; cells primarily involved in the transportation of oxygen to the cells of the body.

hemoglobin:
a complex protein that gives erythrocytes their red color; a molecule that transports oxygen throughout the body.

anemia:
a reduction in number of circulating erythrocytes (red blood cells), the amount of hemoglobin, or the volume of packed red blood cells in a given volume of blood.

Red Blood Cells   White Blood Cells

Red Blood Cells   Neutrophil   Eosinophil   Basophil

Platelets   Monocyte   Lymphocyte

Figure 2-1: Blood-forming Elements

white blood cells: also known as *leukocytes*; blood cells responsible for fighting infection.

There are five different **white blood cells** (leukocytes) in the bloodstream. Some white blood cells ingest materials, such as bacteria, to help battle infection. Others produce antibodies to help the immune system fight invasion. Physicians often wish to know in what proportion the different white blood cells appear in the blood.

platelets: cells found in the blood that assist in clot formation; thrombocytes.

Platelets (also called thrombocytes) aid in blood coagulation, the process in which bleeding is stopped. Platelets help this process by forming a plug to stop blood flow from a damaged vessel and by releasing substances that bring about clotting. These platelets, which are actually parts of cells, are often counted to assess the body's ability to stop bleeding. Blood elements will be discussed in more detail in Chapter Eight.

complete blood count: CBC; a blood test that determines the number of erythrocytes, leukocytes, and platelets that are present in the patient's blood, as well as the hemoglobin and hematocrit, among other determinations.

The **complete blood count** is the hematology test which is most frequently ordered. It is performed routinely using automated instruments (Figure 2-2) that count the cells and calculate results electronically. The clinical laboratory assistant/phlebotomist can operate this instrument under the supervision of a clinical laboratory technologist in many clinical laboratories. Figure 2-3 includes tests that are normally found in the complete blood count.

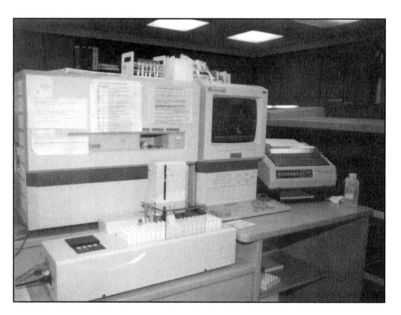

Figure 2-2: The automated cell counter is used most frequently in the hematology department.

Common Components of a Complete Blood Count

red blood cell (RBC) count

white blood cell (WBC) count

hemoglobin (Hbg or Hb)

hematocrit (Hct or Crit)

mean corpuscular volume (MCV)

mean cellular hemoglobin (MCH)

mean cellular hemoglobin concentration (MCHC)

differential white count (Diff) – manual or automated

Figure 2-3: Common Components of a Complete Blood Count (CBC)

The following tests are also frequently performed in the hematology department; they will be discussed in detail later in the textbook:

- cerebrospinal fluid blood cell count
- complete blood count
- eosinophil count
- hemoglobin/hematocrit count
- platelet count
- reticulocyte count
- sedimentation rate (ESR)
- sickle cell testing

coagulation:
the process of
blood clotting.

**prothrombin
time:**
PT; a common
blood test used
to assess a part
of the coagula-
tion system;
commonly used
to monitor oral
anticoagulant
therapy such as
coumadin
therapy.

**activated
partial throm-
boplastin time:**
a frequently
ordered coagu-
lation test that
assesses part of
the coagulation
mechanism in
the body.

urinalysis:
the examination
of urine to
observe the
physical,
chemical, and
microscopic
characteristics to
assess the possi-
bility of infec-
tion, disease, or
damage to the
urinary tract.

turbidity:
the appearance
of cloudiness
in a normally
clear liquid. In
the laboratory,
often due to
the growth of
microorganisms
in the specimen.

Coagulation. Usually, the coagulation section of the clinical laboratory is housed in the hematology department, although some laboratories may recognize this area as a separate department. Coagulation testing involves the study of defects in the blood clotting mechanism and the monitoring of medication given to patients who may be forming blood clots (anticoagulant therapy). A physician may want to "thin" a patient's blood to prevent more blood clots, but at the same time, the blood shouldn't be so thin that the patient bleeds excessively. Other tests done in this department test for special disease conditions in which the blood may not clot normally, such as hemophilia. Common coagulation tests include the **prothrombin time (PT)** and the **activated partial thromboplastin time (APTT)**.

Urinalysis. The urinalysis section of the clinical laboratory is often housed in the hematology or chemistry department. A urinalysis is a test performed on urine involving a physical, chemical, and microscopic description of the urine and its contents. The physical part of the urinalysis is a description of how a urine sample appears, including color and **turbidity**. Chemical tests look for substances in the urine that are not normal, such as excessive amounts of sugar or protein. A microscopic examination identifies the presence or absence of bacteria, crystals, various blood cells, and other substances. The clinical laboratory assistant/ phlebotomist may be asked to prepare urine samples for testing.

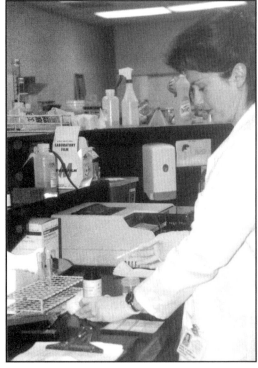

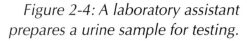
Figure 2-4: A laboratory assistant prepares a urine sample for testing.

Clinical Chemistry

In most clinical laboratories, the **clinical chemistry** department performs the majority of laboratory tests. In larger laboratories, this department may consist of several large automated instruments that can perform multiple testing on one blood sample. This is a very efficient way to produce accurate results and uses as few personnel as possible to run the tests. The following tests are performed commonly in this department:

- bilirubin

- blood gases

- blood urea nitrogen (BUN)

- cholesterol studies

- creatinine

- drug analysis

- electrolytes (sodium, potassium, chloride, bicarbonate)

- enzymes

- glucose testing

- hormone testing

- iron

- magnesium

- total protein

- triglycerides

- uric acid

clinical chemistry: a department of the clinical laboratory in which quantitative analyses of blood and other fluids are performed, including many blood chemistries and drug analyses.

To make ordering in clinical chemistry easier for the physician, chemistry tests are often grouped in **panels**. A physician does not have to order several chemistry tests individually; the physician can instead, order different types of panels depending upon the patient's needs. There are panels that give the physician an overview of the patient's blood chemistry (usually ordered during physical examinations), liver panels that assess liver function, kidney panels to assess kidney function, and many other specialized panels.

Since the chemistry department is highly automated, the clinical laboratory assistant may be asked to prepare large amounts of blood samples for testing, or even to operate some of the equipment.

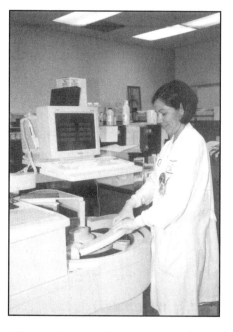

Figure 2-5: A chemistry analyzer is one of the many pieces of equipment that may be found in Clinical Chemistry.

Clinical Microbiology

microbiology:
a department in the clinical laboratory that grows and identifies organisms that can cause infection, disease, or both in humans.

pathogenic:
disease-producing.

Personnel in the **microbiology** department grow and identify microorganisms that may be **pathogenic**. Additionally, microorganisms identified in this department can be tested against various antibiotics to see which drugs will kill the organism. When a physician orders a **culture and sensitivity** on a **specimen** such as urine or sputum (or other body fluids), the physician is asking the microbiology department to put the specimen on **growth media** to see if any pathogenic organisms grow. That is called a culture. Sensitivity testing refers to growing bacteria in antibiotic environments to see which antibiotic will kill the bacteria most effectively.

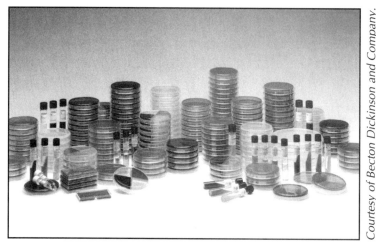

Courtesy of Becton Dickinson and Company.

Figure 2-6: Growth Media in Clinical Microbiology

The clinical laboratory assistant may be asked to set up cultures on various media. Many of the specimens may be infectious, and the clinical laboratory assistant must use extreme caution when handling such specimens. All specimens are handled under the **safety hood** in the microbiology department. The safety hood (Figure 2-7) has built-in suction that draws fumes and aerosols up away from the person setting up the culture.

Another task that the clinical laboratory assistant may perform is the preparation of the **Gram stain**. This test is performed by smearing a small portion of a specimen on a microscope slide (Figure 2-8). After the slide has dried, the specimen is stained with a series of chemicals called the Gram stain. The laboratory technologist then reads the slide under the microscope. Some bacteria are stained purple, and some are stained pink. It is not possible to identify most bacteria this way, but the technologist can see the various shapes of the bacteria (rod-shaped, circular-shaped, and spiral-shaped). The Gram stain gives the physician some idea of what bacteria, if any, might be present.

In addition to bacteria, personnel in the clinical microbiology department may identify pathogenic parasites, fungi, and viruses. Clinical laboratory assistants also might be involved in setting up these specimens for testing.

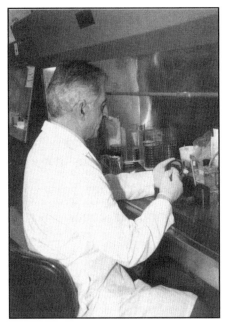

Figure 2-7: Setting up cultures under a safety hood prevents inhalation of certain fumes.

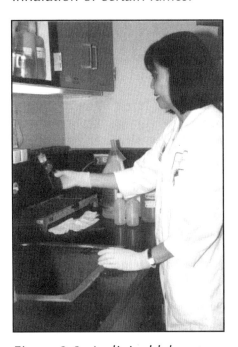

Figure 2-8: A clinical laboratory assistant will be required to perform a Gram Stain on certain blood specimens.

Gram stain: the most common stain performed in the microbiology department of the clinical laboratory; a stain used to observe the gross morphological features of specimens under a microscope.

The following is a list of common tests ordered in the clinical microbiology department:

- acid-fast bacilli (AFB) smear
- anaerobic culture
- blood culture
- culture and sensitivity
- fungus culture
- gonorrhea smear
- Gram staining
- nose/throat culture
- ova and parasites testing
- pinworm preparation
- sputum culture
- stool culture
- urine culture

The Blood Bank

blood bank:
immunohema-
tology;
a clinical
laboratory
department that
processes blood
products for
transfusion.

The **blood bank**, also referred to as the immunohematology department, provides blood products to patients. Before blood is given to a patient, the donor (the one who donates the blood) and the recipient (the one who receives the blood) must have his or her blood typed and tested for compatibility. The clinical laboratory assistant's critical task related to this department is to make sure that all blood drawn for blood bank testing is labeled accurately. Errors in labeling blood to be tested in the blood bank can result in the death of a patient, if the patient receives incompatible blood.

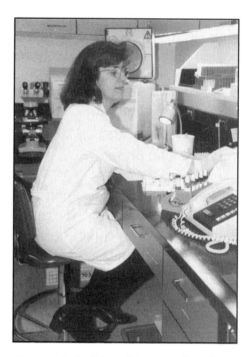

Figure 2-9: Blood is typed and tested for compatibility in the blood bank.

Tests commonly ordered in this department are listed below:

- ABO and Rh typing

- antibody grouping

- antibody titer

- Coombs' test

- hepatitis testing

- HIV testing

Immunology/Serology

The immunology/**serology** department, sometimes located in the blood bank, has the job of performing procedures to identify **antigen-antibody reactions**. These reactions deal with the body's response to the presence of bacterial, viral, fungal, or parasitic diseases. Such diseases may stimulate antigen-antibody reactions (the antigen is the disease, and the antibody is the body's reaction to the disease), which can be demonstrated in the laboratory. Clinical laboratory assistants may perform simple testing here and prepare specimens for testing. Common tests performed in this department include the following:

- antinuclear antibody (ANA)

- ASO screening and titer

- Brucella antibody

- cold agglutinins

- C-reactive protein

- CSF/VDRL testing

- infectious mononucleosis testing

- Lyme disease antibody

- Legionnaires' disease antibody

- Q fever

- rheumatoid factor (RA)

- RPR

- Salmonella agglutinins testing

- syphilis antibody (FTA-ABS)

serology: often a subdepartment of the blood bank; concerned with tests using antigen/antibody reactions.

antigen/ antibody reactions: reactions where a foreign substance (antigen) introduced into the body is attacked by a protein substance (antibody) produced by the body in response to the invader.

Specimen Processing

specimen processing: also known as the *central processing area*; the area of the clinical laboratory where specimens are processed for testing in various departments of the clinical laboratory as well as specimens for transport to other facilities.

Not all clinical laboratories are big enough to have a separate **specimen processing** department. However, larger clinical laboratories may have an extensive department that is dedicated to processing specimens, both for testing in the laboratory and sending out specimens to other laboratories.

The efficient and accurate preparation of specimens for testing is a vital task in the clinical laboratory. Labels often are made for specific tests that have special requirements. Frequently, the requirements will be listed on the label itself. The utmost care must be taken to ensure that each specimen is labeled properly and sent to the correct department. Some specimens may have to be divided up and sent to various departments. Transporting, processing, and distributing clinical specimens is discussed in Chapter Eighteen.

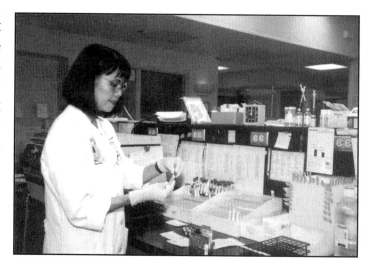

Figure 2-10: Larger clinical laboratories often have a separate specimen processing department.

Chapter Summary

The clinical laboratory assistant/phlebotomist is responsible for an increasing number of tasks inside the departments of today's clinical laboratories. It is important for the clinical laboratory assistant to understand the functions of and the types of tests run in the laboratory departments: hematology, clinical chemistry, clinical microbiology, blood bank, and immunology and serology. In larger clinical laboratories, there is an additional department called specimen processing where the clinical laboratory assistant/phlebotomist may spend a great deal of time.

Name _____

Date _____

Student Enrichment Activities

Circle the letter of the correct answer.

1. The hematology department is involved in testing:

    A. red blood cells.

    B. white blood cells.

    C. platelets.

    D. all of the above.

2. A department that is not a part of the clinical laboratory is:

    A. clinical microbiology.

    B. clinical chemistry.

    C. hematology.

    D. biology.

3. The most common test that is run in the hematology department is the:

    A. cholesterol test.

    B. Gram stain.

    C. complete blood count.

    D. syphilis testing.

4. All of the following tests are run in the clinical chemistry department, except:

    A. BUN.

    B. culture and sensitivity.

    C. electrolytes.

    D. enzyme testing.

5. Tasks that can be performed by a clinical laboratory assistant in the clinical microbiology department include:

   A. Gram staining.

   B. setting up cultures.

   C. using the safety hood.

   D. all of the above.

Match the following numbered items with the appropriate location.

6. _____ syphilis testing

7. _____ platelet counting

8. _____ drug analyses

9. _____ preparing blood

10. _____ determining blood type

A. performed in the immunology/ serology department

B. performed in the hematology department

C. performed in the clinical chemistry department

D. performed in the specimen processing department

E. performed in the blood bank department

Circle T for true, or F for false.

11. T F Coagulation is the process in which bacteria causes disease.

12. T F An urinalysis involves performing chemical tests on urine.

13. T F Immunohematology is another name for hematology.

14. T F Platelets are involved in blood clotting.

15. T F Red blood cells have hemoglobin inside them, which carries oxygen to cells.

Chapter Three
Medical Terminology for the Clinical Laboratory Assistant/ Phlebotomist

Objectives

After completing this chapter, you should be able to do the following:

1. Define and correctly spell each of the key terms.

2. Discuss why it is important for a clinical laboratory assistant/phlebotomist to have a working knowledge of medical terminology.

3. Explain the structure of medical terms, including prefixes, suffixes, word roots, combining vowels, and combining forms.

4. Identify common medical word roots, prefixes, and suffixes.

5. Identify common medical abbreviations encountered in the clinical laboratory.

Key Terms

- combining form
- combining vowel
- prefix
- suffix
- word root

Introduction

Welcome to a world with its own unique language! The medical profession uses a special vocabulary of scientific/technical terms that can sound foreign to the layperson. As a medical professional, the clinical laboratory assistant must be able to understand this language in order to be an effective communicator as well as a valuable employee. In addition to general medical terms used by the medical profession, the clinical laboratory has its own unique terms that must be understood.

Medical terminology is based on many Latin and Greek word elements that form the foundation of nearly all medical terms. These elements include prefixes, suffixes, and word roots. Practice, patience, and experience will be required for the clinical laboratory assistant to become proficient in this unique language.

Word Roots

word root: the body or main part of the word, referring to the primary meaning of a word as a whole.

The **word root** is the foundation of medical terms. The word root is the body or main part of a term, referring to the essential meaning of the word as a whole. Usually, this element refers to the tissue, organ, or body system involved, such as the root *cardi*, meaning heart.

Some terms can have two word roots, such as *cardiopulmonary*, which is made up of the word root *cardi* (heart), the combining vowel *o*, and *pulmonary* (lung). The following table lists common word roots. The clinical laboratory assistant should be familiar with all of these roots, as they form the majority of all medical terms.

Common Word Roots

Root (shown w/combining vowel)	Meaning	Example
aden/o	gland	adenopathy
aer/o	air	aerobic
angi/o	vessel	angioplasty
arteri/o	artery	arteriogram
arthr/o	joint	arthritis
brachi/o	arm	brachial
bronch/o, bronchi/o	bronchial tubes	bronchitis
cardi/o	heart	cardiologist
cephal/o	head	cephalic
chol/e, chol/o	bile; gall	cholecystic
chrom/o	color	polychromatic
cutane/o	skin	cutaneous
cyan/o	blue	cyanotic
cyst/o	fluid-filled sac; urinary bladder; bag	cystogram
cyt/o	cell	cytologist
derm/o, dermat/o	skin	dermabrasion
encephal/o	brain	encephalitis
erythr/o	red	erythrocyte
febr/o	fever	febrile
gastr/o	stomach	gastroenteritis
glyc/o	sugar; glucose	glycogen
gynec/o	woman or female	gynecologist
hemat/o	blood	hematologist
hepat/o	liver	hepatitis
hist/o	tissue	histology
hyster/o	uterus; womb	hysterectomy
lapar/o	abdomen	laparotomy
leuk/o	white	leukemia
lip/o	fat	lipoma
lith/o	stone or calculus	lithotomy
mast/o	breast	mastitis
mening/o	membrane; meninges	meningitis
myel/o	spinal cord; bone marrow	myelocyte

Figure 3-1: Common Word Roots

Common Word Roots (Cont.)

Root (shown w/combining vowel)	Meaning	Example
necr/o	pertaining to death	necrophobia
nephr/o	kidney	nephron
neur/o	nerves or nervous system	neurology
neutr/o	neutral	neutrophil
onc/o	tumor	oncology
orth/o	straight	orthopedic
oste/o	bone	osteopath
path/o	disease	pathologist
ped/o (Latin)	foot	pedicure
ped/o (Greek)	child	pediatrician
phleb/o	vein	phlebotomist
pneum/o	lung	pneumonia
pulmon/o	lung	pulmonary
py/o	pus	pyogenic
ren/o	kidney	renal
scler/o	hardening; sclera	sclerosis
sept/o	poison	septicemia
stomat/o	mouth	stomatocyte
therm/o	heat	thermometer
thorac/o	chest	thoracotomy
thromb/o	clot	thrombosis
tox/o	poison	toxic
ur/o	presence in urine	urinalysis
vas/o	duct; vessel; vas deferens	vasodilator
ven/o	vein	venipuncture

Figure 3-1: Common Word Roots (Cont.)

Prefixes

prefix: a word element placed in front of a root to modify its meaning.

A **prefix** is placed *in front of* a word root to modify its meaning. A prefix can never be a stand-alone term.

Example: Osteo- (prefix) *+ path* (word root) = osteopath

The following table illustrates common prefixes.

Common Medical Prefixes

Prefix	Meaning	Example
a-, an-	without or not	aseptic
ab-	away from; absent	abnormal
ad-	near; toward	addiction
aniso-	unequal	anisocytosis
ante-	before; preceding	antepartum
anti-	against	antiseptic
auto-	self	autotransfusion
baso-	blue	basophil
bi/o-	life	biology
contra-	opposite; opposed; against	contraception
di-	two; twice; double	dimorphic
dis-	to cut apart	dissect
dys-	difficult; painful; bad disordered	dysfunction
e-, ex-	out; outside	excise
endo-	inside; interior; within	endoscopy
epi-	upon; over; upper	epidermis
hemi-	half	hemisphere
hyper-	excessive; above; increased	hyperchromic
hypo-	below; deficient; under	hypoactive
inter-	between	intercellular
intra-	within	intrauterine
iso-	equal, same	isometric
macro-	large; long	macrocyte
mal-	abnormal; bad; disoriented	maladjusted
mega-	enlarged	megaloblast
meta-	after, next	metastasis
micro-	small	microscope
mono-	one; single	mononucleosis
neo-	new	neoplasm
para-	beside; beyond; apart from; near; abnormal; irregular; opposite; adjacent to	paraplegic

Figure 3-2: Common Medical Prefixes

Common Medical Prefixes (Cont.)		
Prefix	**Meaning**	**Example**
peri-	surrounding; around	periodontal
poly-	many	polycystic
post-	following; after	postprandial
pre-	in front of; before	prenatal
pseudo-	false	pseudocyst
semi-	half	semicircular
sten-, steno-	contracted; narrow	stenosis
sub-	under; below	subacute
super-, supra-	over; above	supersaturated
tachy-	fast; rapid; swift	tachycardia
trans-	across; through	transurethral

Figure 3-2: Common Medical Prefixes (Cont.)

Suffixes

suffix:
a word element placed at the end of a root to modify its meaning.

A **suffix** is a word ending, following a root word and either changing the word meaning or adding to the meaning. As with a prefix, the suffix can never be used alone.

Example: mast (root word) + *ectomy* (suffix) = mastectomy

A list of common medical suffixes follows.

Common Medical Suffixes

Suffix	Meaning	Example
-algia	pain	neuralgia
-blast	germ; primitive	lymphoblast
-centesis	puncture to remove fluid	thoracentesis
-cid, -cide	kill or destroy	suicide
-cyte	cell	thrombocyte
-ectomy	surgical removal; excision	hysterectomy
-emia	blood	anemia
-genic	origin or produced by or in	pyrogenic
-gram	record	pyelogram
-graph	instrument used for recording	electrocardiograph
-itis	inflammation	tonsillitis
-logist	specialist; one who studies	cardiologist
-meter	instrument that measures	thermometer
-oma	tumor	lipoma
-osis	abnormal condition	necrosis
-pathy	disease	cardiomyopathy
-penia	lack of; deficiency	leukopenia
-phil	attraction	eosinophil
-plasty	surgical repair	rhinoplasty
-pnea	breathing	apnea
-poiesis	to make	erythropoiesis
-rhage, -rhagia	bursting forth; excessive flow of blood	hemorrhage
-scope	instrument used to examine or look into a part	microscope
-stasis	stopping	hemostasis
-stomy	surgical creation of an opening	colostomy
-tomy	cutting into; incision	phlebotomy
-uria	present in urine	glycosuria

Figure 3-3: Common Medical Suffixes

Combining Vowels

combining vowel:
a vowel that is placed between two word elements to join the two word parts.

A **combining vowel**, usually an "o," is used to join the word root to a suffix or another root word. The combining vowel helps the communicator pronounce the word.

Example: *hemat* (word root) + *"o"* (combining vowel) + *logy* (suffix)
                 Blood (hemat) + "o" + study of (logy) = the study of blood.

Sometimes a combining vowel is not used when the suffix begins with a vowel.

Example: *phleb* (root word) + *itis* (suffix)= phlebitis
                 (no combining vowel)

A combining vowel can come between two root words.

Example: *arteri* (root word) + *"o"* (combining vowel)
                 + *scler* (root word) + *osis* (suffix) = arteriosclerosis

Combining Forms

combining form:
a root word plus a combining vowel.

A root word along with a combining vowel is called a **combining form**.

Example: The combining form *erythro,* meaning "red," combined
                 with the word *cyte,* meaning "cell," forms *erythrocyte,*
                 which means "red cell."

Abbreviations

The following is a list of abbreviations for medical terms that are commonly used in the clinical laboratory.

Common Medical Abbreviations

ABO	blood group system
AIDS	acquired immune deficiency syndrome
aka	also known as
alk phos	alkaline phosphatase
ALL	acute lymphocytic leukemia
ALT	alanine transaminase
AML	acute myelocytic leukemia
ASAP	as soon as possible
ASCP	American Society of Clinical Pathologists
AST	asparate aminotransferase
BID or bid	twice daily
bl	blood
BP	blood pressure
BUN	blood urea nitrogen
c̄	with
Ca	calcium
CA	cancer
CAD	coronary artery disease
CBC	complete blood count
cc	cubic centimeter
CCU	coronary care unit
cm	centimeter
CML	chronic myelogenous leukemia
CNS	central nervous system
CO	carbon monoxide
CO_2	carbon dioxide
COPD	chronic obstructive pulmonary disease
CPR	cardiopulmonary resuscitation
CSF	cerebrospinal fluid
CVA	cerebrovascular accident
diff	differential white blood cell count
dil	dilute
DOB	date of birth
DRG	diagnosis related group
Dx	diagnosis

Figure 3-4: Common Medical Abbreviations

Common Medical Abbreviations Cont.

EBV	Epstein-Barr virus
ECG or **EKG**	electrocardiogram
EEG	electroencephalogram
EENT	eye, ear, nose, and throat
eos	eosinophils
ER	emergency room
ESR	erythrocyte sedimentation rate
FBS	fasting blood sugar
Fe	iron
FUO	fever of undetermined origin
Gm or **gm**	gram
GI	gastrointestinal
GTT	glucose tolerance test
Gtt or **gtt**	drop
GYN or **gyn**	gynecology
h	hour
hb or **hgb**	hemoglobin
HBV	hepatitis B virus
HCG	human chorionic gonadotropin
HCl	hydrochloric acid
Hct	hematocrit
HDL	high-density lipoprotein
HIV	human immunodeficiency virus
ICU	intensive care unit
IM	intramuscular
IV	intravenous
IVP	intravenous pyelogram
K	potassium
Kg	kilogram
L or **l**	liter; left
LD or **LDH**	lactic dehydrogenase
LDL	low-density lipoprotein
LE	lupus erythematosis
MCH	mean corpuscular hemoglobin
MCHC	mean corpuscular hemoglobin concentration

Figure 3-4: Common Medical Abbreviations (Cont.)

Common Medical Abbreviations Cont.

MCV	mean corpuscular volume
mEq	milliequivalents
mg	milligram
Mg	magnesium
MI	myocardial infarction
ml	milliliter
mm	millimeter
mono	monocyte
Na	sodium
neg	negative
NG	nasogastric
nm	nanometer
NPO	nothing by mouth
O_2	oxygen
OB or Obs	obstetrics
OR	operating room
path	pathology
peds	pediatrics
pH	hydrogen ion concentration (potential of hydrogen)
PKU	phenylketonuria
PMNs	polymorphonuclear leukocytes
pos	positive
post-op	after the surgery
PP	postprandial (after meals)
PT	prothrombin time/protime or physical therapy
PTT	partial thromboplastin time
pt	patient
QNS	quantity not sufficient
RBC	red blood cell/count
RIA	radioimmunoassay
R/O	rule out
RT	respiratory therapy
s̄	without
sed rate	erythrocyte sedimentation rate (ESR)
segs	segmented white blood cells

Figure 3-4: Common Medical Abbreviations (Cont.)

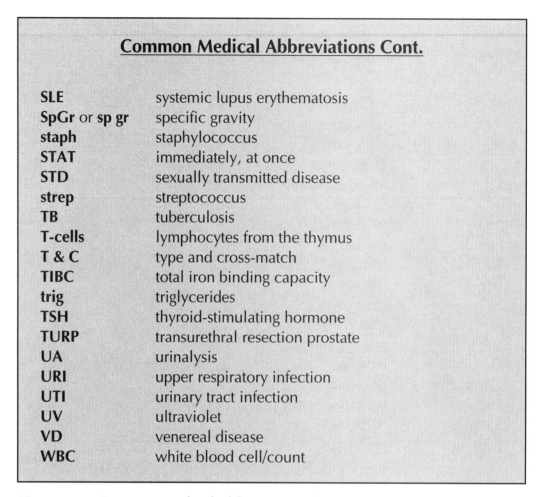

Common Medical Abbreviations Cont.	
SLE	systemic lupus erythematosis
SpGr or **sp gr**	specific gravity
staph	staphylococcus
STAT	immediately, at once
STD	sexually transmitted disease
strep	streptococcus
TB	tuberculosis
T-cells	lymphocytes from the thymus
T & C	type and cross-match
TIBC	total iron binding capacity
trig	triglycerides
TSH	thyroid-stimulating hormone
TURP	transurethral resection prostate
UA	urinalysis
URI	upper respiratory infection
UTI	urinary tract infection
UV	ultraviolet
VD	venereal disease
WBC	white blood cell/count

Figure 3-4: Common Medical Abbreviations (Cont.)

Chapter Summary

The language of medicine is unique. The clinical laboratory assistant/phlebotomist must put much effort into learning the terms that are used in the clinical laboratory and in the hospital. It is especially important to learn the names of the most common clinical laboratory tests. By learning the language of medicine, the healthcare professional becomes a much better employee and communicator.

Name _____

Date _____

Student Enrichment Activities

Complete the following exercises.

1. Name five types of word elements used in medical terminology.

   A. _____

   B. _____

   C. _____

   D. _____

   E. _____

2. Most medical terms are derived from two languages: _____

   and_____.

3. Define the following medical terms.

   A. microscope:_____

   _____

   _____

   B. cytology: _____

   _____

   _____

   C. pathology: _____

   _____

   _____

   D. lipoma:_____

   _____

   _____

   E. pathologist: _____

   _____

   _____

F. lithotomy: _____

_____

_____

G. encephalogram: _____

_____

_____

H. cardiology: _____

_____

_____

I. bronchitis: _____

_____

_____

J. glycosuria: _____

_____

_____

4. What do the following abbreviations mean?

A. BUN: _____

B. STAT: _____

C. ASAP: _____

D. OR: _____

E. Hct: _____

F. Hgb: _____

G. CBC: _____

H. mg: _____

I. ml: _____

J. FUO: _____

Chapter Four
Ethical and Legal Considerations for the Clinical Laboratory Assistant/Phlebotomist

Objectives

After completing this chapter, you should be able to do the following:

1. Define and correctly spell each of the key terms.

2. Explain the terms *unethical* and *illegal.*

3. List some characteristics of professional behavior.

4. Discuss several medical laws that apply to the medical professional.

5. Explain the significance of the *Patient's Bill of Rights.*

6. Identify the importance of patient consent.

7. Discuss issues of confidentiality in the healthcare facility.

Key Terms

- advance directive
- assault
- battery
- confidentiality
- duty of care
- emancipated minor
- ethics
- libel

- malpractice
- medical law
- negligence
- Patient's Bill of Rights
- privileged information
- reasonable care
- scope of practice
- slander

Introduction

Everyone who works in a service profession has a responsibility to those who receive his or her services. Personal and professional rules of performance and conduct are called **ethics**. Ethical decisions involve integrity, honesty, and a strong sense of right and wrong. The healthcare profession has an enormous need for employees who are dedicated to ethical behavior and to using technical skills, knowledge, and training to serve the patient in the best way possible.

ethics: principles of conduct that establish standards and morals that govern decisions and behavior.

medical law: laws that govern the legal conduct of the members of the medical profession; includes local, state, and federal laws.

Medical law focuses on whether the medical professional has acted legally or illegally. If a medical professional acts illegally, the act is always unethical. However, unethical behaviors may not always be illegal. (See *Thinking It Through* in the next section.) Medical law governs the legal conduct of members of the medical profession, involving federal, state, and local laws. Medical professionals who violate such laws can be fined, can have licenses revoked, and can receive prison sentences.

Sometimes it can be difficult to determine the difference between the terms *unethical* and *illegal.* Consider the following discussion.

Thinking It Through...

> Janet, a clinical laboratory assistant, is afraid of contracting AIDS. She feels frightened when she has to draw blood from AIDS patients, but she hasn't shared her feelings with any of her coworkers. When Janet comes into contact with Joseph Jones, a patient who has full-blown AIDS, Janet is rude to him when drawing his blood. She feels his disease is a terrible danger to her.
>
> 1. Is Janet behaving unethically toward Joseph?
>
> 2. Should Janet tell her supervisor how she feels?
>
> 3. How could Janet deal with her fears responsibly?
>
> ***************
>
> Janet knows Joseph from high school. She calls her friend Eileen (who also knows Joseph) when she gets home and tells Eileen that Joseph Jones has full-blown AIDS.
>
> 1. Is Janet's phone call to Eileen unethical?
>
> 2. Could Janet's call be considered illegal?

Professionalism

As part of being an ethical employee, the clinical laboratory assistant must always be aware of acting in a professional manner. The clinical laboratory assistant is often the only representative of the clinical laboratory that the patient will see. The impression that the clinical laboratory assistant/ phlebotomist makes can form the impression that the patient has of the entire laboratory. A sloppy, unpleasant and careless clinical laboratory assistant may cause the patient to question the quality of the laboratory in general.

FRIENDLINESS. Since the clinical laboratory assistant/phlebotomist often interacts with the patient, a friendly manner is necessary. However, this attitude must be tempered with professionalism. Being "too friendly" can feel inappropriate to the patient. So, it's best not to call patients by their first name (except children) unless they request that you do so. Personal relations with patients can interfere with the deliv-

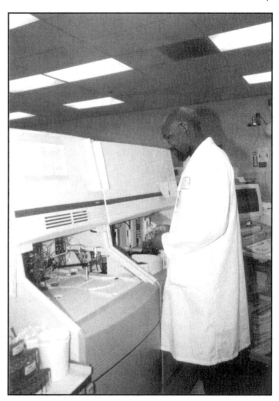

Figure 4-1: A clinical laboratory professional is well-groomed and has an assuring presence.

ery of client care. Patients are not interested in the private life of the clinical laboratory assistant. And in like manner, asking the patient personal questions is not professional. A pleasant, warm, but professional manner is a good balance to achieve with the patient.

PERSONAL APPEARANCE. In addition to conduct, another component of professionalism is to maintain a neat, clean personal appearance. How you look contributes to the image the clinical laboratory assistant conveys to the patient. So, a messy appearance may give the patient the impression that the entire clinical laboratory is disorderly. Conversely, an orderly appearance will inspire confidence in many patients. The following are points to consider about the laboratory assistant's professional appearance:

- Clothing should be clean and free from wrinkles. White uniforms should be a true white, not a dingy off-white. Uniforms and laboratory coats should be in good repair, with all buttons in place. Clothing should fit loosely and should be appropriate for the job.

- Shoes should be in good condition and comfortable. High heels and other inappropriate shoes for an employee on his/her feet much of the day should be avoided.

- Hairstyles should be conservative. Long hair hanging down in the patient's face while the laboratory assistant is drawing blood is not appropriate. Long hair should be tied back. Beards should be trimmed.

- The condition of the clinical laboratory assistant's/phlebotomist's hands is very evident to the patient. So, nails should be clean and well manicured. Chipped nail polish is not appropriate. Long nails are not practical or hygienic for this position.

- Personal hygiene is critical for the laboratory assistant. A strong body odor and bad breath do not make a good impression. Remember, the laboratory assistant is often in very close proximity to the patient.

- The use of cologne and perfume is discouraged by some healthcare facilities because some patients are allergic to fragrances.

- Jewelry should be moderate, as should makeup.

Thinking It Through...

"Hi Ethel! I'm Sherrie. I'm the resident vampire, and I'm going to get your blood," Sherrie exclaims as she enters the blood drawing room, cracking her gum before and after the greeting, her long hair flying behind her.

"Jeez. Am I in a hurry! And now I got another run in these dang nylons. You got any hints, Ethel, for not getting runs? Since my old man ran out on me, I don't have money for more than a few pairs. And with these short skirts I like to wear, more and more leg shows. O.K. Ethel, I'm going to draw your blood now. Wow! I love your diamond ring! Where'd you get this doozy? Bet it cost a fortune. You must be rich! My old man wouldn't have given me the time of day, you know what I mean?"

1. How many unprofessional behaviors does Sherrie perform in this scenario?

2. How would you respond to Sherrie?

3. Should Sherrie be fired?

EFFICIENCY. Today's medical environment calls for greater efficiency on the part of all medical employees. Physicians may want the results of a blood test immediately when a patient is ill. However, the clinical laboratory assistant/phlebotomist should not rush the blood collection process to the point that the patient is treated like an item on an assembly line. So, no matter how much pressure is being applied to hurry and get the sample, carrying out a pleasant, light conversation with the patient is important. Efficiency should never replace accuracy and quality. Hurrying can also result in dropping the blood or sticking one's self with a needle. Professionalism under hurried circumstances requires a delicate balance between treating the patient ethically and getting the job done in a rapid manner.

COMPASSION. Many patients may be very fearful of needles and of healthcare facilities in general. For example, some patients may have had bad experiences having their blood drawn in the past. Patients must be treated with respect, even though time is short. Empathizing with patients (trying to put yourself in their position) should be a goal for all laboratory assistants/phlebotomists during each and every encounter.

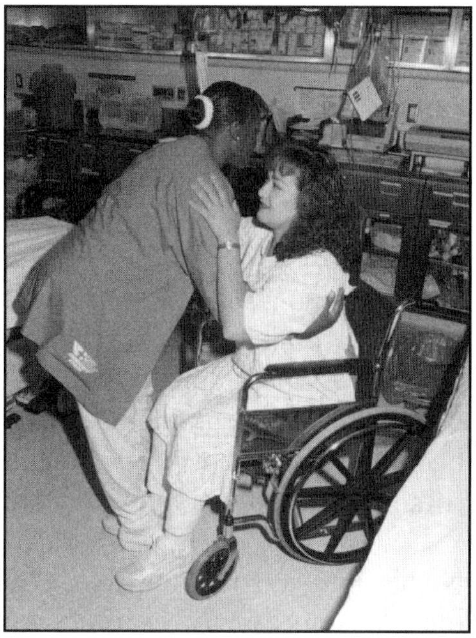

Scope of Practice

Since the early 1980's, there has been a rapid increase in the number of lawsuits against healthcare workers. One of the most successful ways to avoid being involved in a lawsuit is for clinical labo-

Courtesy, K. St. Clair Garber, EMS Options Unlimited, Zephyr Cove, Nevada. Printed with permission.

Figure 4-2: A laboratory assistant helpfully assists a patient from a wheelchair.

ratory assistants to fully understand their **scope of practice**. An employee's scope of practice is what the employee is assigned to do based on his/her educational and training background. Proper education and adherence to procedures will help build a strong defense if an employee is named as a defendant in a lawsuit.

scope of practice: a legal description of what a specific health professional may and may not do.

Medical Law

It is not enough to be aware of acting in a professional, caring manner. All healthcare employees should also be aware of many legal concepts that apply to the medical workplace. In most instances, acting unprofessionally or unethically will not result in immediate job loss. However, when the medical professional acts illegally, immediate job loss, fines, loss of a medical license, and even prison sentences are possible. The following summarizes some laws that apply to the medical workplace.

Lawsuits

malpractice: professional misconduct or lack of professional skill that results in injury to the patient; negligence by a professional, such as a physician or nurse.

Two specific types of lawsuits are common to the healthcare field. Medical **malpractice** is professional misconduct or lack of professional skill that results in injury to the patient. A patient who thinks that a medical worker has failed in diagnosing and treating an illness or accident can file a medical malpractice claim. Most of these claims are made against physicians, but a clinical laboratory assistant can be named in such a suit. Most medical malpractice insurance policies allow pathologists and/or clinical laboratories to cover themselves and employees of the clinical laboratory. In some environments, clinical laboratory assistants have their own insurance policies. When a person becomes employed by a clinical laboratory, the laboratory's management should be questioned immediately about its malpractice coverage.

negligence: the failure to give reasonable care or to do what another prudent person with similar experience, knowledge and background would have done under the same or similar circumstances.

Negligence is defined as the failure to give reasonable care or the giving of unreasonable care. An example of negligence would be when a patient tells you that he or she is prone to fainting and would like to have blood drawn in a prone position. But you are too busy to take the patient into the other room where there is a bed for such a situation. You go ahead and draw blood from the patient, who promptly faints and suffers an injury while you are busy labeling the blood. Given your above actions, you may be found negligent because you have neglected to act in the best interests of the patient.

Intentional Torts

Intentional torts are wrongful acts which are performed intentionally. Several types are listed here:

assault: the threat of an immediate harmful or offensive contact, without actual commission of the act.

battery: the unlawful touching of an individual without consent.

- **Assault** is the threat of an immediate harmful or offensive contact, without the actual commission of the act. An example would be if a clinical laboratory assistant tells a patient something like "If you don't cooperate, I'm going to have to tie you down."

- **Battery** is the unlawful touching of an individual without consent (eg, performing a blood draw after the patient has refused).

- **False imprisonment** is restraining a person against his or her will, either physically or with verbal threats.

- **Abandonment** is the termination of supervision of a patient by a physician without adequate written notice or the patient's consent.

- **Invasion of privacy** is the public discussion of private information (eg, release of medical information without the patient's written consent). Maintaining patient **confidentiality** means being sure everything that is heard, written, or discussed in the hospital STAYS IN THE HOSPITAL. All information about the patient is privileged and should remain confidential.

- **Duty of care** is the understanding that the patient has the assurance of safe care. The healthcare worker must treat the patient according to common or average standards of practice expected in the patient's community.

- **Libel** is defined as a written attack on a person's reputation.

- **Slander** is a spoken attack on a person's reputation. For example, gossiping about a patient's medical condition or private business to an outside party could possibly result in a slander suit by the patient.

- **Reasonable care** is a legal term which protects the healthcare worker if the worker can prove that he or she acted reasonably as compared to fellow workers. If the healthcare worker fails to meet this standard, a charge of negligence may result.

Advance Directives

Another healthcare legal term is the **advance directive.** This is a document prepared while an individual is alive and competent. It provides guidelines to healthcare professionals in the event the patient is no longer able to make decisions. The directive includes the individual's preferences concerning life support measures and organ donation and can give authority to another person to make decisions for the terminally ill patient in event of a coma.

The Patient's Bill of Rights

Patients have the right to expect and receive a certain standard of care when they enter a healthcare facility. The American Hospital Association has developed a **Patient's Bill of Rights** that is posted in facilities in a location readily visible to patients. Patients should receive a copy of these rights upon admission to healthcare services. An example follows.

---

duty of care: a legal term referring to the healthcare worker's duty to treat the patient according to common or average standards of practice expected in the community.

libel: false and malicious writing about another constituting a defamation of character.

slander: a spoken attack on a person's reputation.

reasonable care: care that a healthcare worker is expected to provide to patients.

advance directive: a legal document prepared when an individual is alive, competent, and able to make decisions. It provides guidance to the healthcare team if the person is no longer able to make decisions.

Patient's Bill of Rights: a document that identifies the basic rights of all patients.

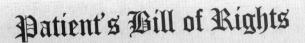

Patient's Bill of Rights

1. The patient has a right to considerate and respectful care.

2. Patients have the right to obtain from their physician complete current information concerning their diagnosis, treatment and prognosis in terms they can be reasonably expected to understand.

3. An informed consent should include knowledge of the proposed procedure, along with its risks and probable duration of incapacitation. In addition, the patient has a right to information regarding medically significant alternatives.

4. The patient has the right to refuse treatment to the extent permitted by law, and to be informed of the medical consequences of his action.

5. Case discussion, consultation, examination, and treatment should be conducted discretely. Those not directly involved must have the patient's permission to be present.

6. The patient has the right to expect that all communication and records pertaining to his care should be treated as confidential.

7. The patient has the right to expect the hospital to make a reasonable response to his request for services. The hospital must provide evaluation, service, and referral as indicated by the urgency of the case.

8. The patient has the right to obtain information as to any relationship of his hospital to other healthcare and educational institutions, insofar as his care is concerned. The patient has the right to obtain information as to the existence of any professional relationships among individuals, by name, who are treating him.

9. The patient has the right to be advised if the hospital proposes to engage in or perform human experimentation affecting his care or treatment. The patient has the right to refuse to participate in such research projects.

10. The patient has the right to expect reasonable continuity of care.

11. The patient has the right to examine and receive an explanation of his bill regardless of the source of payment.

12. The patient has the right to know what hospital rules and regulations apply to his conduct as a patient.

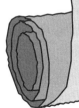

Figure 4-3: The Patient's Bill of Rights

Consent

The concept of patient consent is very important for the clinical laboratory assistant to understand. The law states that each and every patient has the right to determine what shall or shall NOT be done with his/her body. First, the patient must always give verbal consent to any blood drawn. If the consent is not given and the blood is obtained anyway, the laboratory assistant could be accused of battery.

Some procedures, including in some states drawing blood for HIV testing, must be accompanied by a written consent by a patient, a contract that is established between the patient and the healthcare facility. All consents require a witness who is over 21 years old. The treatment of consents by minors can be handled differently from state to state. Be sure to learn your state's laws concerning the treatment of minors and **emancipated minors**.

Confidentiality

Working in any healthcare facility exposes the healthcare worker to special information about patients. This information is called **privileged information** and includes all medical and personal details provided in the medical records and information that the patient has disclosed to the healthcare provider. An important rule to remember as a healthcare professional, as previously stated, is EVERYTHING THAT IS HEARD, WRITTEN, AND DISCUSSED IN THE HOSPITAL STAYS AT THE HOSPITAL. It is often tempting to discuss a difficult patient with a fellow employee when you are at lunch, at the hospital gift shop, or in the parking lot of the hospital. But, conversations can be, and often are, overheard. Any comments made must be confined to the clinical laboratory and to fellow employees who need the information to help them do their job.

emancipated minor: a person under the age of 18 who is financially responsible for himself/herself and free of parental care.

privileged information: confidential data; all data concerning a patient that is disclosed within the healthcare facility.

confidentiality: privacy; refers to the limiting of access to patient information to authorized personnel only.

Thinking It Through...

Peter is a clinical laboratory assistant who often draws blood at the alcohol rehabilitation unit of the hospital. Today, he draws blood from a patient he recognizes as his old geometry teacher, a difficult man who flunked both Peter and his brother Sam. Peter is dying to tell Sam about their former teacher's plight.

1. How should Peter react to his former teacher?

2. Can Peter tell Sam if Sam promises not to tell anyone?

3. Do you think Peter should be fired if his employer finds out that he has discussed this matter outside of the hospital?

4. How often do you think you might recognize a patient at your workplace?

Chapter Summary

Patients have the right to expect competent, highly professional treatment when they seek healthcare. Laboratory professionals must always treat patients with kindness, consideration, and respect. Further, the clinical laboratory assistant must constantly be aware of ethical and legal issues that are relevant to work in the clinical laboratory. Therefore, laboratory employees must also understand their legal scope of practice and the healthcare facility's policies and procedures concerning patient care.

Name _____

Date _____

Student Enrichment Activities

Complete the following statements.

1. Ethics are _____.

2. Medical law focuses upon _____

   _____.

3. Different aspects of behavior to consider when being a professional include

   _____, _____, _____, and

   _____.

4. Scope of practice means _____

   _____.

5. Confidentiality includes _____

   _____.

6. An advance directive is _____

   _____.

Unscramble the following terms.

7. CIHETS   _____

8. RYTTBAE   _____

9. BILLE   _____

10. NERSALD   _____

Circle T for true, or F for false.

11. T   F   It is always easy to determine the difference between medical law and ethics.

12. T   F   There is such a thing as being too friendly with patients.

13. T   F   Long fingernails are not hygienic in the laboratory.

14. T   F   Assault and battery are the same concept.

15. T   F   Written patient consents must sometimes be obtained.

Chapter Five
Infection Control Practices in the Clinical Laboratory

Objectives

After completing this chapter, you should be able to do the following:

1. Define and correctly spell each of the key terms.

2. Identify the role of the Centers for Disease Control and Prevention regarding infectious diseases.

3. Explain the importance of infection control programs in healthcare facilities.

4. Identify the component parts of the infection cycle and the steps taken to break the cycle.

5. Explain what is meant by occupational exposure.

6. Discuss the importance of handwashing and of wearing gloves in the healthcare environment.

7. List some personal protective gear and why it is used in the clinical laboratory.

8. Discuss the importance of Standard Precautions.

9. Describe precautions taken with sharps in the clinical laboratory.

Key Terms

- AIDS
- bloodborne pathogens
- carrier
- Centers for Disease Control and Prevention
- chemotherapy
- hepatitis
- immune globulin
- incident report
- infection control

- infection cycle
- Joint Committee for Accreditation of Healthcare Organizations
- nosocomial infection
- occupational exposure
- Occupational Safety and Health Administration
- resistance
- sharps
- Standard Precautions

infection control: efforts taken to control infectious agents in a healthcare facility.

chemotherapy: the use of drugs or chemicals to treat or control diseases such as cancer.

nosocomial infection: an infection that is acquired during a stay at a hospital.

Introduction

When the body is invaded by pathogenic bacteria, viruses, fungi, or parasites, the resulting condition is called an **infection**. These infections can affect the body seriously. Persons who are particularly susceptible to such infections include people who are already weakened from a disease, are being treated for cancer (such as **chemotherapy**), or are fragile in old age. In the healthcare facility, **infection control** programs are in place to attempt to control and eliminate **nosocomial infections**, infections acquired after admission to a healthcare facility. Efforts are always made to keep both staff and patients in an infection-free state so that there is not cross-contamination between patient and staff, as well as between patient and patient. Clinical laboratory assistants/phlebotomists are in continual contact with patients and must be acutely aware of not spreading infection or acquiring infections themselves.

The Centers for Disease Control and Prevention

The **Centers for Disease Control and Prevention (CDC)** is a governmental agency responsible for protecting public health through the prevention and control of disease. By studying causes and distribution of diseases, employees of this agency provide the public and professional healthcare providers, including employees in the clinical laboratory, with valuable information concerning the prevention and control of diseases.

Standards and regulations established by the CDC and other agencies require all employers to provide ongoing training for employees concerning the management of infectious and hazardous waste products. This is especially important in the clinical laboratory where hazardous waste products such as blood, urine, other body fluids, and stool are handled on a regular basis. This also refers to the disposal of contaminated products such as body fluid containers, needles, scalpels, and other products.

Centers for Disease Control and Prevention: CDC; the government agency responsible for protecting public health through the prevention and control of disease.

Infection Control Programs

Healthcare institutions must have a procedural infection control program that is designed to prevent infection in the workplace. The patients are of prime concern to the infection control department in a healthcare facility, but so are the employees, visitors, and any other people who come into contact with the institution. An infection control program includes the monitoring and collecting of data on infections within the healthcare facility. The infection control department also works with the facility to ensure that all employees are protected from infectious and hazardous waste products. The clinical laboratory has a close association with the infection control department.

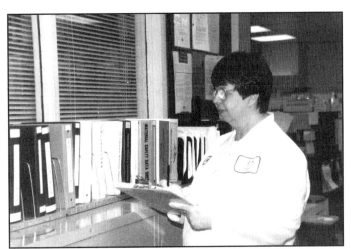

Figure 5-1: The infection control department monitors infections within the healthcare facility.

Occupational Safety and Health Administration: OSHA; a government agency that develops safety standards and establishes maximum levels of exposure to many biohazardous materials.

Joint Committee for Accreditation of Healthcare Organizations: JCAHO; a voluntary nongovernmental agency charged with establishing standards for the operation of hospitals and other health-related facilities and services.

infection cycle: a pattern that describes the origin and transmission of a disease or illness.

carrier: a human or animal who is infected with a pathogen, and who can spread the disease to others, but who does not show any outward signs or symptoms of disease.

When an outbreak of infection does occur in a facility, the infection control department takes special precautions to prevent the infection from spreading. These programs follow regulations and guidelines established by the CDC, the **Occupational Safety and Health Administration (OSHA)**, and the **Joint Committee for Accreditation of Healthcare Organizations (JCAHO)**, in addition to other state and local regulatory agencies.

The Infection Cycle

As a clinical laboratory assistant/phlebotomist, you will be expected to be an active part of the healthcare facility's effort to control and eliminate the spread of infection in the workplace. Since you may be in constant contact with patients—some with and some without infectious disease—you must do all you can to prevent the spread of infection to yourself, to other employees, and especially to other patients.

As a part of a team that works continually to prevent the spread of infection, it is helpful to understand the various ways that infection can be transmitted, as well as the various methods that break the **infection cycle**. This cycle can be visualized as a chain of events that can allow infection to get inside the human body. Six components make up the infection cycle (Figure 5-2).

1. INFECTIOUS AGENT: any disease-causing microorganism (pathogen).

2. RESERVOIR HOST: the individual in which the infectious microorganisms reside. Examples include animals, water, air, soil, and human beings. Humans or animals who do not show any outward signs or symptoms of a disease but are still capable of transmitting the disease are known as **carriers**.

3. PORTAL OF EXIT: the route by which a pathogen leaves the body. Examples of portals of exit are breaks in the skin, respiratory secretions, reproductive secretions, and blood.

4. ROUTE OF TRANSMISSION: the method by which the pathogen gets from the reservoir to the new host. Transmission may occur through direct contact, air, insects, etc.

5. PORTAL OF ENTRY: the route through which the pathogen enters its new host. The respiratory, gastrointestinal, urinary, and reproductive tracts, and breaks in the protective skin barrier are common points of entry.

6. SUSCEPTIBLE HOST: a person capable of being affected or infected by invading microorganisms, depending on the degree of that person's **resistance**. Some examples of susceptible hosts are people who are malnourished, people who have suppressed immune systems, or people who are in poor health.

resistance: the ability to fight off a particular force, such as an infection.

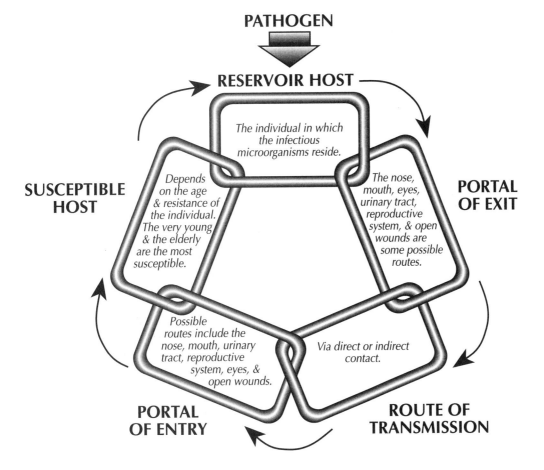

Figure 5-2: The Infection Cycle

Interrupting the Infection Cycle

The infection control department of a hospital is particularly interested in how to interrupt the infection cycle before the infection spreads in the hospital. For each component of the infection cycle, there are methods used to interrupt that part of the cycle. These methods follow.

1. INFECTIOUS AGENT: the infectious agent (pathogen) must be identified rapidly by the physician and appropriate treatment started promptly.

2. RESERVOIR HOST: the employee must maintain proper personal hygiene and **asepsis**. The working environment must be disinfected and sanitized.

3. PORTALS OF EXIT: employees must wear proper attire such as laboratory coats and uniforms; take **Standard** or **Transmission-based Precautions**; control body secretions (eg, sneeze into a tissue); and wash hands frequently according to protocol.

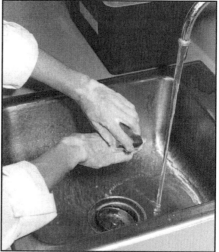

Courtesy K. St. Clair Garber, EMS Options Unlimited, Zephyr Cove, Nevada.

Figure 5-3: Proper handwashing can interrupt the infection cycle.

4. ROUTE OF TRANSMISSION: the employee must practice good handwashing, disinfection, and sterilization techniques; properly dispose of all potentially infected materials; isolate infected patients from others; and REFRAIN FROM WORKING IF INFECTIOUS!

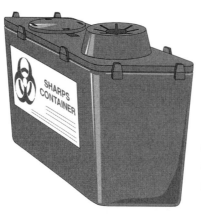

Figure 5-4: Always dispose of needles and other sharp instruments in a special sharps container!

5. PORTALS OF ENTRY: employees must practice good asepsis, disinfection, and sterilization.

6. SUSCEPTIBLE HOST: employees must identify high-risk patients and take appropriate action to avoid unnecessary exposure.

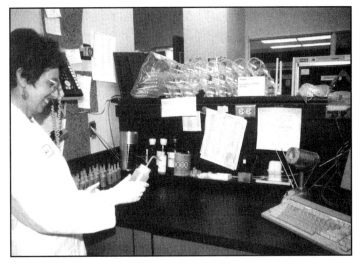

Figure 5-5: Work surfaces in the clinical laboratory are often cleaned with a strong disinfectant.

Occupational Exposure

The clinical laboratory assistant/phlebotomist must be constantly aware of the risk of infection to the laboratory worker. **Occupational exposure** refers to reasonably anticipated exposure to infectious materials that can occur during the course of a healthcare worker's employment.

Two serious diseases that can cause significant risk to the medical laboratory assistant/phlebotomist are **hepatitis** and **acquired immune deficiency syndrome (AIDS).** Hepatitis is an inflammation of the liver, caused by a variety of physical or chemical agents. Viral hepatitis is the main concern of the clinical laboratory employee. There are several strains of the hepatitis virus, including hepatitis A, B, and C.

Hepatitis A is the most common form of viral hepatitis occurring in children and young adults. The spread of hepatitis A is by fecal-oral routes, usually by people who fail to wash their hands after using the bathroom. Infection with hepatitis A can be debilitating but usually clears up in a few weeks with no lasting effects.

occupational exposure: exposure to infectious materials that can be reasonably anticipated to occur during the course of one's work; exposure can be to the eye, skin, mucous membranes, or through needle sticks or breaks in the skin.

hepatitis: inflammation of the liver.

Hepatitis B is the most common cause of infection in healthcare workers. Also a viral disease, it is spread through contact with infected blood products and sexual contact. There is an effective vaccine against hepatitis B that all healthcare workers should receive. This vaccine must be made available free-of-charge to every employee who has the potential for occupational exposure to the virus. The vaccine is given in three doses over a six-month time period.

Hepatitis C, spread by the same routes as hepatitis B, is also a viral disease. It is a serious threat to the healthcare worker, and no vaccination for this type of hepatitis exists. Clinical healthcare workers in contact with blood and body fluids must wear gloves at all times and must practice careful and frequent handwashing to reduce the risk of contracting this disease.

AIDS:
acquired immune deficiency syndrome; a viral disease caused by the human immu-nodeficiency virus (HIV), which damages the immune system leaving the patient susceptible to other infections. It is contracted through infected blood and other body fluids and sexual contact.

AIDS can be transmitted through blood and sexual contact. The AIDS virus, known as HIV or Human Immunodeficiency Virus, attacks the immune system (blood cells and other immune system components that work together to fight off infections and disease).

Handwashing and Wearing Gloves

Perhaps the most effective precautions that the clinical laboratory assistant/phlebotomist can take to prevent the spread of infection to oneself or to patients is to wash hands and wear gloves whenever procuring specimens or working with specimens. Hands should be washed before putting on gloves. After taking the gloves off and disposing of the gloves properly, the hands should be washed again. Proper handwashing technique is demonstrated on the following pages.

Handwashing Technique

Materials needed:

✔ liquid soap
✔ paper towels

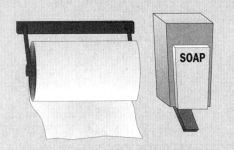

1. <u>Procedural Step:</u> Turn on the faucet. Adjust the temperature of the water to warm, not hot.
   Reason: Warmer water helps kill possible contaminants and hot water may burn.

2. <u>Procedural Step:</u> Always wet your hands with the fingertips pointing down into, but not touching, the sink.
   Reason: Keeping your hands down keeps your forearms dry and prevents contaminated water on your forearms from running over your clean hands. (In most cases, your hands will be dirtier than your arms anyway, so concentrate on getting your hands clean.)

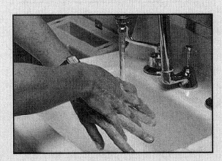

3. <u>Procedural Step:</u> Use a liberal amount of soap and rub the palms of your hands together several times.
   Reason: This friction will create a lather and help remove any unwanted microorganisms from the skin surface.

4. <u>Procedural Step:</u> Put the palm of one hand over the back of the other hand and briskly rub them together.
   Reason: All parts of the hands are capable of carrying germs.

5. <u>Procedural Step:</u> Repeat step #4 using the opposite hands.
   Reason: To clean the other hand.

6. <u>Procedural Step:</u> Interlock the fingers of both hands and vigorously rub them together. You should scrub your hands for a total of two minutes.
   Reason: To remove harmful microorganisms.

7. <u>Procedural Step:</u> Use an orange (cuticle) stick to clean under each nail. If a cuticle stick is not available, use a hand brush.
   Reason: To remove dirt and microorganisms from under the nails.

8. <u>Procedural Step:</u> Rinse all soapy lather from the wrists and hands, continuing to point the hands downward.

Handwashing Technique (cont.)

Reason: *To prevent contaminated water on your forearms from running over your clean hands.*

9. Procedural Step: Leave the water running and dry all areas of the hands using a paper towel.
Reason: *Paper towels are disposable and prevent the spread of pathogenic microorganisms.*

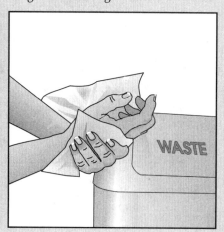

10. Procedural Step: Dispose of the wet paper towel. Obtain another paper towel and, placing the paper towel on the faucet handles, turn off the water.
Make sure the towel is dry.
Reason: *A wet paper towel allows microorganisms to pass through the towel and back to your clean hands. The dry paper towel will shield your hands from germs on the faucet. THE FAUCET AND SINK ALWAYS ARE CONSIDERED TO BE CONTAMINATED.*

11. Procedural Step: Discard all debris and leave the sink and surrounding area clean, taking care not to recontaminate your hands.
Reason: *The area must be ready for the next person who wants to wash.*

Gloves are the most frequently used form of personal protective equipment. The clinical laboratory assistant must wear gloves when contacting blood, potentially infectious material, mucous membranes, or non-intact skin. All specimen collection procedures must include gloves. Bandage any cuts before wearing gloves. If gloves are damaged or contaminated in any way, they should be replaced immediately. Disposable gloves are never washed for later use. Removal of contaminated gloves should be done carefully so as not to contaminate hands and clothes.

Removing Contaminated Gloves

Materials needed:

✓ a trash can lined with a red biohazard bag

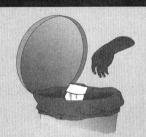

1. Procedure: Hold your gloved hands over a trash can.
   Reason: You will throw away your used gloves.

2. Procedure: Without touching the bare skin of your forearm, grasp the contaminated (or outside) area of the dominant glove cuff (approximately 1 to 2 inches from the top) with your nondominant gloved hand.
   Reason: To avoid contamination.

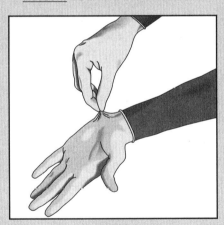

3. Procedure: Pull the glove off. It will now be inside out. Do not snap gloves when removing them.
   Reason: Microorganisms on the gloves could become airborne.

4. Procedure: Discard the glove directly into the trash container lined with a red biohazard bag.

Reason: Gloves cannot be reused. They are considered hazardous waste, and therefore must be disposed of in the proper manner.

5. Procedure: Place the bare fingertips of the dominant hand inside the other glove, and grasp it near the top. Don't let your bare hand touch the contaminated portion of the glove.
   Reason: To avoid contamination.

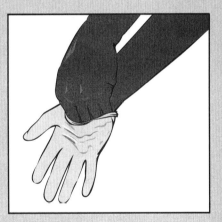

6. Procedure: Pull the second glove off. It also will be inside out. Discard it in the trash can lined with a red biohazard bag.
   Reason: Gloves cannot be reused.

7. Procedure: Wash your hands thoroughly before touching anything.
   Reason: Standard Precaution.

Personal Protective Gear

Clinical laboratory assistants should have at their disposal the following protective equipment.

- GLOVES: As explained above, gloves are essential when handling potentially infectious and hazardous materials.

- MASKS: Masks are worn to prevent transmission of airborne infectious agents, often when a patient has an immune system that is compromised. Masks can also be worn during procedures that are likely to create droplets or blood or other body fluids. Masks must be changed between each patient contact and discarded in hazardous waste receptacles.

- LABORATORY COATS: Laboratory coats (lab coats) are worn to prevent the soiling of clothes with potentially infectious materials as well as hazardous materials such as acids that can be used during collection or testing procedures. Lab coats should never be worn when the clinical laboratory assistant is not on duty, such as in the cafeteria.

- GOWNS: Gowns are worn when the clinical laboratory assistant goes into a situation, such as a bedside of an immune system-compromised patient, where the laboratory coat could be a potential source of infection for the patient. Gowns may also be worn for certain procedures in the laboratory, when going into a recovery room to obtain blood from a patient, or in other situations that require special attention to infection control.

- APRONS: Aprons can also be used to protect clothing from soiling. Aprons are often worn when dealing with materials in testing that may be radioactive or corrosive.

- FACE SHIELDS: Face shields are used to protect the face from droplets of infectious or corrosive materials.

- GOGGLES: Goggles are worn to protect the eye from splashes of infectious or corrosive materials.

Standard Precautions

Formerly called Universal Precautions, **Standard Precautions** refer to recommendations made by the Centers for Disease Control and Prevention to prevent both healthcare workers and patients from contracting diseases spread by **bloodborne pathogens** — especially hepatitis and AIDS. These precautions advise that ALL PATIENTS SHOULD BE TREATED AS IF THEY HAVE AN INFECTIOUS BLOOD-BORNE DISEASE. It is possible to be infected and capable of transmitting a disease without showing any symptoms. OSHA regulates and enforces Standard Precautions.

Standard Precautions: guidelines developed by The Centers for Disease Control and Prevention for protecting healthcare workers from exposure to bloodborne pathogens in body secretions.

bloodborne pathogens: the disease-causing micro-organisms that are present in human blood. Examples include the human immuno-deficiency virus (HIV) and the hepatitis B virus (HBV).

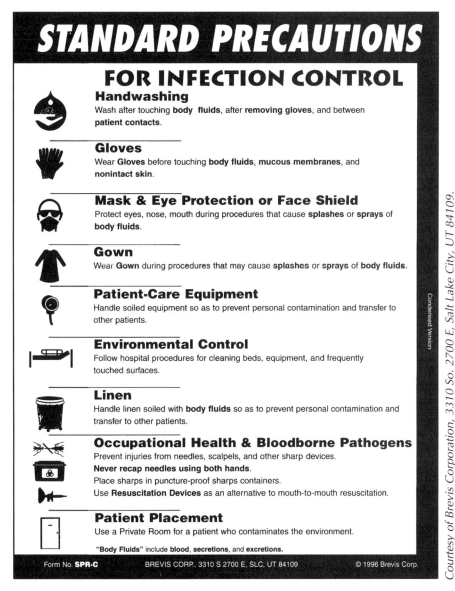

Figure 5-6: Standard Precautions

Treating each patient as if he or she were infected with a serious blood-borne disease is a skill that must become routine to the clinical laboratory assistant/ phlebotomist. The greatest care must be taken to handle all blood and body fluids with gloves, assuming that each and every specimen is potentially infectious. This kind of caution will reduce the risk of the employee contracting an infection. Of course, using this kind of caution does not mean that you should not continue to treat all patients with care and concern! This is the primary duty for all healthcare workers. Remember to treat the disease as potentially infectious — not the patient!

Sharps Precautions

sharps:
a general term given to all items in the operating room that are sharp; includes scalpel blades, needles, and glass items.

For the clinical laboratory assistant/phlebotomist, following proper procedures for the disposal of **sharps** — needles, syringes, or other implements designed to puncture the skin — is critical. Sharps present the double hazard of physical injury and disease transmission. After use, sharps are to be placed in rigid, biohazard-labeled, leakproof, and puncture-proof containers (Figure 5-4), kept at the site of blood collection or at any site where sharps are routinely used.

Needles are NOT to be recapped, bent, broken, or manipulated by hand. If sharps disposal units are not immediately available, a one-handed recapping technique may be used. This technique that must only be used when no other safe disposal method is available.

One-Handed Recapping Method

1. Place the needle cap on a flat surface where the cap cannot roll away.

2. Put the needle unit on the same plane as the cap, lining up the needle and cap.

3. Scoop up the cap with the needle unit. Using only one hand prevents accidental needle punctures of the other hand.

4. Press the cap on a flat surface to secure the cap to the needle unit, again preventing a needle stick to the other hand.

5. Dispose of the recapped needle as soon as possible.

Dispose of sharps containers when they are about 80% full because if they are overfilled, contaminated needles will protrude from the units. The full units are collected and disposed of by the facility along with other biohazardous materials each day. Many facilities hire disposal companies to handle such materials.

If you stick yourself with a contaminated needle or come into direct contact with contaminated fluids by experiencing, for example, a splash from contaminated fluid which contacts the mucous membranes of the eyes or mouth, the incident must be reported immediately to a supervisor. An **incident report** is prepared by the employee stating the exact sequence of events that led to the incident, as well as preventive measures to be taken in the future.

incident report: a report made by a healthcare worker when an event occurs that is not consistent with the routine operation of the healthcare facility.

Thinking It Through ...

Jamie has been a clinical laboratory assistant at Swellcare Hospital for 3 months. She has just finished her training and is eager to please the supervisor.

One morning while drawing blood, Jamie sticks herself with a needle just after she draws blood from an elderly woman. The needle barely sticks her finger, but she does have slight bleeding.

Jamie is embarrassed. No one has seen her stick herself. The elderly woman seems to be no health threat as she is a stroke patient with no other problems. Jamie is also afraid her supervisor will be angry. The needlestick was also shallow. She decides not to report the incident.

1. Is Jamie doing the right thing?

2. Could a shallow needlestick cause any harm?

3. Is Jamie correct in thinking that the elderly woman is not infectious?

4. Could Jamie get fired for this accident?

5. What if Jamie gets sick and has not reported the incident?

OSHA requires employers to provide free medical evaluation and treatment to any employee in the event of an exposure incident. Immediately after a needle stick, the clinical laboratory assistant/phlebotomist must decontaminate the needlestick site with alcohol or flush the mucous membrane contact site with water. The employee then directly reports to a healthcare provider for an immediate medical evaluation and counseling, as well as any other necessary treatment. An evaluation could include the following:

- The employee's blood may be tested for HIV.

- The patient whose body fluid was the source of contamination may be tested for HIV and for hepatitis, providing permission is granted by the patient.

- If the patient refuses any testing and is hepatitis or HIV positive or is in a high-risk category, the employee may be given either **immune globulin** or a hepatitis B vaccination.

- If the source patient is HIV positive, the employee is counseled and evaluated for HIV at periodic intervals. Medications may also be given to the employee.

- The employee is counseled to watch for acute viral symptoms within 12 weeks of exposure. Fortunately, needlesticks rarely lead to HIV infections.

immune globulin: a preparation injected into an individual to boost the immune system; often given to employees who have just stick themselves with a contaminated needle.

Additionally, work practices to prevent infection should include the following:

- Do not eat, drink, smoke, apply cosmetics or lip balm, or handle contact lenses while in the work areas where exposure to infectious materials can occur.

- No food and drink should be stored in areas were potentially infectious materials are present. Refrigerators used to store specimens should not contain food and drink.

- Never use a **pipette** by drawing fluid up with the mouth.

- Take EVERY precaution when performing procedures involving possible infectious materials; minimize splashes or spraying. Goggles, face shields, and splash screens should be available for use in such situations.

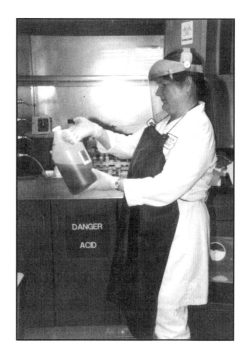

Figure 5-7: A clinical laboratory assistant should use goggles or a splash guard when splashes of potentially infectious materials might occur.

Chapter Summary

There has never been greater emphasis put on infection control in the healthcare facility than there is today. Extraordinary efforts are taking place to keep healthcare facilities as free from infection as possible for both the patients and the employees. It is important for the clinical laboratory assistant/phlebotomist to understand the significance of the infection cycle and how to break this cycle.

Bloodborne pathogens such as viral hepatitis and AIDS make it critical for the laboratory employee to adhere to Standard Precautions continually, remembering that ALL PATIENTS SHOULD BE TREATED AS IF THEY HAVE AN INFECTIOUS BLOOD-BORNE DISEASE. Care must be taken with all body fluids, and the clinical laboratory assistant should wear as much protective gear as is necessary to be protected against infection.

Name _____

Date _____

Student Enrichment Activities

Circle T for true, or F for false.

1.   T F   Viral hepatitis is the form of hepatitis that is of most concern to the clinical laboratory worker.

2.   T F   OSHA regulates and enforces Standard Precautions.

3.   T F   Hepatitis C is not a threat to the healthcare worker.

4.   T F   AIDS is an example of a blood-borne disease.

5.   T F   An incident report is not necessary after a needle stick.

6.   T F   All needles must be placed in sharps containers.

7.   T F   Sharps containers should only be 50% filled.

8.   T F   Standard Precautions were formerly known as Universal Precautions.

9.   I F   Lab coats are not usually contaminated and can be worn in the cafeteria.

10. T F   There is not a vaccine for hepatitis B.

Complete the following exercises.

11. Name three agencies that are involved in protecting both patient and employee
     from infections in the workplace.

     _____

12. What should an employee do after sticking him or herself accidentally with
     a contaminated needle?

     _____

     _____

     _____

     _____

13. Provide two examples of blood-borne pathogens.
     A. _____   B. _____

14. List five categories included in Standard Precautions, and briefly explain each one.
     A. _____

         _____

         _____

     B. _____

         _____

         _____

     C. _____

         _____

         _____

     D. _____

         _____

         _____

     E. _____

         _____

         _____

15. Name five types of personal protective gear worn by clinical laboratory assistants.

     _____

Chapter Six
General Safety Issues in the Healthcare Environment

Objectives

After completing this chapter, you should be able to
do the following:

1. Define and correctly spell each of the key terms.

2. Discuss general issues related to clinical laboratory safety.

3. Explain the importance of safety manuals.

4. Identify uses for the safety hood in the clinical laboratory.

5. Explain why a safety shower and emergency eye wash station are located in the clinical laboratory.

6. Explain key aspects of fire safety regulations in the healthcare facility.

7. Describe how a clinical laboratory assistant can minimize electrical accidents in the healthcare facility.

8. Explain how to identify and avoid undue exposure to radiation in the healthcare facility.

9. Identify key aspects of a chemical safety program in the healthcare facility.

Key Terms

- aerosol
- cardiopulmonary resuscitation
- caustic materials

- material safety data sheet
- safety hood

Introduction

Chapter Five covers the safety issues related to handling infectious materials. In addition to such materials, there are other potential safety hazards that impact the clinical laboratory as well as other areas of the healthcare facility.

General Clinical Laboratory Safety

The goal of safety in the healthcare facility is to recognize and eliminate hazards so that employees can work in a healthy environment. Safe working conditions must be ensured by the employer and have been mandated by law under OSHA standards. Knowledge of OSHA requirements is necessary for both the employer and its employees; and cooperation between the employer and employee concerning these requirements is necessary in all healthcare facilities. Therefore, the employer must provide information concerning safety education to each employee . Personal as well as patient safety must always be a priority as a healthcare employee performs each daily task.

The Safety Manual

Every department in a healthcare facility should have its own safety manual. When you go to work in a clinical laboratory, part of your training should include familiarizing yourself with the location and the contents of the laboratory safety manual. Within the laboratory, individual departments will have their own specific rules for safety. The following list of rules appears in most safety manuals in the clinical laboratory setting:

- While working on the job, nothing should be put into one's mouth. This includes food, pencils, fingers, and so on.
- Hands must be washed frequently throughout the day.
- Cosmetics should not be applied on the job.

- NO food should be placed in any laboratory refrigerator unless the refrigerator is designated as a "For Food Only" refrigerator.

- Loose clothing and long hair should not be worn in the clinical laboratory as they can get caught in machinery, especially in centrifuges.

- Open-toed shoes are prohibited in most areas of the healthcare facility. In the laboratory, chemicals and glassware can be dropped, putting unprotected toes at risk.

- **Caustic materials**, as well as biohazardous materials, should be disposed of properly. OSHA regulations dictate that biohazardous liquid materials such as blood and body fluids may be poured down a sink if permitted by local ordinances. Caustic substances may have to be disposed of in their own sealed container.

caustic materials: materials destructive to living tissue.

The Safety Hood

One of the most important safety measures which prevents biohazardous and caustic accidents is the use of the **safety hood** (Figure 6-1). Throughout the healthcare facility, safety hoods are used to prevent **aerosol** contamination.

Opening a specimen or caustic materials can produce splashes and release aerosols that can reach mucous membranes. To avoid such accidents, a safety hood is turned on and allowed to run for a few minutes. Inside the hood, the air is pulled up into the top of the hood and vented to the outside. The employee then sits down with hands inside the hood while handling potentially hazardous materials.

safety hood: a device that separates a laboratory employee from a specimen or potentially toxic materials by a glass in front of the face. Fumes and aerosols are drawn through the top of the hood and away from the employee.

aerosol: a substance released in the form of a fine mist.

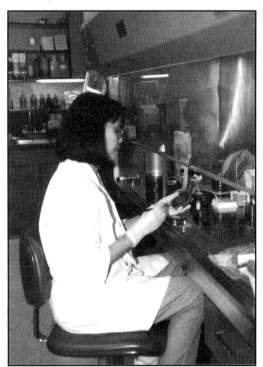

Figure 6-1: A clinical laboratory assistant works with a specimen under a safety hood.

Safety Showers and Eyewash Stations

Acids are used in the clinical laboratory, often as preservatives for tests such as 24-hour urine specimens. Safety showers are installed in areas where a possibility of a chemical accident exists, such as when an employee comes into contact with an acid. Permanent damage to the skin can result from a chemical burn. For this reason, a victim of a chemical spill should rinse immediately in the safety shower for at least 15 minutes after removing contaminated clothing.

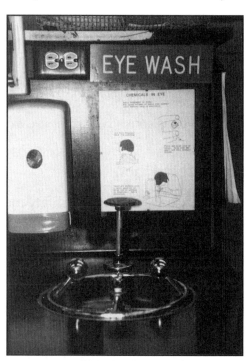

If chemicals are splashed into the eye, the victim should rinse the eye at an eyewash station (Figure 6-2) for a minimum of 15 minutes. Contact lenses can be a further complication in this instance. The lenses should be removed prior to the rinsing in order to cleanse the eyes thoroughly. The injured employee should never rub his or her eyes.

After rinsing the affected area following a chemical accident, the victim should be taken to the emergency department for treatment.

Figure 6-2: An Eyewash Station

Chemical Spill Cleanup

Chemical spills should not be simply wiped up with paper towels. Healthcare facilities have spill cleanup kits in areas where chemicals are used. The kit includes absorbents and neutralizers to clean up acid, alkali, mercury, and other types of spills. In some cases with toxic spills, a specially-trained team from maintenance might have to be called in to handle the spill.

Disinfection in the Healthcare Facility

Disinfection of the healthcare facility is the constant duty of the housekeeping staff of the hospital. Additionally, each department must strive continually to keep its department as free from infectious and other potentially dangerous materials as possible.

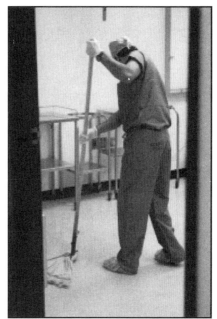

In the clinical laboratory, specimen collection areas are regularly **decontaminated** with a 1:10 bleach solution or other strong disinfectant to render the areas free from pathogenic microorganisms. Many benches in the clinical laboratory are covered daily with paper that has a special plastic undercoating. This paper is thrown away at the end of each day in a biohazard waste container.

Fire Safety

Fire safety is considered the responsibility of ALL employees in a healthcare facility. Clinical laboratory employees should know the exact location of fire extinguishers and their use (Figure 6-4). Extinguishers are usually classified according to the type of fire they can put out.

Figure 6-3: It is each department's responsibility to maintain an environment as free from pathogens as possible.

- CLASS A: This extinguisher puts out paper, wood, fabric, rubber, and certain plastic material fires.

- CLASS B: This extinguisher is for flammable liquids, oil, paint, fat, and gasoline fires.

- CLASS C: This extinguisher is used for fires caused by electrical equipment such as motors, appliances, and switches. The clinical laboratory is full of electrical equipment.

- CLASS D: This extinguisher is used for combustible metals such as sodium, magnesium, potassium, uranium, and powdered aluminum.

Note: Not an official picture symbol.

Figure 6-4: Classes of Fire Extinguishers

In many facilities, multipurpose extinguishers, called ABC extinguishers, are installed to reduce the confusion associated with operating and maintaining different types of extinguishers.

Operating a fire extinguisher is easy. Hold it upright, pull the pin, and direct the spray at the base of the fire. Figure 6-5 illustrates the proper use of the extinguisher.

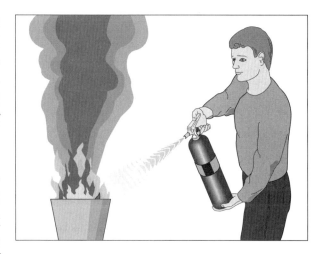

Figure 6-5: Make sure you are trained in the proper use of a fire extinguisher.

While in training, you will be given directions about your specific role in the event of a fire. General directions include the following:

1. Immediately find the nearest alarm box and pull the lever.

2. Call the switchboard of the healthcare facility, and report the fire.

3. If the fire is very small, attempt to extinguish it by using an extinguisher.

4. If you are with a patient, such as drawing blood in an outpatient area, make sure that the patient is taken safely out of the fire area.

5. Unplug any electrical equipment you are using immediately.

6. If evacuation becomes necessary, do not use elevators. Use the stairwell if necessary.

7. Close all doors and windows before leaving.

8. If your clothing is on fire, drop to the floor and roll, preferably in a fire blanket, which should be stored in a visible location in the clinical laboratory.

9. If caught in a fire, crawl to the exit. Smoke rises, and breathing is easier at the floor level. Breathing through a wet towel also helps.

10. Do not panic, run, abandon patients, reenter the building, or block entrances!

Electrical Safety

It is always possible that you could get an electrical shock while operating equipment. The clinical laboratory has many pieces of equipment powered by electricity. Injuries can include moderate burns, severe skin damage, unconsciousness, and even death. Observance of safety guidelines concerning electricity can help reduce the risk of electrical shock.

1. Follow all safety regulations dictated in your clinical laboratory safety manual.

2. Participate in all laboratory and facility-wide safety drills.

3. Never use a piece of equipment until you have been properly instructed and supervised as to its correct use.

4. Inspect electrical cords on any piece of equipment you use. Do not use the equipment if a cord is damaged or frayed.

5. All equipment used in a healthcare facility must be equipped with a three-prong plug. The third plug is used for grounding purposes. If a third prong has been removed, do not use the plug.

6. Report any damaged or malfunctioning piece of equipment to the supervisor immediately. Do not attempt a repair.

7. Make sure your hands, the patient's hands, and the floor are dry!

8. Do not do any routine maintenance on a piece of equipment until you are sure it is unplugged.

Thinking It Through ...

Larry is a clinical laboratory assistant who has a talent for fixing mechanical objects. Larry is working in the laboratory outpatient department drawing blood. He is supposed to spin down blood samples using the centrifuge in the blood drawing room. After he spins down the blood, he must take the processed samples to the laboratory for testing.

Today is a busy day, and Larry has many samples to centrifuge. He hears a "clunk" soon after he starts the centrifuge, which was recently purchased. Larry opens the centrifuge and sees that the problem is a fairly simple mechanical one. It should take Larry only a few minutes to fix the machine.

Larry decides to go ahead and make the repair so that he can get the blood processed as quickly as possible.

1. Is Larry wise to attempt the repair?

2. Are patients better served by having Larry make the repair?

3. Could the warranty on the new centrifuge be compromised by Larry's repair?

If an electric shock accident does occur, shut off the electrical power source immediately. If you cannot reach the power source, remove the electrical contact from the injured person. Use something that does not conduct electricity, such as asbestos gloves or glass, to separate the electrical contact from the person. Call for medical assistance immediately. If the heart has stopped or if the victim is in cardiac arrest, start **cardiopulmonary resuscitation (CPR)** at once. Keep the victim warm until help comes.

**cardio-
pulmonary
resuscitation:**
CPR; the basic
lifesaving
procedure
of artificial
ventilation
and chest
compressions
that is done in
the event of a
cardiac arrest.

Radiation Safety

Radiation hazards are present in the healthcare facility. The clinical laboratory assistant can encounter such hazards, indicated by the sign illustrated in Figure 6-6, in many areas. For instance, radiation hazards may be encountered when handling specimens collected from patients who have been injected with radioactive dyes and from other radiology procedures. Also, care must be taken when delivering specimens to areas of the clinical laboratory where testing with radioactive materials is done.

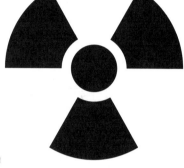

As a clinical laboratory assistant/phlebotomist, you should be aware of the healthcare facility's radiation safety procedures. Pregnant employees should avoid areas displaying the radiation symbol. If you have continual exposure to radiation for a period of time, you must wear a badge that records exposure. The badge is checked periodically to make sure that you are not exposed to potentially damaging levels of radiation.

Figure 6-6: The Radiation Hazard Symbol

Chemical Safety

Chemical injuries such as those caused from inhaling toxic fumes or splashing acid into the eye are possible in the health-care facility. Housekeeping, janitorial, laboratory, dietary, and pharmacy assistants are just a few of the employees that may be at risk of chemical injury.

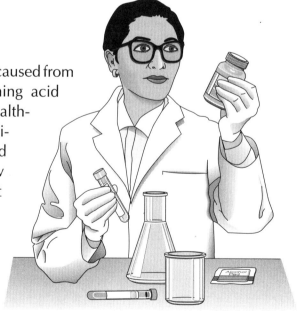

Figure 6-7: Safety precautions must be used when dealing with chemicals.

The most common chemical injury is a burn. Simple redness may be the only result, but proper first aid must be applied immediately. As discussed in the section on emergency showers and eye washes, the site of the chemical contact should be flushed with water at once. Harmful gases also may be produced by various chemicals, causing burns to the respiratory tract, shortness of breath, a type of pneumonia, or other respiratory distress. These simple guidelines will reduce the risk of chemical injury greatly.

1. Always wear gloves when using chemical solutions.

2. Always read the label on the chemical container at least three times (Figure 6-7). Read the label when you first pick up the container, before you pour or mix the solution, and immediately after you have poured the chemical.

3. Do not use chemicals in containers with no labels.

4. Use chemicals in a well-ventilated area.

5. Clean up all spills immediately, using a special spill kit.

6. If the skin or the eyes come in contact with a chemical, immediately flush the affected area with water, and continue to do so for up to 10 minutes.

7. When using chemicals, read the **material safety data sheet** that should be provided for each chemical used in a healthcare facility. The sheet contains information concerning the chemical makeup, possible hazards, first aid treatment, and appropriate dilution and mixture concentration, as well as indications and uses.

material safety data sheet: MSDS; an official required document that identifies all the chemicals that are used in a specific department and that details important information regarding those chemicals.

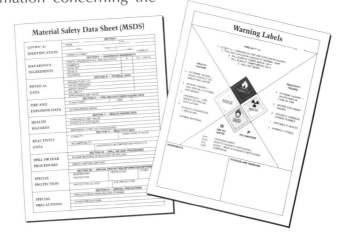

Figure 6-8: Information concerning chemicals is provided on material safety data sheets.

Chapter Summary

There are many potential hazards throughout the healthcare facility. As a clinical laboratory assistant, you must be aware of the safety of patients, fellow employees, and yourself continually.

It is your responsibility to read any safety manuals in the areas where you will be working in the healthcare facility. You must familiarize yourself with the use of the safety hood in the clinical laboratory, as well as the use and location of the safety shower and of the emergency eye wash.

Disinfection of your work area will be required on a regular basis. You will also be required to understand the requirements to maintain fire, electrical, radiation, and chemical safety in the workplace.

Name _____

Date _____

Student Enrichment Activities

Complete the following exercises.

1. Explain how to operate a standard fire extinguisher.

   _____

   _____

2. What is the significance of a material safety data sheet?

   _____

   _____

3. Name three places where the clinical laboratory assistant could come into contact with radiation in the clinical healthcare facility.

   A. _____

   B. _____

   C. _____

4. Name four rules that appear in most safety manuals.

   A. _____

   B. _____

   C. _____

   D. _____

5. If your clothing catches on fire, what should you do?

   _____

   _____

   _____

Circle T for true, or F for false.

6. T F   ABC extinguishers can be used for several types of fires.

7. T F   Three-pronged plugs are not necessary in the clinical laboratory.

8. T F   A 1:20 dilution of bleach is used for disinfecting laboratory benches.

9. T F   If a person is receiving an electrical shock, you should grab his or her hand and drag the person away from the electrical source.

10. T F   The third prong in a three-pronged electrical plug is for grounding purposes.

Complete the following statements.

11. You can put food in a laboratory refrigerator labeled _____

_____.

12. Loose hair can get caught in laboratory _____.

13. Safety hoods are used to prevent _____ contamination.

14. If a chemical acid is splashed in the eye, rinse the eye in an emergency eye wash for _____ minutes.

15. The most common chemical injury is a _____.

Chapter Seven
An Introduction to Blood Drawing: The Circulatory System

Objectives

After completing this chapter, you should be able to
do the following:

1. Define and correctly spell each of the key terms.

2. Explain the anatomy of the heart.

3. Describe the function of arteries, veins, and capillaries.

4. Identify the various components of blood.

Key Terms

- anticoagulant
- artery
- atria
- buffy coat
- capillaries
- circulatory system

- erythrocyte
- leukocytes
- oxygenated blood
- plasma
- vein
- ventricles

Introduction

Clinical laboratory testing is designed to assess the status of all of the body's systems: the circulatory, lymphatic, digestive, endocrine, integumentary, muscular, nervous, reproductive, sensory, and urinary systems. As a clinical laboratory assistant/phlebotomist, you should possess a general knowledge of the structure and function of all of these systems in order to understand more fully why each test is being ordered. Because the circulatory system is the primary system with which you will work, the circulatory system will be featured in this textbook. However, you are encouraged to do further reading and study of all of the body systems.

circulatory system: the network of vessels that carries blood to all parts of the body.

The **circulatory system** is made up of the heart, the blood vessels (including **arteries, veins,** and **capillaries**) and the blood. This system plays a vital role in transporting nutrients, gases, hormones, and waste products through the body. The circulatory system also plays an important role in the immune response and temperature regulation of the body.

The Heart

The heart is a muscled organ approximately the size of a man's fist. You can visualize the heart as a system of two pumps. One pump sends the blood flow from the right ventricle of the heart through the lungs where oxygen and carbon dioxide are exchanged. Then the blood is directed to the left atrium, where the other pump sends the blood to the rest of the body. The **pulmonary circulation** is the blood flowing to the lungs. The blood flowing to the rest of the body is called the **systemic circulation**. Your heart pumps about 5 liters of blood per minute, contracting approximately 70 times per minute.

Four chambers make up the heart: two **atria** and two **ventricles.** The right **atrium** receives blood returning from the tissues of the body. This blood has given up most of its oxygen to the body's cells and is carried back to the heart by the veins. The right ventricle pumps the venous blood received by the right atrium into the lungs. Then the left atrium receives the blood from the lungs that is now carrying oxygen, also referred to as **oxygenated blood**. The left ventricle pumps the oxygenated blood back to the body's tissues. This blood going from the heart to the body is carried by the arteries.

atria:
the upper left and right chambers of the heart; also known as the receiving chambers.

ventricles:
the pumping chambers of the heart, located inferior to the atria.

oxygenated blood:
blood that contains a sufficient level of oxygen necessary for proper functioning of the body systems.

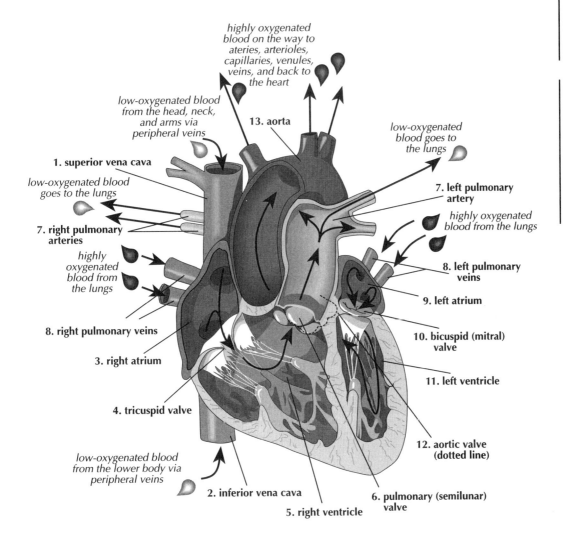

Figure 7-1: The Circulatory Path

The left and right sides of the heart work together. The heart's contractions push the blood through its chambers. Contractions beginning in the atria are followed by contractions in the ventricles. The atria rest while the ventricles contract. When a chamber contracts, the blood is forced out. When a chamber rests, the blood comes into the chamber.

Blood Vessels

The combination of the pulmonary circulation and the systemic circulation together are called the **peripheral circulation.** Blood flows in a closed system through the blood vessels and the four chambers of the heart. There are three main types of blood vessels in this system: the arteries, veins, and capillaries.

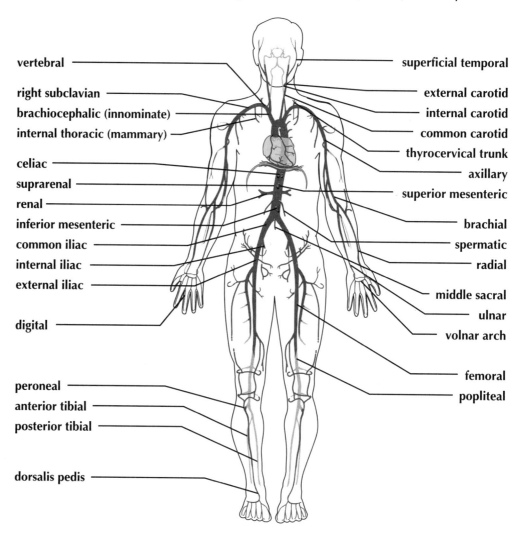

Figure 7-2: The Major Arteries of the Body

The Arteries

Arteries are blood vessels that carry highly oxygenated blood away from the heart to all other parts of the body. The largest artery in the body is the **aorta,** originating at the heart, arching upwards, and then descending through the body (see Figure 7-2). Major arteries branch off the aorta at various points. Arteries contain three muscular layers, allowing them to receive the blood that is being pumped under high pressure from the heart. Arteries further subdivide into smaller branches called **arterioles**. Figure 7-2 illustrates the major arteries of the human body.

Because the arteries are thick-walled and under pressure, they present a special challenge to the blood drawer who must take blood from an artery (blood is most often obtained from a vein). Arteries are buried deeper in the body than are veins, often making access more difficult when taking an arterial sample. The arterial puncture can also be more painful because nerves surround the arteries. Chapter Eleven describes the arterial puncture.

The Veins

Veins are composed of three layers, but the total thickness of the wall of the vein is significantly thinner than the wall of an artery. Veins are not under the pressure that is present in arteries. Since veins are transporting blood back to the heart, they contain one-way valves that keep blood from flowing backwards. Because of the low concentration of oxygen in the veins, the blood is a deep, dark red. This color is in contrast to arterial blood, which is bright red due to the heavy concentration of oxygen.

When veins are cut, blood flows out in a stream. When arteries are cut, blood spurts out due to the force of blood in the arteries. The differences in the force of blood through the different vessels are due to the pumping action of the heart. Pulses are only felt in arteries, not veins.

Venous blood is more accessible than arterial blood for testing. Venous blood is closer to the surface of the skin and can be used for almost every test in the clinical laboratory. Arterial blood is primarily tested for oxygen content, usually as a lung function test. Figure 7-3 illustrates the major veins of the body.

artery:
a blood vessel that transports highly oxygenated blood away from the heart to the tissues.

vein:
a blood vessel that carries low-oxygenated blood to the heart.

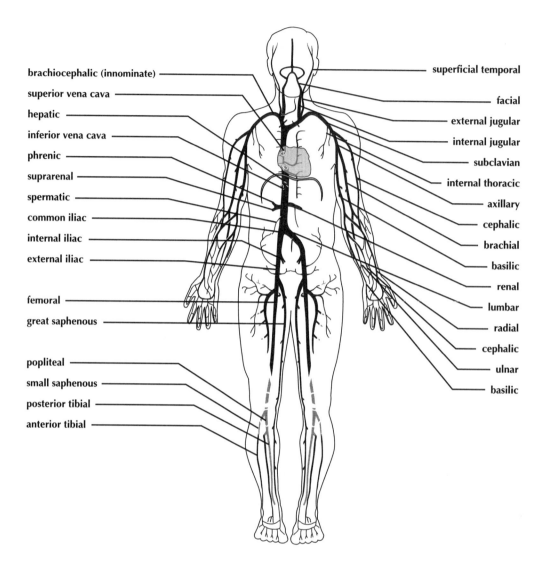

Figure 7-3: The Major Veins of the Body

The Capillaries

capillaries:
tiny blood
vessels in the
circulatory
system that link
arteries and
veins.

Capillaries are the smallest of the major blood vessels in the body. A capillary has only one thin wall that allows oxygen and nutrients to pass through into each cell. Gas exchange occurs at this level. Cells receive oxygen from the blood, and in turn release carbon dioxide and other waste products. One end of a capillary is joined to the arteriole, and the other end is joined to one of many small veins, known as **venules**.

When a blood drawer is having difficulty obtaining blood from veins, an alternative that is discussed in Chapter Ten is to puncture **capillary beds** (as in the finger tip) and obtain a small sample from that site.

The Blood

The components of blood are important for the clinical laboratory assistant to know. This knowledge will help you understand why many blood tests are performed — especially the most common blood test, the **complete blood count**.

Blood is composed of fluid, several types of blood cells, and many different chemical substances. Blood is approximately 78% water and 22% various solids. Three important cell types in the blood are erythrocytes, leukocytes, and platelets (Figure 7-4).

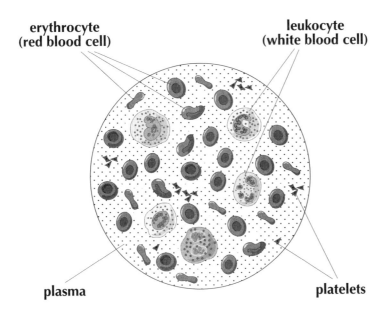

erythrocyte
(red blood cell)

leukocyte
(white blood cell)

plasma

platelets

Figure 7-4: Types of Blood Cells

Erythrocytes

Erythrocytes, or red blood cells as they are more commonly known, form the largest part of the solids that are in the blood. Red blood cells live about 120 days. They are continually being produced in the bone marrow. Their main function is to carry oxygen and carbon dioxide. They are red because of a complex protein contained within the red blood cell called **hemoglobin**. Approximately two-thirds of the body's iron is found in hemoglobin.

erythrocyte:
a red blood cell.

Erythrocytes are shaped like concave disks, thinner at the center than at the edges. The red blood cell count for men is approximately 5.4 million cells per cubic microliter (one-millionth of a liter) of blood, and women have approximately 4.8 million red blood cells per cubic microliter of blood.

Leukocytes

leukocytes:
white blood
cells that are
responsible
for fighting
infection.

Leukocytes (white blood cells) are another formed element in the blood. They lack hemoglobin and are colorless in appearance. Leukocytes are larger than red blood cells in general. One clinical laboratory test (the **differential cell count**) involves counting five different types of white blood cells: the **neutrophil**, **eosinophil**, **basophil**, **lymphocyte**, and **monocyte** (Figure 7-5). The main function of white blood cells is to fight various infections. They act as scavengers and destroy bacteria, viruses, fungi, and other pathogens.

White Blood Cells

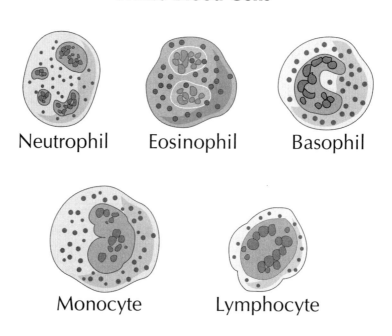

Figure 7-5: Five Types of White Blood Cells (Leukocytes)

Neutrophils (also called polymorphonuclear leukocytes) are the most common white blood cells and are classified as **granulocytes** along with eosinophils and basophils because they contain granules inside. Lymphocytes are formed mostly in the lymph nodes. They do not contain granules, so they are classified as **agranulocytes**. Lymphocytes are involved in fighting infection, most often viruses, and they are the main cells attacked by the AIDS virus. Monocytes are also agranulocytes and are also fighters of infection.

Categories of Leukocytes		
White Blood Cell (Normal Count)	**Category**	**% of Total WBCs**
Neutrophil (polymorphonuclear leukocytes)	Granulocyte	50-70%
Eosinophil	Granulocyte	0-3%
Basophil	Granulocyte	0-1%
Lymphocyte	Agranulocyte	20-35%
Monocyte	Agranulocyte	2-6%

Figure 7-6: Categories of Leukocytes

White blood cells are an integral part of the immune system and are necessary for good health. When a body is under a great deal of stress, the white blood count can actually fall (**leukopenia**), leaving the immune system less able to fight infection. When certain white cells are increased in the blood stream (**leukocytosis**), a physician may suspect an infection in the patient.

Platelets

Platelets (also known as **thrombocytes**) are the third element in the blood. Platelets are not cells but rather fragments of cells called **megakaryocytes**, which are found in the bone marrow. Platelets are the smallest of the blood elements. They number from 150,000 to 400,000 per cubic microliter of circulating blood, and they live for approximately eight days.

Platelets are essential to blood coagulation, which means that they are part of the formation of a blood clot. Platelets get activated by a tear in the connective tissue. Platelets then accumulate around the tear and form a plug that seals the damaged area of the blood vessel. When platelets fall below a normal level in the blood (thrombocytopenia), the danger of uncontrolled bleeding increases. For example, chemotherapy can destroy platelets, as can several physical disorders. Much less often, patients can experience thrombocytosis, a condition in which platelets increase above normal, causing an increased possibility of blood clots.

Aspirin can interfere with the ability of platelets to clump together. So, people who are prone to blood clots often take a small daily dosage of aspirin as a preventive measure against blood clots. If a patient is being measured for platelet function, the patient must not have taken aspirin for several days. The clinical laboratory assistant/phlebotomist needs to be aware of these conditions concerning platelet function and the effects of aspirin usage.

Plasma

plasma:
the fluid part of the blood that contains serum, proteins, solids, chemical substances, and gases; collected using an anti-coagulated tube.

The liquid portion of the blood, without the various cells, is called **plasma**. If a chemical agent called an **anticoagulant** is added to a blood collection tube to prevent clotting, a blood sample can be separated by **centrifugation** into the various cell types and plasma. Centrifugation is the rapid spinning of material to separate a solid from a liquid by use of a centrifuge (Figure 7-6). Plasma is made up of about 90% water and 10% dissolved substances such as glucose, amino acids, fats, wastes, gases, hormones, enzymes, minerals, antibodies and other substances.

anticoagulant:
a substance that prevents blood from clotting.

The cellular portion of the blood contains white and red blood cells and platelets. The red blood cells will sink to the bottom if allowed to settle or if centrifuged. The white blood cells and platelets will form a thin white layer above the red blood cells called a **buffy coat**. The plasma portion remains on top and can be removed easily for testing of various substances.

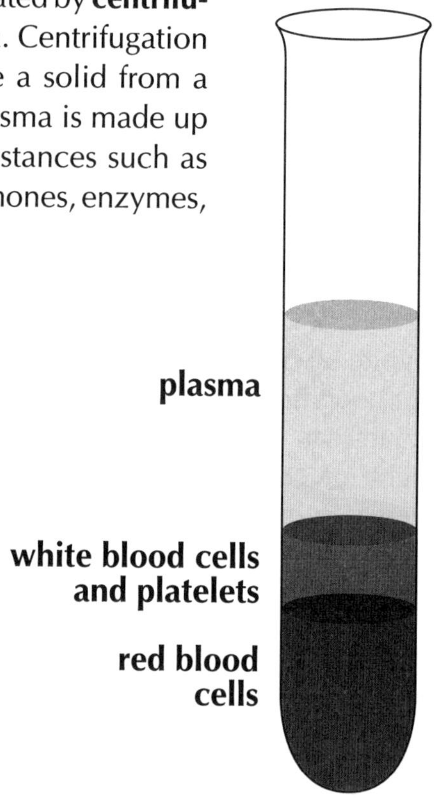

buffy coat:
in a coagulated blood sample, the layer of white blood cells and platelets that settles between the plasma and the red blood cell layer.

plasma

white blood cells and platelets

red blood cells

Chapter Summary

As a clinical laboratory assistant/phlebotomist, you should make every effort to understand the various components of the

Figure 7-7: A Blood Specimen Separated into Component Parts

circulatory system, including the heart, the blood vessels, and the blood. It is especially important to understand the location and function of the blood vessels used in obtaining a blood sample. It is also helpful to have knowledge of the components of blood, which are all tested frequently in the clinical laboratory.

Name _____

Date _____

Student Enrichment Activities

Circle T for true, or F for false.

1. T (F) Platelets are involved with carrying oxygen.

2. T (F) The heart pushes the blood to the lungs through the right atrium.

3. T (F) Arteries carry blood toward the heart.

4. T (F) Erythrocyte is another word for platelet.

5. T (F) Veins are bigger than arteries.

6. (T) F Plasma is the liquid portion of the blood.

7. T (F) There is more pressure on veins than on arteries.

8. (T) F Venous blood is used most frequently for blood tests.

9. (T) F The buffy coat is made up of white blood cells and platelets.

10. (T) F Blood coming out of an artery generally spurts out.

Circle the correct answer.

11. The three main blood vessels of the body are:
    A. the veins, arteries, and capillaries.
    B. the aorta, veins, and arteries.
    C. the arteries, arterioles, and veins.
    D. the veins, arteries, and venules.

12. Systems of the body include:
    A. the circulatory system.
    B. the integumentary system.
    C. the skeletal system.
    D. all of the above.

13. Platelets are actually fragments that come from:
    A. neutrophils.
    B. lymphocytes.
    C. megakaryocytes.
    D. monocytes.

14. Blood can be drawn from:
    A. veins.
    B. arteries.
    C. capillary beds.
    D. all of the above.

15. All of the following are names of arteries except:
    A. brachial.
    B. radial.
    C. venules.
    D. carotid.

Name _____

Date _____

Complete the following statements.

16. Neutrophils, eosinophils, and basophils are all categorized as _WBC_ .

17. Arteries carry blood _away_ _from_ the heart.

18. Veins carry blood _to_ the heart.

19. The parts of the circulatory system include the heart, blood vessels, and the _blood_

20. The walls of an artery are _thicker_ than the walls of a vein.

Chapter Eight
Preparing for Blood Collection

Objectives

After completing this chapter, you should be able to do the following:

1. Define and correctly spell each of the key terms.

2. Describe the components of the vacuum tube system.

3. Explain the unique design of the multi-sample needle.

4. Discuss the different types of evacuated blood tubes available.

5. Explain the "order of draw" for evacuated blood tubes.

6. Discuss when to use a syringe for drawing blood.

7. Explain the use of blood drawing accessories such as tourniquets, gloves, antiseptic, gauze pads and bandages, various needles, microscope slides, blood drawing trays, and blood drawing chairs.

Key Terms

- bevel
- butterfly infusion set
- cannula
- centrifugation
- evacuated tubes
- gauge

- heparin
- serum
- serum separator tubes
- syringe
- tourniquet
- vacuum tube system

Introduction

The primary duty of many clinical laboratory assistants/phlebotomists is to collect blood specimens for laboratory analysis. Venous blood is used for most tests, with venipuncture equipment making up 95% of blood-drawing items in a clinical laboratory. This chapter will discuss venipuncture equipment, which is designed to allow the venipuncturist to collect blood accurately and safely. Collection tubes are produced carefully to protect and preserve the blood specimen so that tests will provide an accurate picture of the patient's blood status. The vacuum tube system is the most efficient, safest, and easiest method of collecting a venous blood sample, especially when multiple tests are ordered.

The Vacuum Tube System

Virtually all clinical settings where blood is drawn use the vacuum tube system. This system features a multiple-sample needle, allowing the venipuncturist to put many blood tubes on the needle system. Prior to the development of this system, patients who had more than one test ordered had to have multiple needlesticks.

evacuated tubes: premeasured vacuum tubes that receive the patient's blood during venipuncture.

There are several names for the vacuum tube system, including the **evacuated tube** system (all air is removed or evacuated from the tubes), and the Vacutainer™ system. Many laboratories call the system the Vacutainer™ system because the manufacturer Becton-Dickinson originally developed this system. The Monoject™ system by Sherwood Medical Company is a similar product.

The **vacuum tube system** includes the following:

- a **multiple-sample needle** specifically designed for the vacuum tube system

- a variety of evacuated tubes

- a vacuum tube **adapter** (also called tube holder)

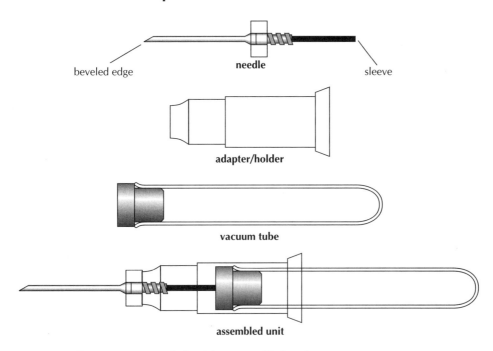

Figure 8-1: Components of the Vacuum Tube System

vacuum tube system:
a system used for blood collection; contains a disposable needle, an adapter (holder), and various types of blood collection tubes.

Vacuum Tube System Needles

The multiple-sample needle is generally 1″ long, but can come in 1½″ sizes also. The needle gauge (the size of the interior bore of the needle) is generally between 20 and 23. Both ends of this needle are **beveled**, meaning that there is an angular cut at each end of the needle for a smoother entry into the skin. (See the angled tip of the needle shown in Figure 8-1.) One end of the needle pierces the patient's vein. The other end, which pierces a vacuum tube is covered with a hollow rubber sleeve that can move up and down. When the needle is engaged in the tube, the sleeve is down, allowing blood to flow into the vacuum tube. When the tube is removed, the sleeve covers the needle end so that blood does not leak into the tube holder while another tube is prepared. The sleeve is a safety measure to help keep blood exposure to a minimum.

bevel:
the point of a needle that has been cut on a slant for ease of entry.

cannula:
a tube or
sheath.

Another safety innovation to avoid needlestick injuries involves the point of the multiple-sample needle that is used to penetrate the patient's vein. When the needle is engaged and the tube is pushed forward, the pressure of the tube locks a hollow metal **cannula** within the needle beyond the point of the bevel. When the needle comes out, there is no longer a sharp point as the cannula extends beyond the needle tip, eliminating the risk of needlestick injury. The Bio-Plexus Puncture-Guard™ needle is an example of this type of needle.

Several states have drafted new regulations in attempts to eliminate the risk of a needlestick injury. Healthcare facilities are being required to use needles with engineered sharps injury protection, such as the Bio-Plexus Puncture-Guard™ needle. These regulations extend to other sharps as well, such as scalpels.

Evacuated Tubes

Evacuated tubes (Figure 8-2) can be used both in the vacuum tube system and in the syringe method of blood drawing. Using these tubes, the phlebotomist can collect the blood directly into the tube during the actual venipuncture process. Evacuated tubes fill immediately because of the vacuum that exists inside the tube. The vacuum in each tube is premeasured exactly so that the tube will draw a precise amount of blood. The vacuum is guaranteed by the manufacturer until its expiration date. However, the vacuum can be lost by opening the tube before drawing blood, dropping the tube, pushing the tube too far into the needle holder, or pulling the needle partially out of the skin during a blood draw.

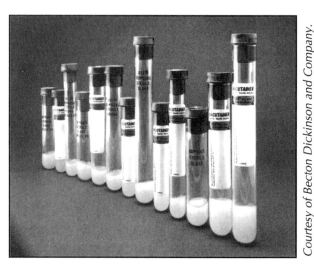

Courtesy of Becton Dickinson and Company.

Figure 8-2: Evacuated Tubes Used in Vacuum Tube Collection

The vacuum tube system includes vacuum tubes in a range of different sizes (from 2 to 15 ml). Sizes are selected with the amount of blood required in mind. Also, the size of the tube is related directly to the amount of vacuum or strength with which blood is drawn out of the vein. Larger tubes have more vacuum and may not be appropriate for use on fragile veins. Smaller tubes are often used for pediatric specimens and for small and fragile veins of adults. This system also features tubes with or without additives.

1. NONADDITIVE TUBES: Vacuum tubes are not only distinguished by size and strength, but they also come with and without substances (additives) inside of the tubes. The rubber stoppers on each tube indicate the contents of the tube. When blood is collected into tubes without additives, the blood will clot on **centrifugation.** The liquid part of the specimen that is recovered (on top of the cells) is called **serum.** Serum is used in many laboratory analyses. The stoppers traditionally used to designate nonadditive vacuum tubes are brick-red, marbled-red, or yellow-marbled. A gold plastic cap is found with the Hemogard™ safety tubes (Figure 8-3). These safety tubes are unique because they have a plastic shield that covers the rubber stopper to prevent blood from spraying when the stopper is removed.

centrifugation: the application of centrifugal force to spin and separate substances of different densities.

serum: the liquid portion of the blood after blood coagulation.

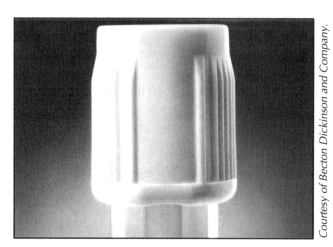

Courtesy of Becton Dickinson and Company.

Figure 8-3: Hemogard™ Safety Tubes

2. ADDITIVE TUBES: Additive tubes are described as vacuum tubes that have an additive in them that plays a specific role in specimen collection. Some additive tubes simply have a substance added to speed up and enhance clot formation. **Serum separator tubes** can contain thixotropic gel, which forms a physical barrier of separation, glass particles that accelerate clotting, and a filter that separates the cellular components from the liquid components of blood. Examples include Corvac™ and SST™ tubes, which often are orange-colored or black and orange-stippled.

An **anticoagulant** is a chemical that can prevent blood from clotting. Most additives to vacuum tubes are a variety of anticoagulants used to produce plasma after centrifugation. Plasma is used for testing in many laboratory departments.

serum separator tubes: vacuum tubes that can contain thixotropic gel that forms a physical barrier of separation, glass particles that accelerate clotting, and a filter that separates the cellular from the liquid components of blood.

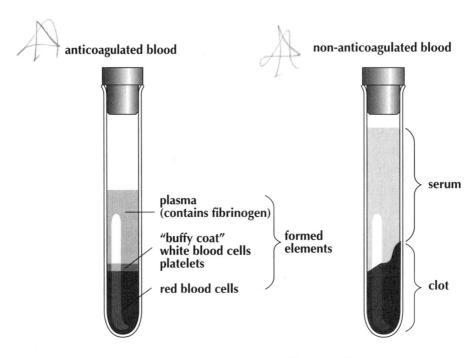

Figure 8-4: Blood Centrifuged in Anticoagulated Tubes and Non-anticoagulated Tubes

Commonly used anticoagulants are discussed below.

EDTA: Ethylenediaminetetraacetic acid, more commonly known as EDTA, is used for whole blood hematology studies. EDTA prevents the blood from clotting by binding calcium in the form of a potassium or sodium complex. The stopper on an EDTA-additive tube is lavender (also referred to as purple). Commonly drawn tests in EDTA include the complete blood count, sedimentation rate, and the reticulocyte count.

heparin:
a natural blood thinner produced by the liver; also used as a medication of patients who are prone to abnormal blood clotting.

HEPARIN: Vacuum tubes with **heparin** in them have a green stopper. These tubes contain either sodium or lithium heparin. Heparin is a natural anticoagulant. It stops the blood from clotting by inactivating two substances involved in the clotting process: thrombin and thromboplastin. Heparin is the most common anticoagulant used in the chemistry department for plasma determinations and is frequently used in STAT determinations to save time required for a serum specimen to clot. Tests commonly drawn in heparin tubes include electrolyte and ammonia testing.

SODIUM CITRATE: Sodium citrate is the anticoagulant used for coagulation studies using plasma. This anticoagulant works by binding calcium, an integral part of blood clotting. The stopper color is blue (royal blue). Tests commonly drawn in sodium citrate tubes include the prothrombin time and the activated partial thromboplastin time.

SODIUM FLUORIDE: Sodium fluoride is used as an anticoagulant primarily for glucose testing. It inhibits the coagulation process by binding calcium, as does sodium citrate. The stopper is gray for this tube.

ACD: ACD (acid-citrate-dextrose) is an anticoagulant present in yellow-stoppered tubes. ACD maintains red blood cell integrity. Yellow-stoppered tubes can also contain sodium polyanetholesulfonate (SPS). These tubes with SPS are often the tube of choice for blood culture collections, in which blood is specially collected to determine if there is an infection (usually bacterial) in the blood.

There are also tubes with other colored stoppers, such as black and dark blue. These tubes may contain a variety of additives. The clinical laboratory assistant/phlebotomist must be aware of tubes that are used less frequently. Appendix E in the back of this textbook gives an overview of the use of vacuum tubes in different laboratory departments. Appendix B includes the amount of specimen required and the type of vacuum tube required for some frequently ordered laboratory tests.

The Vacuum Tube Adapter

The vacuum tube adapter is the device that has the multiple-sample needle screwed into one end of the adapter and the vacuum tube placed inside the other end. (Refer to the diagram of the assembled unit in Figure 8-1.) Adapters have been developed recently with increased safety in their design. The Safety-Lok™ adapter shields the needle for disposal, and other designs allow the release of the needle into a sharps container without unscrewing the needle from the adapter. Clinical laboratory employees should always be looking for products that increase safety and minimize the risk of blood-borne pathogen exposure.

Order of Draw for Vacuum Tubes

One of the most important aspects of the vacuum tube system is the ability of the system to allow multiple blood draws. One venipuncture can produce samples drawn in a variety of evacuated blood tubes for a variety of blood tests. The clinical laboratory assistant/phlebotomist can use a series of anticoagulated blood tubes, but an "order of draw" is recommended to avoid contamination of nonadditive tubes from additive tubes, as well as cross-contamination between different types of additive tubes.

Manufacturers recommend the following order of tubes to be drawn, the first one on the list being the first tube used after the needle is securely in the vein.

1. Blood culture tubes (a test requiring sterile specimens).

2. Red-stoppered tubes (no additive).

3. Red/gray-stoppered tubes (any tubes containing gel separator additives or other additives to help the separation of serum from the clot).

4. Blue-stoppered tube (sodium citrate) used for coagulation studies.

5. Green-stoppered tube (heparin) used for several chemistry studies.

6. Purple-stoppered tube (EDTA) used for hematology studies.

7. Gray-stoppered tube (sodium fluoride) used most often for glucose studies.

[handwritten annotation: "Old Order of Draw" with renumbering 1, 2, 3, 3, 4, 5, 6, 7]

The Syringe System

syringe:
a device used to inject fluids or medications into the body or withdraw them from the body.

Another apparatus used for drawing blood from veins is the **syringe** system (Figure 8-5). This system is preferred for veins that can collapse (constrict) under a vacuum. Such veins may be those of small children or fragile, small, or otherwise difficult veins on any patient. The syringe system consists of a hypodermic needle attached to a sterile, disposable plastic syringe.

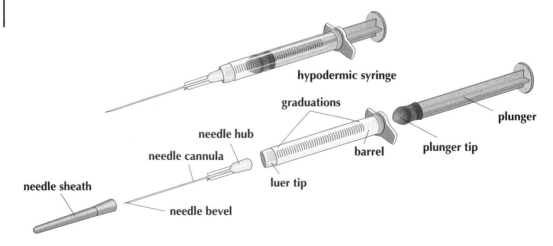

Figure 8-5: A Common Syringe System

Syringe Needles

The syringe needle is a sterile needle designed for single use. This needle comes in a variety of **gauges**. The needle gauge is the measure of the diameter of a needle, with smaller numbers indicating larger diameters. For example, a 20-gauge needle is larger in diameter than a 23-gauge needle. In general, 21 to 23-gauge needles are used. These needles also come in different lengths; 1" to 1$\frac{1}{2}$" lengths most commonly are used in venipunctures. Multiple-draw needles in the vacuum collection system also come in the variety of gauges.

gauge: a standard for measuring the diameter of the lumen of a needle.

Syringes come in a range of sizes, with 3 ml to 10 ml syringes being used for phlebotomy most frequently. The syringe has two parts: a barrel with graduated markings in either milliliters or cubic centimeters, and a plunger that fits in the barrel of the syringe. When drawing blood with the aid of a syringe, the plunger is slowly pulled back by the blood drawer, allowing the barrel to fill with blood. Blood specimens are then transferred from the syringe to evacuated blood tubes. This process has several problems, including the additional step of transferring blood, which is not done with the vacuum collection system, adding more opportunity for a needlestick injury. The transfer can also damage blood cells if the blood from the syringe is forced into the vacuum tube too rapidly. Cells can also be damaged if blood does not flow quickly and evenly into the syringe.

The Butterfly Infusion Set

A **butterfly infusion set** consists of a $\frac{1}{2}$ to $\frac{3}{4}$-inch stainless steel needle connected to a 5 to 12-inch length of tubing. It is called a butterfly because of its wing-shaped plastic extensions used for gripping the needle.

butterfly infusion set: a needle and tubing connected with a plastic wing-shaped holder; used for fragile veins when a small volume of blood is sufficient.

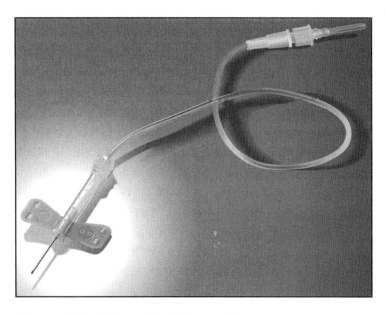

Figure 8-6: A Butterfly Infusion Set

The butterfly infusion set is an important tool for collecting blood from small or difficult veins, such as hand veins or veins from both elderly or pediatric patients. Because of the design of the set, it is much more flexible and precise than a syringe system. A 23-gauge needle is the most common size used with this set. A smaller needle can run a risk of hemolyzing (breaking down red blood cells) the blood specimen.

Blood Drawing Accessories

In addition to the equipment mentioned previously, several other accessories are integral to the process of the venipuncture. Because of the number of supplies necessary to perform a safe and efficient blood draw, the clinical laboratory assistant/phlebotomist must be well organized and knowledgeable about each piece of equipment used. Chapter Nine includes exact procedures for using these accessories correctly while performing a venipuncture.

The Tourniquet

tourniquet: a device, often a rubber band at least $1/2$ inch wide, that reduces the flow of blood in the veins and allows the veins to become more prominent.

The **tourniquet** is used to increase resistance in the venous blood flow. When a tourniquet is applied before the blood is drawn, veins become distended and a venipuncture location can be determined more easily. However, the tourniquet should be kept on the patient for no longer than 1 minute because prolonged use will affect the test results (the blood can become more concentrated due to the constriction) and will be uncomfortable for the patient. A variety of tourniquets are available, including blood pressure cuffs, rubber straps, and velcro tourniquets.

Gloves

Gloves are MANDATORY for all blood collections. Gloves provide a protective barrier between you and infectious agents that could enter the body through a cut or abrasion. They do not, however, protect against an accidental needlestick.

Usually gloves are made of latex, vinyl, or nitrile. Vinyl gloves are not snug fitting and, therefore, are not often used. Latex gloves are most commonly used because they conform more completely to the blood drawer's hand. Nitrile gloves have gained acceptance with a wide range of laboratory employees because they are tear resistant and comfortable, but they are more expensive.

Some gloves are available with talcum powder inside to aid in taking the gloves on and off. However, some employees are allergic to the powder and need to wear powder-free gloves. Employees must change gloves before working with each new patient. Handwashing is required between each removal and reapplication of gloves. Gloves must always be discarded in a biohazardous waste container.

Antiseptics

Antiseptics are substances or solutions used to prevent infection of the venipuncture site during a blood draw. Certain antiseptics are safe to use on human skin and are used to clean the skin prior to a puncture.

The most common antiseptic used for routine blood drawing is 70% isopropyl alcohol in the form of individually-wrapped pads. Antiseptics that are stronger include povidone iodine in several forms, including Betadine™. This type of antiseptic comes in individually-wrapped packets and has the antiseptic pre-applied on swabsticks and pads.

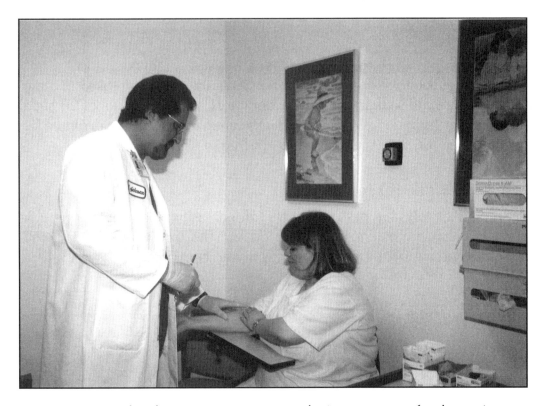

Figure 8-7: A safe, clean venipuncture results in no trauma for the patient.

Gauze Pads and Bandages

Sterile gauze pads (2 x 2) folded in fourths are used to hold pressure over the venipuncture site after completion. The patient may be alert enough to apply pressure, or you may have to apply appropriate pressure yourself to make sure that the wound has stopped bleeding.

After pressure is held on the wound (up to 5 minutes and more for a person who is taking anticoagulants), adhesive bandages are used to cover the site once the bleeding is finished. Paper, cloth, or knitted tape over a gauze square can be used, especially for patients who are allergic to bandages. Some people are also allergic to certain types of tape and refuse bandaging on their puncture site. In this case, the clinical laboratory assistant should make sure the site has stopped bleeding completely before releasing the patient. These patients should also be warned not to carry a purse or anything heavy with the arm of the unbandaged wound site for at least an hour.

Bandages should not be used on children under 2 years of age because of the danger of **aspiration** and suffocation (choking) from a loose bandage.

Microscope Slides

Precleaned glass microscope slides are used to make blood films for certain hematology department tests. Generally, slides are used that are frosted on one end so that the clinical laboratory assistant can label the slide properly with the patient's name and identification number. The procedure for making slides after the venipuncture is covered in Chapter Eleven.

Blood Drawing Tray

Blood drawing trays are designed to be carried easily. They contain enough space to carry equipment for several draws. The tray must be kept well organized and clean, and should be replenished continually.

The following materials may be on a blood drawing tray:

- vacuum collection system components: 1 or 2 adapters, evacuated tubes (both with additives and without), and several multiple-draw needles

- sterile gauze

- alcohol sponges individually-wrapped

- paper tape and/or bandages

- a few syringes/butterfly systems

- a few syringe needles

- glass slides

- marking pen for labeling if necessary

- a tourniquet

- gloves

- a small sharps container for clipping and disposing of needles

- capillary stick equipment if necessary (including scalpels and collection containers)

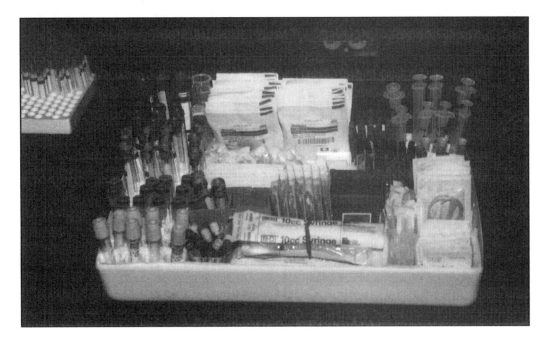

Figure 8-8: A blood drawing tray must be organized and free from contaminated materials.

Blood Drawing Station

When the clinical laboratory assistant/phlebotomist is not drawing blood on inpatients in a healthcare facility (using a blood collection tray), he or she may be assigned to a blood drawing station in a special area of the laboratory equipped for performing venipunctures, mostly on outpatients.

A blood drawing station includes a table for supplies and a chair (and hopefully a bed) for the patient. The table should be next to the chair or bed for convenient use and with space for the equipment used in the blood draw. The chair should be comfortable for the patient, and it should have an armrest that will lock in place to prevent the patient from falling out of the chair should he or she become faint.

A bed or reclining chair should be available to patients who inform the laboratory assistant in advance that fainting from venipuncture is a possibility.

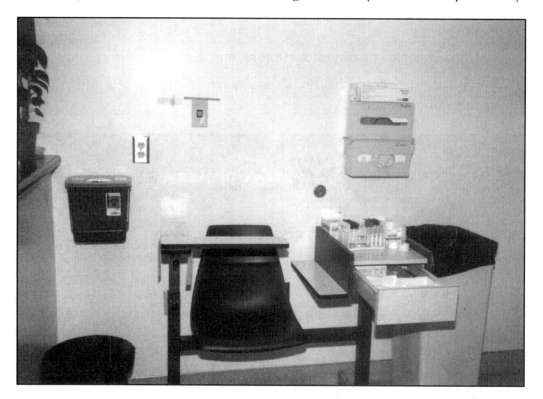

Figure 8-9: A blood drawing station should be pleasant, tidy, and well-stocked with blood drawing supplies.

Other supplies that might be stocked in a blood drawing station include ammonia salts (in a disposable ampule) that can be used to revive a fainting patient, equipment for obtaining tiny amounts of blood (discussed in Chapter Ten), pencils and pens, and a variety of bandages.

Chapter Summary

Clinical laboratory assistants/phlebotomists must be thoroughly comfortable and proficient in using all of the equipment involved in performing a venipuncture. The vacuum tube system makes it possible to collect many blood specimens at the same time. Care must be taken to use the correct evacuated blood tube in this system. This involves knowing the different anticoagulants and other additives in each tube in order to collect the correct plasma, as well as knowing the tubes that collect serum for testing.

In addition to the vacuum tube system, you must also be familiar with the use of the syringe system and the butterfly needle collection technique. The clinical laboratory assistant must use all other accessories for the blood draw with efficiency and safety in mind for both the patient and the employee.

Name _____

Date _____

Student Enrichment Activities

Complete the following exercises.

1. Name the three components of the vacuum tube system.

    A. _____

    B. _____

    C. _____

2. Describe the unique construction of the vacuum tube system needle.

    _____

    _____

    _____

    _____

    _____

3. Explain why a vacuum exists in an evacuated tube.

    _____

    _____

4. Name three evacuated tube additives.

    A. _____

    B. _____

    C. _____

5. List the "order of the draw" for evacuated tubes.

    A. _____   E. _____

    B. _____   F. _____

    C. _____   G. _____

    D. _____

Circle T for true, or F for false.

6. T   F   An adapter for a vacuum tube system is also called a vacuum tube holder.

7. T   F   Blood drawn in a nonadditive tube and centrifuged yields plasma.

8. T   F   An anticoagulant prevents blood from clotting.

9. T   F   A syringe can be used to obtain blood when large amounts of blood need to be drawn.

10. T   F   As the gauge on a needle gets bigger, the interior bore of the needle gets bigger.

Complete the following statements.

11. Often, a butterfly infusion set is used for getting blood from _____ veins.

12. The anticoagulant ethylenediaminetetraacetic acid is abbreviated _____.

13. Heparin as an anticoagulant is often used for tests in the _____ department of the clinical laboratory.

14. An example of an antiseptic used to cleanse the site before a venipuncture is _____.

15. Bandages should not be used on children under 2 years of age because of the danger of _____ and _____.

Name _____

Date _____

Match the anticoagulant with the correct stopper color.

16. _____ EDTA   **A.** blue stopper

17. _____ heparin   **B.** red stopper

18. _____ no additive   **C.** lavender stopper

19. _____ sodium citrate   **D.** yellow stopper

20. _____ ACD   **E.** green stopper

Chapter Nine

Performing the Venipuncture

Objectives

After completing this chapter, you should be able to
do the following:

1. Define and correctly spell each of the key terms.

2. Discuss three methods of obtaining venipunctures.

3. Identify important aspects of preparing the patient
    for a venipuncture.

4. Explain how to apply and release a tourniquet.

5. Explain how to cleanse a venipuncture site.

6. Describe the anchoring of a vein before the venipuncture.

7. Briefly describe the procedure for a venipuncture using the
    vacuum tube system.

8. Explain the procedure for performing a venipuncture using
    a syringe.

9. Describe the procedure for a venipuncture using a butterfly
    infusion kit.

Key Terms

- anchoring
- antecubital space
- edema
- hematoma

- hemoconcentration
- Luer adapter
- NCCLS
- thrombosed

Introduction

Venipuncture is the primary method of blood collection for most laboratory tests. Chapter Eight describes the equipment used for various blood collections, including the vacuum tube system, the syringe method, and a butterfly infusion set venipuncture. This chapter will discuss the procedures for each of these methods of performing a venipuncture.

Selecting a Venipuncture Method

There are three commonly used methods by which a clinical laboratory assistant/phlebotomist obtains venous blood. Figure 9-1 summarizes each method, as well as its advantages and disadvantages.

Method	Advantages	Disadvantages
Vacuum Tube Collection (method of choice for most venipunctures)	Fast, generally safe, best for quality and quantity of venous blood specimens.	Can fail with fragile and small veins, hand veins, small children.
Syringe Collection (use with difficult veins, adequate hand veins)	Veins may not collapse due to controlling the draw; good specimen quality.	Tube transfers can be awkward, limited amount of blood at one time; risk of clotting with larger volumes if blood comes slowly.
Butterfly Infusion Set (use with small children and fragile veins)	Less pain; less likely to collapse small veins; can attach to syringe.	Difficult to use when blood comes slowly due to loss of blood in tubing; potential hemolysis when draw is difficult; cannot draw large amounts.

Figure 9-1: Venipuncture Collection Methods

The vacuum tube collection method, the syringe collection method, and the butterfly infusion set method are all important techniques for the clinical laboratory assistant/phlebotomist to master. The vacuum tube system will be used most of the time, especially if the patients are healthy adults. It provides the best overall specimen, presumably free from clots and hemolysis. Therefore, it is considered the method of choice by most healthcare facilities. Furthermore, there is no additional risk of needlestick injury as there is when blood is transferred from the syringe to various tubes.

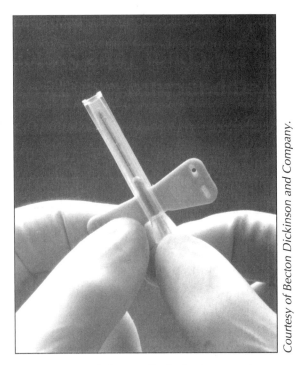

Courtesy of Becton Dickinson and Company.

Figure 9-2: A butterfly infusion set is often the method of choice for drawing blood on small patients.

The butterfly infusion set is a less painful method of drawing blood and is often the technique of choice for drawing blood from a squirming, fearful, small child. The design of the tubing allows for greater flexibility of movement and can often be used on tiny veins (Figure 9-2).

Preparing the Patient for the Venipuncture

Even before you decide upon a method of venipuncture to use, there are important procedures to follow with the patient before a venipuncture can be performed. These procedures generally apply when obtaining blood using other methods as well (skin puncture, arterial stick, and so on). These steps are very important and must be completed before a blood sample is obtained.

Entering Patient Information Into the Computer System

Patient information must be entered into an organized system of identification, such as the computer systems of the hospital and clinical laboratory. Patient identification should be linked to test results. In an outpatient setting, the clinical laboratory clerical worker usually will have registered the patient into the computer system. The patient may arrive at your blood drawing station with test requisitions and even computer labels for the specimens. For inpatients, the tests have already been ordered in the computer system by the nursing staff or the health unit coordinator, and labels have been printed for the specimens.

If you are required to do patient registration, you must follow the procedures for patient registration and for test requisition spelled out in the facility's clinical laboratory clerical procedures manual.

Greeting and Identifying the Patient

You should greet the client in a pleasant manner and introduce yourself. Explain that you are going to draw blood as ordered by the physician. Assure the patient that the procedure will be quick and only slightly uncomfortable. Appear professional so that the patient immediately has some confidence that you know what you are doing. If the patient is sleeping, awaken the patient gently and explain the procedure.

Identify patients by asking them their name. Do not ask them "Are you Mrs. Jones?" A confused or sleepy patient may agree to anything you say. For inpatients, check the identification band on their wrist (Figure 9-3). Make sure that the patient's name is exactly as it appears on the test requisition. Duplicate names are common.

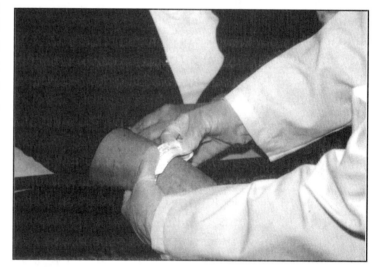

Figure 9-3: You must identify inpatients correctly by checking the identification band located on the wrist.

Verify Orders and Possible Dietary Restrictions

You must verify the orders for blood drawing. There may be some special considerations in drawing certain tests, such as keeping the specimen cold and protected from the light. You need to know how much blood is needed (you never want to take excessive amounts of blood, especially on people who have many tests), and you want to select correctly which tubes you will need to fill for the tests.

The patient may need to comply with dietary restrictions before you draw the blood. Ask the patient if he or she has been **fasting** (not taking in food or drink for a period of time) or has followed a special diet if it is required for that test. If there is a question, consult your supervisor. It may be necessary to contact the physician to see if he or she wants the test drawn even though the patient has not followed a special diet.

Assembling Supplies and Positioning Equipment

Supplies for venipuncture are discussed in Chapter Eight. It is very important to assemble your supplies and position them so that you can easily reach every piece of equipment during the blood draw. When drawing blood from inpatients, you will have a collection tray with you that should be placed next to the patient's bed. An outpatient facility will have an equipment area next to the blood drawing chair, often built into the chair itself. Vacuum tubes should be organized in the order of draw.

Wash Your Hands and Put On Gloves

After the patient has been identified, you have explained the procedure to the patient, and you have assembled your equipment based on what kind of venipuncture you wish to perform (see Figure 9-1), you should then wash your hands and put on gloves that fit well. Loose fitting gloves can be hazardous and clumsy.

Position the Patient

If you are dealing with an outpatient, the patient should be seated comfortably in a chair with an armrest. A chair that reclines is best for protection against fainting. Position the arm in a straight line from the shoulder, not bending the elbow. The arm should be positioned slightly downward.

The Tourniquet

Applying a **tourniquet** is an important part of the venipuncture. An inexperienced blood drawer will have a difficult time applying a tourniquet without fumbling. Practice is necessary to become proficient at putting on and releasing the tourniquet.

A tourniquet is applied to the arm to slow the blood flow and make the veins more prominent. It should be placed 3 to 4 inches above the venipuncture site. If the patient has sensitive skin, the tourniquet may be applied over a sleeve or a dry washcloth may be wrapped around the arm.

Usually, latex strips are used as tourniquets. The most comfortable tourniquet is about 1 inch (2.5 cm) wide and about 15 to 18 inches (45 cm) long. Figures 9-4A, 9-4B, and 9-4C illustrate the correct way to apply a tourniquet.

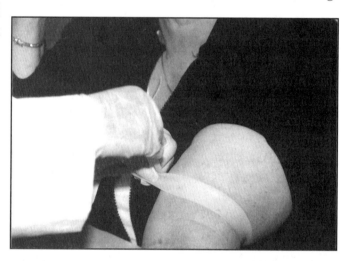

Figure 9-4A: Place the tourniquet around the arm about 3 to 4 inches above the venipuncture site.

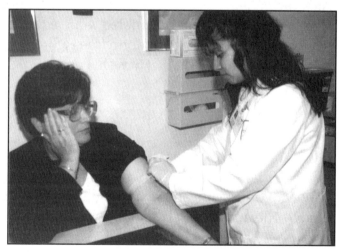

Figure 9-4B: Stretch the tourniquet, crossing both straps securely. Hold the tourniquet tightly near the surface of the arm where the straps overlap. Tuck one strap of the tourniquet under and to the front, forming a loop.

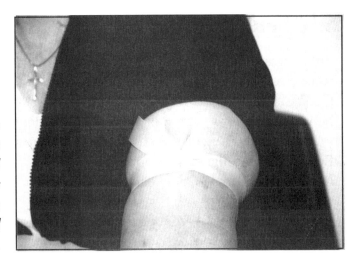

Figure 9-4C: Check the tourniquet to make sure it is secure and tight enough to slow blood flow. Both tourniquet ends should be pointed upward.

Tourniquet Precautions

In addition to being able to put the tourniquet on quickly and without difficulty, you must be aware of the following precautions when applying the tourniquet:

- A tourniquet should not be applied for more than one minute. If kept on longer, blood can get concentrated in the veins (**hemoconcentration**) and cause blood tests to be incorrect. A **hematoma** can also occur. The tourniquet pressure also can make the patient more uncomfortable, which may make the client jerk and create potential for a needlestick injury.

- Do not apply a tourniquet over an open sore. Use another site.

- Do not apply a tourniquet to an arm on the side of the body on which a mastectomy has been performed without the permission of the patient's physician.

- The tourniquet should feel slightly tight to the patient. It should not be rolled or twisted. It should not hurt the patient or pinch the arm. The arm should not be turning red or purple.

- A tourniquet that is applied too tightly may restrict flow completely. A tourniquet that is too loose will be ineffective.

- Sometimes a clinical laboratory assistant will apply a tourniquet solely for the purpose of site selection. If this is the case, the tourniquet should be released if the entire venipuncture will take longer than 1 minute from the initial application of the tourniquet. The site can be cleansed, and then the tourniquet can be placed back on the arm after 2 minutes. The veins should be back to normal by then.

hemo-concentration: an increase in the concentration of formed blood elements caused by lack of fluid in the blood; often caused by a tourniquet too tightly applied to the arm or left on too long.

hematoma: a blood-filled swollen area; a goose egg caused by bleeding under the tissues.

Site Selection for the Venipuncture

The clinical laboratory assistant has to make a preliminary assessment of the best veins on the patient's arms. Most of the time, a venipuncture can be accomplished in the **antecubital space** (the area at the bend of the elbow) using the vacuum tube system. Needle size is also determined at this time. You will probably have three or four sizes to choose from, from a gauge of 20 to 23. (Remember: the higher the number, the smaller the diameter of the needle.) As the needle gets smaller, the chance of hemolysis of the red blood cells increases.

The veins used most frequently for venipuncture are the superficial veins located in the forearm, extending to the hand (Figure 9-5). Of those, the larger **median cubital** and **cephalic** veins, located in the antecubital space, are used most often. Other veins in the anterior surface of the forearm, as well as in the wrist and hand, are acceptable, provided that the selected site has no scarring, hematomas, burns, or swelling (**edema**).

In times past, clinical laboratory employees have been allowed to draw blood from sites other than the arms and hands, such as the feet and legs. However, there is a much larger risk of blood clots forming in these sites and, therefore, they are no longer areas to consider. Extracting blood from ear lobes is not productive for any draws that need more than a few drops. If blood is impossible to draw from hands and arms, a physician may take more dramatic measures and draw blood from scalp veins of infants or from arterial sites on the body.

antecubital space: the area of the arm located in the vicinity of the bend of the elbow where the major veins for venipuncture are located.

edema: swelling due to fluid in the tissues; fluid retention.

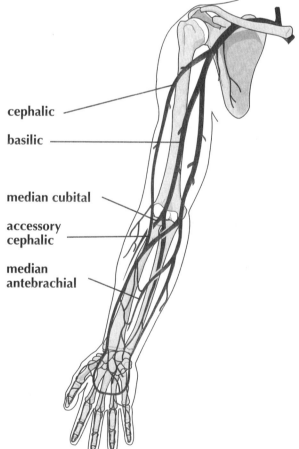

cephalic

basilic

median cubital

accessory cephalic

median antebrachial

Figure 9-5: The Major Veins of the Arm

Generally, you do not draw blood from an arm on the side of a mastectomy (breast removal) or on an arm receiving intravenous infusions. You should depend on touch, not sight, to locate the proper vein. A healthy vein will be bouncy to the touch when it is palpated. A **thrombosed** vein, which should not be selected, will feel cord-like, will be hard, and will have no spring. The selected vein should not be so superficial that it rolls around when touched. It is better to choose a vein that is well-anchored by surrounding tissues.

thrombosed: clotted with blood.

If a vein is not obvious, you can ask the patient to open or close his or her fist without a pumping action. Pumping is the process of tightly opening and closing one's fist which tightens muscles, and can jeopardize the quality of the blood specimen. Veins can become more prominent after opening and closing the fist. Some laboratory assistants also may pat the area to bring veins to the surface.

If you do not feel a vein, remove the tourniquet and try the other side. Patients may have information about where blood was successfully drawn previously. Follow patient suggestions if you can't find a vein.

Cleansing the Venipuncture Site

Once you have found a vein, the next step is to clean the area with a 70% isopropyl alcohol pad. The **National Committee for Clinical Laboratory Standards (NCCLS)** recommends that the tourniquet be released after a venipuncture site has been found and that the site be cleaned and dried. Cleanse the area by applying friction and moving in a circle from the inside out (see Figure 9-6). The site must be air-dried before continuing with the venipuncture. The time allowed for the alcohol to dry gives the antiseptic time to kill microorganisms. Additionally, a wet site can cause hemolysis of the specimen and can make the patient uncomfortable. Blowing on the site to hurry the drying process can contaminate the area, as can wiping the area with an unsterile gauze pad. One of the most important things to remember here is DO NOT TOUCH THE VENIPUNCTURE AREA AFTER CLEANSING.

NCCLS: National Committee for Clinical Laboratory Standards; a national organization that develops standards for the accurate performance of laboratory procedures based on voluntary consensus.

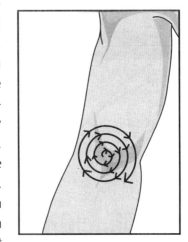

Figure 9-6: Cleanse the venipuncture area with an outward circular motion.

Anchoring the Vein Before Venipuncture

anchoring:
holding a
vein in
position
before
performing a
venipuncture.

One of the most important aspects of securing a good venipuncture is the **anchoring** of a vein. Anchoring consists of firmly securing a vessel in place during the venipuncture. Elderly patients and heavily muscled individuals can have veins that are easy to see but have a tendency to roll. A vein can be anchored by the two-finger method illustrated in Figure 9-7.

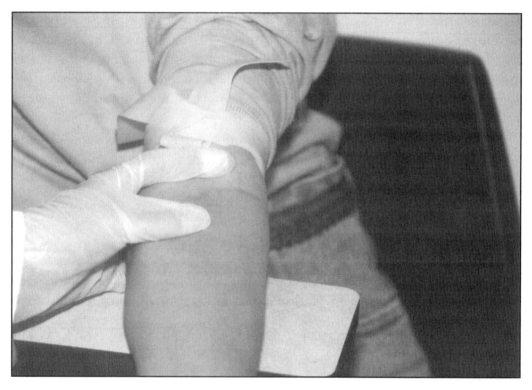

Figure 9-7: A Two-fingered Method of Anchoring a Vein for Venipuncture

The thumb of the nondrawing hand can be placed about 1 to $1\frac{1}{2}$ inches below the venipuncture site, right over the vein. The index finger can be placed above the venipuncture site, again directly over the vein.

Venipuncture Using the Vacuum Tube System

The following procedure has been approved by the NCCLS. Although clinical laboratories may allow for slight variation, you should adhere to the methods in this approved procedure for using the vacuum tube system.

Venipuncture By Vacuum Tube

Materials needed:
- ✓ fresh, clean gloves
- ✓ goggles (may be used for training in case of splash)
- ✓ laboratory coat (preferable OSHA-approved)
- ✓ vacuum tubes (extras of each - noting their expiration date)
- ✓ disposable multidraw needles for vacuum system (usually 20, 21 and 22 gauge)
- ✓ adapter for vacuum system
- ✓ alcohol prep pads (70% isopropyl)
- ✓ clean 2 x 2 gauze pads
- ✓ clean tourniquet
- ✓ adhesive bandage or paper tape (preferred by many patients)
- ✓ permanent marker or pen
- ✓ fresh solution of 10% bleach or comparable solution (required for cleaning spills and so on)

1. Procedural Step: Make sure the patient information and tests are entered into the computer system of the healthcare facility and/or the clinical laboratory.
   Reason: A record must be kept of the patient information and test results.

2. Procedural Step: Greet and identify the patient. Introduce yourself, and explain what you intend to do.
   Reason: The patient MUST be identified correctly. Also, to get the best cooperation from the patient, you want him or her to feel comfortable.

3. Procedural Step: Verify the orders for the patient.
   Reason: You want to make sure that the necessary amount and type of blood is drawn.

4. Procedural Step: Make sure the patient has been following dietary restrictions, if required for a specific test.
   Reason: If the patient has not been following a special regimen for the test, probably the blood should not be drawn as the results will not be accurate.

5. Procedural Step: Assemble all supplies and equipment and position them correctly.
   Reason: If the proper equipment is not assembled nearby and positioned correctly, you might have to redo the venipuncture because you cannot reach the equipment.

6. Procedural Step: Wash hands and apply gloves.
   Reason: Standard Precautions.

Venipuncture By Vacuum Tube (Cont.)

7. <u>Procedural Step:</u> Position the patient for the venipuncture. Make sure the arm is straight and slightly downward.
   Reason: The correct position of the arm facilitates a successful venipuncture.

8. <u>Procedural Step:</u> Apply the tourniquet, making sure that it is not on more than 1 minute. The tourniquet should be tight enough to slow down blood flow, but not so tight as to stop arterial blood flow (the arm may lose color) and cause discomfort. If applied just for site selection, remove it before the venipuncture and apply again in 2 minutes to perform the venipuncture.
   Reason: A tourniquet left on too long can cause hemoconcentration and unnecessary discomfort.

9. <u>Procedural Step:</u> Select a vein. Have the patient open and close the fist if necessary.
   Reason: A successful venipuncture depends on a well-selected vein.

10. <u>Procedural Step:</u> Cleanse the site, releasing the tourniquet and letting the alcohol dry.
    Reason: The site should be cleansed with 70% isopropyl alcohol to kill microorganisms that could cause infection. Letting the alcohol dry further facilitates the killing process and causes less pain to the patient.

11. <u>Procedural Step:</u> Reapply the tourniquet, and remove the needle cover from the needle after putting the needle in an adapter.
    Reason: The tourniquet can only be on 1 minute, and the needle cover should only be removed right before the puncture.

12. <u>Procedural Step:</u> Anchor the vein.
    Reason: The vein must be held in place to prevent rolling.

13. <u>Procedural Step:</u> Insert the needle at a 15° angle with the bevel up (Figure 9-8), following the direction of the vein, threading the needle ¹/₄" within the vein. Be sure that the needle does not move.
    Reason: This position is best for adequate penetration into the vein without going through a vein.

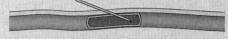

Figure 9-8: Correct Needle Insertion Technique

14. <u>Procedural Step:</u> Fill the vacuum tubes following the correct order of draw. Use the nondrawing hand to insert each tube into the adapter, gently pushing the tube forward while pushing against the edge of the adapter so the needle doesn't move forward. Remove each tube after filling by grasping the end of the tube, inverting additive tubes 10 to 12 times to mix anticoagulant.

Venipuncture By Vacuum Tube (Cont.)

Reason: The correct order of drawing anticoagulated tubes is designed to make sure that there is no cross contamination and that certain sensitive tests are drawn first. The vacuum tubes should be inserted carefully to avoid repositioning the needle. Tubes should be mixed immediately to circulate the anticoagulant. Shaking vigorously may rupture red blood cells.

15. Procedural Step: Release the tourniquet when you have finished the blood draw.
Reason: The tourniquet should not be on more than 1 minute.

16. Procedural Step: Withdraw the needle carefully, applying gauze to the puncture with pressure for 3 to 5 minutes.
Reason: When the puncture site is exposed after the needle is removed, bleeding will occur. For that reason, pressure must be put on the site with clean gauze for 3 to 5 minutes. If the patient is not capable of holding the gauze, you must apply the pressure yourself to help prevent a hematoma.

17. Procedural Step: Dispose of the needle immediately into a sharps biohazard container, which must be within reach. Some containers are designed for the needles to be clipped. Others allow the blood drawer to drop the needle directly into the container.
Reason: For protection against needle sticks, you must not recap the needle.

18. Procedural Step: Label all tubes immediately. If no computer label is available, label the tubes with at least the patient's name, identification number, date, time of collection, AND YOUR INITIALS.
Reason: The blood MUST be carefully identified. Labeling is critical. You must always initial all blood tubes you draw in case there is a question about the blood drawn.

19. Procedural Step: Examine the patient's arm for bleeding, and apply a bandage if necessary.
Reason: The patient should not be dismissed before bleeding has stopped. Large, painful hematomas can result if a wound does not have proper pressure applied.

20. Procedural Step: Thank the patient and say good-bye.
Reason: Customer service should always be a top consideration.

21. Procedural Step: Remove and discard all contaminated items into the biohazard container, wiping up any spills with the 1:10 bleach solution.
Reason: Standard Precautions

22. Procedural Step: Wash your hands.
Reason: Standard Precautions

Venipuncture Using the Syringe

Although the vacuum tube method is the preferred and most frequently used method of venipuncture, use of the syringe for a venipuncture is a valuable skill to learn. As discussed previously, the syringe can be useful with difficult draws involving collapsing veins, hand veins, and assisting with blood draws from a patient's indwelling line (see Chapter Eleven). Except for the equipment used, there are few differences between the vacuum tube method of venipuncture and the syringe method. Figure 9-9 addresses these differences.

SYRINGE	VACUUM TUBE
1. When assembling equipment, pop the plunger to release the seal and insure easy movement by completely pushing the plunger forward. The syringe needle is then placed on the syringe.	1. When assembling the equipment, the needle is placed on (screwed onto) the adapter.
2. It is obvious immediately if the needle is in place as blood appears in the syringe as soon as the needle is in the vein.	2. Blood is not evident until the tube is placed in the holder and the stopper punctured by the multi-sample needle.
3. The plunger is pulled back slowly to control the blood flow.	3. The vacuum is controlled by the volume of the tube.
4. If a large amount of blood is needed, a new syringe can be put on the needle, but not without leakage as the syringes are changed, risking bloodborne pathogen exposure.	4. Any amount of blood is collected directly into the vacuum tubes without blood leakage.
5. To get blood into the tubes from the syringe, great care MUST be taken to avoid a needlestick injury during the transfer and to avoid blood clots at the same time.	5. Blood is collected immediately in the vacuum tubes before it can clot.

Figure 9-9: Differences in Procedure Between the Syringe and the Vacuum Tube System

Transferring blood to vacuum tubes from syringes and needles is one of the riskier procedures that is performed by the clinical laboratory assistant/phlebotomist. The NCCLS discourages syringe collection for that reason. You must consider this method CAREFULLY before proceeding.

The safest way to transfer blood is to place the tubes upright in a rack, transferring the blood into the tubes while they are in the test tube rack. Do not hold the tubes with your other hand while transferring the blood as that is the most common source of needlestick accidents. Do not force the blood through the tube after the syringe needle penetrates the rubber stopper of the vacuum tubes. Hemolysis easily results from forcing blood.

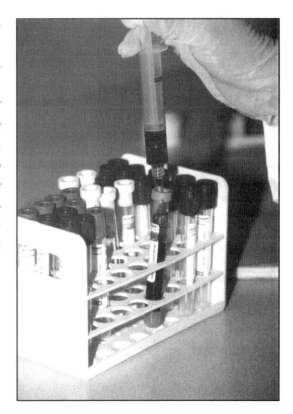

Figure 9-10: To avoid a needlestick, you must be extremely careful when transferring blood from a syringe to a vacuum tube.

Venipuncture By Syringe

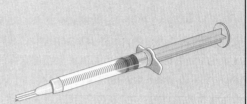

Materials needed:
- ✓ fresh, clean gloves
- ✓ goggles
- ✓ laboratory coat
- ✓ vacuum tubes
- ✓ disposable covered needle
      for syringe system (20 to 23 gauge)
- ✓ alcohol prep pads
- ✓ clean 2 x 2 gauze pads
- ✓ tourniquet
- ✓ adhesive bandage or paper tape
- ✓ permanent marker or pen
- ✓ approved sharps biohazard container
- ✓ fresh solution of 10% bleach or comparable solution
- ✓ ammonia inhalant

1. Procedural Step: Make sure the patient information and tests are entered into the computer system of the healthcare facility and/or the clinical laboratory.
   Reason: A record must be kept of the patient information and test results.

2. Procedural Step: Greet and identify the patient. Introduce yourself, and explain what you intend to do.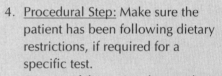
   Reason: The patient MUST be identified correctly. Also, to get the best cooperation from the patient, you want him or her to feel comfortable.

3. Procedural Step: Verify the orders for the patient.
   Reason: You want to make sure that the necessary amount and type of blood is drawn.

4. Procedural Step: Make sure the patient has been following dietary restrictions, if required for a specific test.
   Reason: If the patient has not been following a special regimen for the test, probably the blood should not be drawn, as the results will not be accurate.

5. Procedural Step: Assemble all supplies and equipment, making sure to arrange the tubes in the correct order of draw in a test tube rack.
   Reason: After the blood draw, you need to take as many precautions as possible during the transfer of the blood to the tubes from the syringe. Do not hold the tubes while putting blood in them.

6. Procedural Step: Position the equipment, assembling the needle and syringe and popping the barrel of the syringe to force all air out of the barrel. Make sure the barrel moves easily.

Venipuncture By Syringe (Cont.)

Reason: Equipment must be within easy reach. The barrel of the syringe must be popped to prevent air from being injected into the patient.

7. Procedural Step: Wash hands and apply gloves.
Reason: Standard Precautions.

8. Procedural Step: Position the patient for the venipuncture. Make sure the arm is straight and slightly downward.
Reason: The correct position of the arm facilitates a successful venipuncture.

9. Procedural Step: Apply the tourniquet, making sure that it is not on more than 1 minute. The tourniquet should be tight enough to slow down blood flow, but not so tight as to stop arterial blood flow (the arm may lose color) and cause discomfort. If applied just for site selection, remove it before the venipuncture and apply again in 2 minutes to perform the venipuncture.
Reason: A tourniquet left on too long can cause hemoconcentration and unnecessary discomfort.

10. Procedural Step: Select a vein. Have the patient open and close the fist if necessary.
Reason: A successful venipuncture depends on a well-selected vein.

11. Procedural Step: Cleanse the site, releasing the tourniquet and letting the alcohol dry.
Reason: The site should be cleansed with 70% isopropyl alcohol to kill microorganisms that could cause infection. Letting the alcohol dry further facilitates the killing process and causes less pain to the patient.

12. Procedural Step: Reapply the tourniquet, and remove the needle cover from the needle after putting the needle in an adapter.
Reason: The tourniquet can only be on 1 minute, and the needle cover should only be removed right before the puncture.

13. Procedural Step: Anchor the vein.
Reason: The vein must be held in place to prevent rolling.

14. Procedural Step: Insert the needle at a 15° angle, threading the needle ¼ inch inside the vein. Make sure that the needle is not moving. If blood is being obtained, blood will appear in the hub of the syringe (Figure 9-11).
Reason: The 15° angle is best for adequate penetration into the vein, as is the ¼ inch penetration.

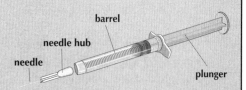

Figure 9-11: Parts of a Syringe

Venipuncture By Syringe (Cont.)

15. Procedural Step: Release the tourniquet once there is evidence in the hub that blood was obtained.
Reason: The blood is now flowing and will not be enhanced by the tourniquet remaining on.

16. Procedural Step: Fill the syringe by slowly and firmly pulling the plunger with the nondrawing hand.
Reason: Slowly pulling back keeps the blood from becoming hemolyzed and reduces the chance that the vein might collapse from too much pull.

17. Procedural Step: Withdraw the needle and immediately apply pressure to the wound for 3 to 5 minutes.
Reason: When the puncture site is exposed after the needle is removed, bleeding will occur. Pressure must be put on the site with clean gauze to stop the bleeding.

18. Procedural Step: Transfer the blood into vacuum tubes immediately, using caution to avoid a needlestick injury. Do not force the blood into the tubes.
Reason: An immediate blood transfer into tubes that are sitting in a rack will decrease the blood clotting in the syringe and will reduce the possibility of needlestick in the transfer, if the free hand does not hold the tubes. The possibility of hemolysis is reduced if blood is not forced into the tubes.

19. Procedural Step: Dispose of needle syringe assembly immediately in one piece into a sharps container.
Reason: Disposing of the whole syringe/needle assembly reduces the chance of an accidental needle stick.

20. Procedural Step: Label all tubes immediately. If no computer label is available, label the tubes with at least the patient's name, identification number, date, time of collection, AND YOUR INITIALS.
Reason: The blood MUST be identified carefully. Labeling is critical. Always initial all blood tubes you draw in case there is a question about the blood drawn.

21. Procedural Step: Examine the patient's arm for bleeding and apply a bandage if necessary.
Reason: The patient should not be dismissed before bleeding has stopped. Large, painful hematomas can result if a wound does not have proper pressure applied.

22. Procedural Step: Thank the patient and say good-bye.
Reason: Customer service should always be a top consideration.

23. Procedural Step: Remove and discard all contaminated items into the biohazard container, wiping up any spills with the 1:10 bleach solution.
Reason: Standard Precautions.

24. Procedural Step: Wash your hands.
Reason: Standard Precautions.

Venipuncture by the Butterfly Infusion Set

Venipuncture by the butterfly infusion set (also called the "winged infusion set")
is a safe and valuable alternative for all healthcare workers. This method is
particularly useful for obtaining blood from hand veins and for drawing blood
from children (see Figure 9-1 to review).

The preferred winged infusion equipment has a **Luer adapter** that can be
attached either to a syringe or to a vacuum tube adapter. The vacuum tube
adapter is preferred because of the risks involved in transferring blood from a
syringe to vacuum tubes.

It is important to use small tubes for collection (pediatric sizes) with a vacuum
tube adapter so that the vacuum will be minimal for the small vein.

Luer adapter:
a device
for connecting
a syringe to
the needle
and when
locked into
place gives a
secure fit.

Venipuncture By Butterfly Infusion Set

Materials needed:
- ✓ fresh, clean gloves
- ✓ goggles
- ✓ laboratory coat
- ✓ pediatric vacuum tubes
- ✓ disposable winged infusion set
     (usually 23 gauge)
- ✓ adapter for vacuum system
- ✓ alcohol prep pads, 70% isopropyl
- ✓ clean 2 x 2 gauze pads
- ✓ a tourniquet
- ✓ adhesive bandage or paper tape
- ✓ permanent marker or pen
- ✓ approved sharps biohazard
     container
- ✓ fresh solution of 10% bleach
     or comparable solution
- ✓ ammonia inhalant

1. Procedural Step: Make sure the patient information and tests are entered into the computer system of the healthcare facility and/or the clinical laboratory.
   Reason: A record must be kept of the patient information and test results.

2. Procedural Step: Greet and identify the patient. Introduce yourself, and explain what you intend to do.
   Reason: The patient MUST be identified correctly. Also, you want to make the patient feel comfortable with the procedure for the best cooperation.

3. Procedural Step: Verify the orders for the patient.
   Reason: You want to make sure the necessary amount and type of blood is drawn.

4. Procedural Step: Make sure the patient has followed dietary restrictions, if required for a specific test.
   Reason: The results will not be accurate. If the patient has not followed a required regimen, the blood probably should not be drawn.

5. Procedural Step: Assemble the butterfly apparatus, with uncoiled tubing and Luer adapter attached to a tube holder or syringe (tube holder is recommended).
   Reason: You must be prepared before the venipuncture takes place.

6. Procedural Step: Wash your hands and put on gloves.
   Reason: You must follow all Standard Precautions.

7. Procedural Step: Position the patient. For a hand draw, have the client hold onto a rolled washed cloth or similar material. Make sure that tubes are positioned slightly lower than the puncture site.
   Reason: Correct positioning of the patient makes it easier to do a good blood draw.

8. Procedural Step: Apply the tourniquet. A tourniquet should be applied just above the wrist bone for a hand draw.

Venipuncture By Butterfly Infusion Set (Cont.)

Reason: The tourniquet slows down blood flow and makes veins more prominent.

9. Procedural Step: Select a vein. For hand draws, have the client grasp a rolled washcloth and locate a suitable vein between the knuckle and the wrist bone. Be careful not to stick a bone.
Reason: Although hand veins are usually quite easy to see, the skin is fairly thin on the hand, and frequently, the veins are close to many bones in the hand.

10. Procedural Step: Cleanse the site and release the tourniquet.
Reason: The site is cleansed to remove microorganisms that might infect a puncture wound. The tourniquet is released to prevent hemoconcentration.

11. Procedural Step: Apply the tourniquet again after 2 minutes. Remove the needle cover from the needle assembly on the butterfly infusion set.
Reason: The tourniquet is put on again after 2 minutes to allow the blood flow to recover from the first tourniquet application. In order to reduce the risk of contamination, the needle cover is removed just before the vein is punctured.

12. Procedural Step: Anchor the vein again.
Reason: The vein is anchored to hold the vein in place during the venipuncture.

13. Procedural Step: Insert the needle at a 15° angle with the bevel up, following the direction of the vein. Thread the needle ¼ inch within the vein. Be sure that the needle does not move.
Reason: All methods of venipuncture use these steps.

14. Procedural Step: Release the tourniquet once there is evidence that there is blood obtained, signified by blood in tubing. Pull the looped free end downward.
Reason: The tourniquet is no longer needed when blood is flowing properly; pulling the loop down will facilitate a better blood flow through the tubing.

15. Procedural Step: Fill the pediatric vacuum tubes following the correct order of draw. Invert anticoagulated tubes 10 to 12 times immediately after the draw.
Reason: Following a prescribed order of vacuum tube draws reduces contamination of blood tubes with other anticoagulants. Inverting tubes disperses anticoagulant.

16. Procedural Step: Withdraw the needle. Some blood drawers put a piece of tape on the butterfly assembly after the needle is in the vein. In that instance, take the tape off before removing the needle, and apply pressure with a clean gauze pad to the puncture site for 3 to 5 minutes.
Reason: Pressure must be placed on the wound as soon as it is exposed to prevent excess bleeding, bruising, and hematoma formation.

Venipuncture By Butterfly Infusion Set (Cont.)

17. Procedural Step: Immediately dispose of the winged infusion set (including needle) while holding the vacuum tube adapter. This entire set should go into a sharps biohazard container immediately. Some laboratories may ask you to save the vacuum tube holder.
    Reason: Contaminated materials must be disposed of in a biohazardous waste container as soon as possible.

18. Procedural Step: Label all tubes immediately. If no computer label is available, label the tubes with at least the patient's name, identification number, date, time of collection, AND YOUR INITIALS.
    Reason: The blood MUST be identified carefully. Labeling is critical. Always initial all blood tubes you draw in case there is a question about the blood drawn.

19. Procedural Step: Examine the patient's arm for bleeding, and apply a bandage if necessary.
    Reason: The patient should not be dismissed before bleeding has stopped. Large, painful hematomas can result if a wound does not have proper pressure applied.

20. Procedural Step: Thank the patient and say good-bye.
    Reason: Customer service should always be a top consideration.

21. Procedural Step: Remove and discard all contaminated items into the biohazard container, wiping up any spills with the 1:10 bleach solution.
    Reason: Standard Precautions.

22. Procedural Step: Wash your hands.
    Reason: Standard Precautions.

Chapter Summary

Probably no skill is more important for you to master than the venipuncture. Whether you choose the vacuum tube method, modify the method with a butterfly infusion kit, or find it necessary to use a syringe method, you must always keep the patient uppermost in your mind. These procedures are designed to provide the highest level of customer service, and include welcoming and correctly identifying the patient, keeping the patient as calm and as free from pain as possible, and drawing just enough blood to run all of the tests ordered.

After properly labeling all blood, all biohazardous materials must be disposed of in the sharps biohazard container promptly. Every precaution must be taken to avoid a needlestick. Standard Precautions are to be followed during every step of the venipuncture.

Name _____

Date _____

Student Enrichment Activities

Complete the following statements.

1. The venipuncture procedure that is considered the method of choice by most health-care facilities is the _____.

2. A tourniquet is applied to __stop__ blood flow and to make veins more __prominent__.

3. A vein selected for venipuncture should be _____ to the touch.

4. A tourniquet should not be left on an arm for more than __1__ minute(s).

5. Usually, an antiseptic such as _____ is used to cleanse the venipuncture site.

Circle T for true, or F for false.

6. T F Keeping the tourniquet on for too short a time can cause hemoconcentration.

7. (T) F Pumping the fist can help raise a vein and produce a good sample.

8. T (F) The time that must elapse between tourniquet applications to the same patient is 2 minutes. 3

9. (T) F Alcohol coming into contact with blood can cause hemolysis.

10. (T) F Letting alcohol dry after cleansing a venipuncture site allows the alcohol to kill microorganisms.

11.   T   F   A thrombosed vein is often chosen for a venipuncture.

12.   T   F   Anchoring a vein before venipuncture prevents a vein from rolling
              during a venipuncture procedure.

13.   T   F   The order of draw of vacuum tubes during a venipuncture is not important.

14.   T   F   Tubes should be labeled after the blood is drawn.

15.   T   F   Pressure should be applied to a venipuncture site for at least 3 to 5 minutes.

Circle the correct answer.

16.   The angle of a needle penetrating a vein for venipuncture should be:
      A. 10 degrees.
      B. 12 degrees.
      C. 15 degrees.
      D. 90 degrees.

17.   One of the riskier procedures for the clinical laboratory assistant/phlebotomist
      while performing a venipuncture is:
      A. applying the tourniquet.
      B. changing tubes during a vacuum tube draw.
      C. applying pressure to a patient's wound.
      D. transferring blood from a syringe to vacuum tube.

Name _____

Date _____

18. The butterfly infusion set is an alternative to other venipuncture procedures when:

   A. children have small veins.

   B. a patient is afraid of pain and the butterfly infusion needlestick is less painful.

   C. a patient has tiny, fragile veins that tend to collapse.

   D. all of the above.

19. Two preferred methods of venipuncture include:

   A. the syringe and the vacuum tube system.

   B. the vacuum tube system and the butterfly infusion set.

   C. the butterfly infusion set and the syringe.

   D. none of the above.

20. All of the following are recommended for use in a venipuncture procedure except:

   A. 70% alcohol pads.

   B. tourniquets.

   C. cotton balls.

   D. needles.

Chapter Ten
Performing the Skin Puncture

Objectives

After completing this chapter, you should be able to do the following:

1. Define and correctly spell each of the key terms.

2. Discuss why a skin puncture might be preferable to obtaining blood from a venipuncture.

3. Identify situations where a skin puncture would not be appropriate.

4. List the components of skin puncture blood.

5. Describe sites selected for a skin puncture.

6. Explain why certain areas are dangerous for a skin puncture due to the possibility of puncturing a bone.

7. Identify various types of equipment used to perform a skin puncture.

8. Describe techniques used to obtain a free-flowing, well-drawn skin puncture specimen.

Key Terms

- arterial blood gas
- capillary action
- capillary tubes
- cyanotic
- interstitial fluid

- osteochondritis
- osteomyelitis
- phenylketonuria testing
- skin puncture

Introduction

skin puncture:
also known as
a capillary
puncture;
collecting
blood after
puncturing the
skin with a
lancet or similar
skin puncture
device.

Most laboratory tests are performed on venous blood, but there are situations when a venipuncture is not possible or appropriate. **Skin punctures**, also called **microcapillary** blood collections, fingersticks, and capillary punctures or sticks, are performed when a patient has no adequate veins for venipuncture.

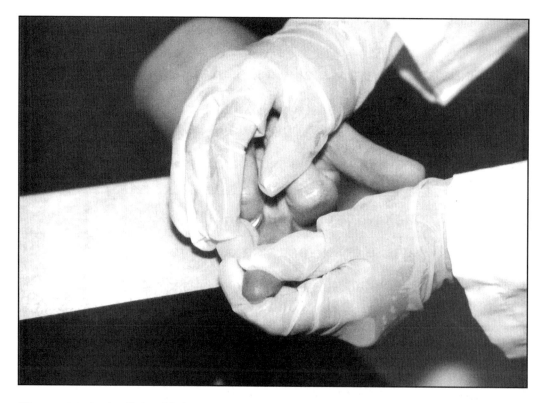

Figure 10-1: A clinical laboratory assistant/phlebotomist performs a skin puncture on an adult patient.

When to Choose the Skin Puncture

There are several occasions when the clinical laboratory assistant/phlebotomist may decide to take blood from a skin puncture rather than from a venipuncture. Examples of such situations are listed below:

- The patient has fragile, superficial veins.

- The patient is an infant who has had many blood tests, and his or her blood volume is too low for larger amounts of blood to be taken.

- The patient is an infant or a small child with no adequate veins found for a venipuncture.

- A patient will not cooperate with you for a venipuncture and requests a skin puncture.

- If the patient is a child, the parent may request a skin puncture instead of a venipuncture.

- The test or tests ordered require only a few drops of blood, such as **phenylketonuria (PKU) testing** for the newborn.

- The patient has burns in venipuncture sites.

- A nurse has requested that the only available vein be reserved for intravenous lines.

- The patient has **thrombotic** problems.

- The patient is **morbidly obese**, and no vein can be felt.

phenylketo-nuria testing: PKU testing; testing on a newborn for a recessive, inherited disease in which a body is unable to break down the amino acid phenylalanine.

A skin puncture is not recommended when the following situations are present:

- The patient's extremities are very cold.

- The patient is severely dehydrated.

- A patient is seriously **edematous**.

- Laboratory tests ordered require far more blood than can be obtained by a skin puncture.

- The patient has poor circulation, especially to the extremities.

- The patient is in shock.

- The patient refuses a skin puncture.

Thinking It Through ...

> Mrs. Ramirez is a lovely old lady who is occasionally very confused. Josh has drawn her blood many times and enjoys talking with her.
>
> Today Mrs. Ramirez is tired and confused. She wants to go home to take a nap. Her doctor has ordered a stat blood test on her. Josh is not finding a vein and tells Mrs. Ramirez he wishes to take blood from her finger as the test ordered does not require much blood.
>
> Mrs. Ramirez has never had blood taken from her finger. She becomes agitated in her confusion and begins to yell at Josh, even giving him a swat. She refuses to have her blood drawn, even though the doctor is insisting that the results are needed urgently.
>
> 1. If you were Josh, what would you do?
>
> 2. Would you try to talk Mrs. Ramirez into the test?
>
> 3. Would you get help?

The Composition of a Skin Puncture Specimen

As discussed in Chapter Seven, veins and arteries narrow into venules and arterioles. The smallest vessels are the capillaries. When skin is punctured for blood collection, the composition of the blood differs from venous blood. This blood is a combination of capillary, arteriole, and venule blood. Values may differ slightly from those obtained from venous blood.

interstitial fluid: the fluid outside the cell (extracellular fluid), excluding the fluid within the blood and lymph vessels.

One of the complications of a skin puncture is the fact that the tissue is damaged during the puncture. **Interstitial fluid** is the fluid present between tissues that is released during the trauma of a skin puncture. The first drop obtained from a skin puncture should be wiped away because it will be diluted with this fluid. If the puncture does not render a free-flowing stream of blood, the clinical laboratory assistant/phlebotomist may have to squeeze the site repeatedly, which can result in excessive **dilution** of the blood sample with interstitial fluid.

Selecting a Site for a Skin Puncture

Generally, the three sites selected for a skin puncture are the fingertips, heels, or toes. Earlobes have also been used, but the earlobe has poor capillary access. It is recommended only when a drop or two of blood is needed. In general, a puncture site on the skin should be warm, colored, and free of cuts, bruises, scars, or rashes. Avoid fingersticks if fingernails are cyanotic. Edema in the hands will interfere with the fingerstick as well, due to potential dilution of fluid from the swollen tissue.

cyanotic: affected by cyanosis; the bluish discoloration of the skin and mucous membranes due to a decrease in oxygen.

The Fingertip

The fingertip is the most common site chosen for the skin puncture, especially for older children and adults. The puncture should be made in the central, fleshy portion of the finger, to the side of center and perpendicular to the grooves of the fingerprint (Figure 10-2).

Additional warnings about puncturing the finger for a blood specimen are listed below:

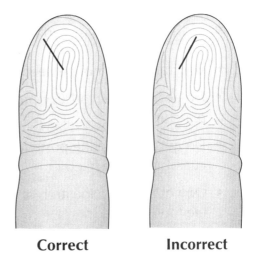

Correct   **Incorrect**

Figure 10-2: The Site and Direction of a Finger Puncture

- Do not puncture fingers of infants and very young children. Bone injury is possible since there is not much tissue between the skin and the bone. Penetrating the bone with a puncture can lead to serious bone infection.

- Do not puncture the index finger; it may be more callused and harder to penetrate than other fingers. Because the index finger is used continually, a wound on this finger takes longer to heal.

- Do not puncture the fifth (pinkie) finger. This finger has the thinnest amount of tissue between the skin and bone.

- Avoid a puncture to the side or tip of the finger. The distance between the skin and the bone is half as much at the side and tip as it is in the central portion of the end of the finger.

- Do not puncture parallel to the grooves of the fingertip. This angle will cause the blood to run down the finger grooves and make collection difficult.

The Heelstick

The heel is a recommended skin puncture site for children less than 1 year-old (infants). The most important thing to consider when performing a heelstick on a small child is to avoid puncturing bone. Puncturing a bone can cause painful **osteomyelitis**, a serious bone infection. **Osteochondritis** (bone and cartilage inflammation) can also result from puncturing a bone. Additional punctures through previous puncture sites (newborns are often punctured several times in the nursery) can also cause infection. Figure 10-3 illustrates areas that are recommended for an infant heel puncture.

Additional precautions for performing heel sticks include the following:

- Punctures must not be deeper than 2.4 mm.

- Do not puncture through previous puncture sites.

- Do not puncture the posterior curvature of the heel.

- Do not puncture the arch of the foot.

osteomyelitis: severe inflammation of bone and bone marrow, resulting from a bacterial infection.

osteochondritis: inflammation of the bone and cartilage.

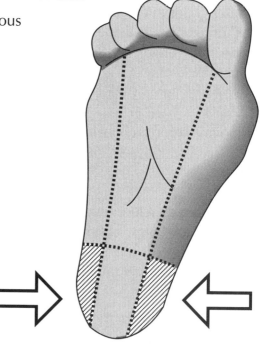

Figure 10-3: Patterned regions indicate recommended areas on an infant heel for a heel puncture.

Skin Puncture Equipment

Equipment for performing a skin puncture has changed over the years as has venipuncture equipment, reflecting the growing attention to the safety of both the patient and blood drawer. For the skin puncture, you will need the following supplies.

The Lancet

A disposable sterile lancet (Figure 10-4) is the most common way to puncture the skin for skin puncture collection. For newborns, the lancet must have a tip of 2.4 mm or less to avoid penetrating bone.

Many lancets today are fully automated, single-use, disposable devices that are designed to protect both the patient and the health-care worker. These lancets are spring-loaded devices that lie on the surface of the skin and make an automatic puncture. The devices have a button that, when pressed, releases the lancets into the skin. The patient does not see the blade penetrate the

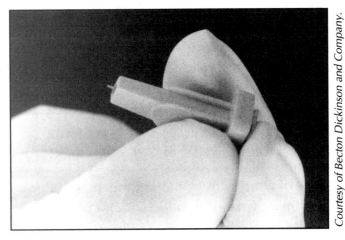

Courtesy of Becton Dickinson and Company.

Figure 10-4: A Disposable, Sterile Lancet for Performing a Skin Puncture

skin. Other lancets that are used are simply sterile blades that the clinical laboratory assistant/phlebotomist pushes into the skin. However, spring-loaded devices are recommended as being safer and easier to use than the sterile blade.

Other devices that are more complicated include an Autolet™ device by Ulster Scientific. This device is a spring-activated puncture device that allows easy ejection of the lancet and platform, providing safety for the patient and the laboratory assistant. The platforms are available in three depths: 1.8 mm, 2.4 mm, and 3.0 mm. Lancets used with this system have been developed with a slimmer needle and a bevel that allows for smooth and easy skin penetration, providing more comfort for the patient. The lancets are disposable and the rest of the device is reused. This system is often used by diabetics who must perform their own skin punctures on a regular basis.

Collection Devices

Once a good puncture is made that allows blood to flow easily, the clinical laboratory assistant/phlebotomist must collect the blood carefully in some type of container for later testing. The following are containers that are commonly used for blood collection.

MICROCOLLECTION TUBES: Plastic micro-collection devices for general laboratory collections have tops that are colored coded with the same colors found on the stoppers of the evacuated tubes described in Chapter Eight. Anticoagulant is included in certain tubes (green top representing heparin inside, and so on). There are several different manufacturers of these tubes,

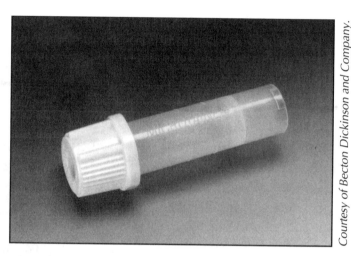

Figure 10-5: A Microtainer® for Collecting Blood from Skin Punctures

some of which can contain as much as 600 microliters of blood. Tubes come with their own blood collector, self-contained serum separator, and plastic top (Figure 10-5). These tubes provide for easy measuring, color coding, stoppering, centrifugation, and storage of the blood obtained by a skin puncture.

THE UNOPETTE®: The Unopette® is a system of collection and dilution for blood samples. These devices are prefilled with specific amounts of **diluents** or **reagents** (or both) for several different types of tests, including the white and red blood cell count, platelet count, hemoglobin determination, red blood cell fragility, sodium and potassium determinations, and so on. The Unopette® contains a disposable,

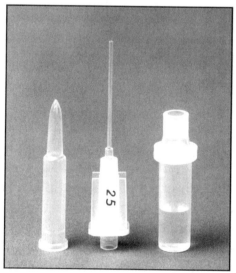

Figure 10-6: The Unopette®, a Collection and Dilution Unit for Blood Samples

Courtesy of Becton Dickinson and Company.

self-filling, diluting pipette that consists of a glass capillary tube fitted into a plastic holder. It also contains a plastic reservoir that contains a premeasured volume of reagent for diluting.

CAPILLARY TUBES: Before the development of blood collection tubes described above, **capillary tubes** were the only option for collecting blood through a skin puncture. The blood flows directly from the site into the tube by **capillary action**. Capillary tubes are disposable narrow-bore pipettes that hold only tiny amounts of blood. These tubes can be color coded as well to indicate if there is anti-coagulant coating the inside of the pipette.

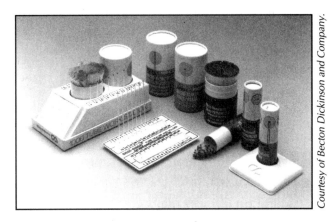

Courtesy of Becton Dickinson and Company.

Figure 10-7: Capillary Tubes

capillary tubes: tubes used to collect blood obtained during a skin puncture.

capillary action: a process by which blood is drawn up by contact only into a small tube.

ARTERIAL BLOOD GAS MICROCOLLECTIONS: Devices are continually being developed to make the microcollection of blood much easier. When an **arterial blood gas** is ordered on a patient who has difficult arterial access (see Chapter Eleven for more information on blood gases), there are systems developed to collect a microsampling of arterial blood. Such a device is known as an AVL microsampler, which has a 26-gauge **microneedle** and tubes for collection of two 120 microliter samples. The tubes are coated with heparin to prevent clotting. These devices are used on a radial, brachial, or femoral artery.

arterial blood gas: any of the gases that normally occur in the blood, such as oxygen and carbon dioxide, when analyzed from the artery rather than from a vein.

Additional Skin Puncture Accessories

In addition to the specialized lancets used for the skin puncture and the microcollection tubes used to collect the blood, you must also have the following items on hand:

- ANTISEPTIC CLEANSER: This is used to clean the skin puncture site. It is usually in the form of 70% alcohol sterile pads or an iodine preparation.

- WARMING DEVICE: Warming the designed puncture area prior to making a skin puncture can increase the blood flow as much as sevenfold. This is especially important on newborns. Several devices are commercially available. A towel or diaper wet with warm tap water can also be used to wrap the hand or foot before puncture. Always be careful not to burn the skin. Keep the warming device warm, not hot!

- STERILE GAUZE/BANDAGES: Use gauze while applying pressure on the wound after obtaining blood. Usually, bandages are not used on children under the age of two in case of aspiration of the loosened bandage. Round spot bandages can be used on larger children and adults.

- GLOVES: These are always mandatory for all blood collection, whether by vein, artery, or skin puncture. The skin puncture can be particularly bloody.

- BIOHAZARD CONTAINER: This should be within easy reach for the clinical laboratory assistant. There are often several disposable materials that must be put in biohazardous containers when the skin puncture procedure is complete.

Finger and Heelstick Technique

Obtaining a skin puncture specimen is done much the same way as the venipuncture is accomplished. The patient must be approached in the same manner, with consideration and a positive attitude. You must assemble all the necessary equipment before the patient is called to have his or her blood drawn.

Performing a Fingerstick Procedure

Materials Needed:
- ✓ gloves
- ✓ alcohol swabs
- ✓ sterile gauze
- ✓ puncture devices
- ✓ blood collection devices
- ✓ bandages (optional)
- ✓ biohazard container
- ✓ fresh solution of 10% bleach or comparable solution
- ✓ ammonia inhalant (in case of fainting)
- ✓ pen or permanent marker

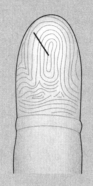

1. Procedural Step: Wash your hands.
   Reason: Standard Precautions.

2. Procedural Step: Greet and identify the patient.
   Reason: Making the patient feel welcome is an important part of customer service. Identifying the patient correctly is MANDATORY.

3. Procedural Step: Make sure you read any orders carefully. Make sure you know what tests are ordered and how much blood must be collected in order to have enough for each test.
   Reason: If you hurry through the orders and forget to draw blood for a test, the patient may have to come back for an additional blood draw. Failure to draw enough blood for a test can also delay results that could affect the treatment of the patient.

4. Procedural Step: Explain the procedure to the patient if he or she is capable of understanding. The explanation should be done in a calm, quiet voice to instill the patient's confidence in your ability as a blood drawer. Your patient will often be a child, and your calm voice can do a great deal to still the anxiety of the patient.
   Reason: Usually, patients are more relaxed if they know what you are about to do. Your calm voice is reassuring.

5. Procedural Step: Have all equipment ready: gloves, puncture device, alcohol pads, gauze, collection device(s).
   Reason: The patient will feel that you are organized and professional in your manner; it is also very awkward to be reaching for more equipment during the procedure.

Performing a Fingerstick Procedure (Cont.)

6. Procedural Step: Select a puncture site.
   Reason: Care must be taken in selecting the site to make sure that you avoid any previous punctures, you avoid scars, rashes, and burns, and you puncture the correct area of the correct finger.

7. Procedural Step: Massage or warm the puncture site.
   Reason: A good blood flow into the site produces a better specimen.

8. Procedural Step: Put on new gloves that fit snugly and are fully intact. GLOVES ON
   Reason: You should protect your skin from being contaminated by the patient's blood; your covered hands will provide a clean environment so that the patient is less likely to have the puncture site contaminated.

9. Procedural Step: Cleanse the fingertip with the alcohol pad to prevent microbiological contamination of the patient and the specimen. Dry the alcohol with sterile gauze.
   Reason: The alcohol on the potential puncture site cleans off bacteria that could cause infection; drying the area after the alcohol is put on prevents the alcohol from mixing with the blood flow and causing the breaking up (hemolysis) of cells.

10. Procedural Step: Remove the cover from the lancet or other device being used.
    Reason: The cover should not be removed from the puncture device until you are ready to use it, in order to avoid contamination of the blade or an accidental stick.

11. Procedural Step: Grasp the patient's finger, placing your thumb at the base of the fingernail. Wrap your fingers around the side of the finger .
    Reason: This position gives the blood drawer the most leverage for obtaining the best specimen.

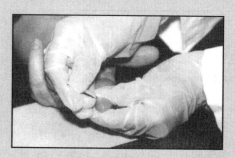

Figure 10-8: A patient's finger must be secured before a skin puncture is done.

12. Procedural Step: Penetrate the site with a lancet or other collection device with one firm and quick puncture.
    Reason: Repeating a puncture because of inadequate penetration causes unnecessary pain for the patient.

13. Procedural Step: Squeeze the patient's finger gently to release the first drop of blood, which is wiped away to avoid unnecessary tissue fluid dilution.
    Reason: Take all precautions to maintain the integrity of the sample, which ensures correct results.

14. Procedural Step: Squeeze the finger again with a milking motion from the base of the finger to the tip, and fill the collecting device(s).
    Reason: Fill the collecting device(s) as quickly as possible before the puncture site clots.

Performing a Fingerstick Procedure (Cont.)

15. Procedural Step: Collect hematology samples first to minimize the possibility of platelets clumping in the collection device.
Reason: Make every effort to assure the integrity of each specimen and of the corresponding tests ordered on the specimen.

16. Procedural Step: Slide your hand to the base of the patient's finger. Milk the finger by firmly sliding your grasp back toward the patient's fingernail.
Reason: Excessive squeezing can cause tissue fluid dilution of the sample.

17. Procedural Step: If the blood flow starts to decrease, wipe the puncture site with alcohol. Alcohol can inhibit clotting. Dry with gauze thoroughly, and squeeze the finger again. Do not squeeze the finger until the alcohol has been dried off.
Reason: Maintain a good flow of blood when at all possible to insure a proper specimen; alcohol can hemolyze blood cells.

18. Procedural Step: After collection, place a clean, dry piece of gauze on the puncture site. Have the client apply pressure (or do it yourself if the patient is unable to do so.) Bandage only if the patient is over 2 years old or according to policy.
Reason: Failure to hold pressure on a wound can result in excessive bruising and bleeding.

19. Procedural Step: Mix all anticoagulated collection devices.

Reason: Mixing disperses the anticoagulant so that the blood will not clot.

20. Procedural Step: Make sure all collection devices are labeled properly after the draw — not before the draw.
Reason: It is CRITICAL that you properly identify specimens with patients. Labeling tubes after the draw assures that all tubes labeled are functioning properly and are filled adequately.

21. Procedural Step: Dispose of all contaminated equipment in a proper biohazard waste container.
Reason: Contaminated equipment can cause a biohazard to patients and to employees.

22. Procedural Step: Remove gloves and dispose of them in a biohazard container.
Reason: Contaminated gloves can pose a biohazard.

23. Procedural Step: Dismiss the patient after you are sure that the bleeding has stopped.
Reason: It is your responsibility to make sure the patient's bleeding has stopped completely; failure to stop the bleeding can result in painful bruising.

24. Procedural Step: Wash hands.
Reason: Standard Precautions.

Performing a Heelstick Procedure

Materials Needed
✓ gloves
✓ alcohol swabs
✓ gauze
✓ puncture devices, not penetrating over 2.4 mm
✓ blood collection devices
✓ biohazard container
✓ fresh solution of 10% bleach or comparable solution
   (if you are obtaining blood at a blood-drawing station)
✓ permanent marker or pen
✓ warming device, if necessary

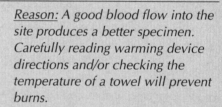

1. Procedural Step: Wash your hands. *Reason: Standard Precautions.*

2. Procedural Step: Properly identify the infant with the tests ordered. *Reason: The careful identification of a patient with the correct test is MANDATORY.*

3. Procedural Step: Assemble your supplies. Supplies are similar to those used with the fingerstick, but the lancet cannot penetrate over 2.4 mm. Open the gauze, alcohol pad and lancet packages, leaving everything inside the packages to assure sterility. *Reason: You must be adequately prepared for each procedure.*

4. Procedural Step: Warm and/or gently massage the heel. If you are warming the heel with a warming device, read the directions on the package completely before proceeding. If you are wrapping the heel with a warmed towel, make sure it will not cause a burn.

Reason: A good blood flow into the site produces a better specimen. Carefully reading warming device directions and/or checking the temperature of a towel will prevent burns.

5. Procedural Step: Select an appropriate puncture site, avoiding any previous puncture sites and the heel curvature. *Reason: Care should be taken in selecting the puncture site to make the puncture as easy and safe for the patient as possible.*

6. Procedural Step: Put on gloves. *Reason: Protect your skin from contamination from blood and also protect the patient's puncture site from bacterial contamination.*

7. Procedural Step: Grasp the infant's heel firmly. Put your forefinger over the arch of the baby's foot and your thumb below the puncture site. Your remaining fingers should rest on top of the infant's foot. The foot should be resting between your index finger and your third finger.

Performing a Heelstick Procedure (Cont.)

Reason: A firm hold on the heel will help prevent sudden movement; a comfortable grasp should help to extract the blood from the heel.

8. Procedural Step: Clean the area thoroughly with alcohol.
Reason: The alcohol on the potential puncture site cleans off bacteria that could cause infection.

9. Procedural Step: Dry the site with sterile gauze.
Reason: Drying the area after an alcohol wipe prevents the alcohol from mixing with the blood flow and causing hemolysis to the cells.

10. Procedural Step: Puncture the skin in a firm, down-and-up motion, similar to the fingerstick procedure. The puncture should be perpendicular to the heelprint lines.
Reason: A good puncture facilitates a good blood flow; making a perpendicular puncture allows the blood to flow easily.

11. Procedural Step: Wipe away the first drop of blood, minimizing tissue fluid dilution.
Reason: You must always do everything to assure the integrity of the blood specimen.

12. Procedural Step: Fill the appropriate collection device(s), using the hematology device first.
Reason: The order of filling the devices is important to obtain the best specimen for each test.

13. Procedural Step: When finished, elevate the infant's foot while placing sterile gauze over the site. Press firmly until bleeding stops. For newborns, you may be asked to put a tiny bandage on the foot.
Reason: Stopping bleeding rapidly minimizes bruising to the site.

14. Procedural Step: Mix collection devices containing anticoagulant.
Reason: Mixing disperses the anticoagulant.

15. Procedural Step: LABEL ALL SPECIMENS. You do not want to have to explain to the nursery nurses or to frantic parents why you have to do the procedure again because of mixed up labeling of specimens!
Reason: It is critical that you properly identify specimens with patients.

16. Procedural Step: Dispose of contaminated equipment immediately. You do not want to leave a lancet in a baby's bed.
Reason: Contaminated equipment can endanger both patient and employee.

17. Procedural Step: Remove gloves and put them in a biohazardous container.
Reason: Contaminated gloves can pose a biohazard.

18. Procedural Step: Wash your hands.
Reason: Standard Precautions.

Chapter Summary

A skin puncture may be needed instead of a venipuncture for several reasons. For instance, patients who are very young or very old and have small and/or fragile veins, or patients who are uncooperative with a venipuncture may require a skin puncture. A skin puncture may also be needed if a test only requires a few drops of blood, a patient is burned at venipuncture sites, or the only available vein is being used for an IV. Obese patients who have no palpable veins and patients with thrombotic problems are also good candidates for skin punctures.

A skin puncture should not be performed when a patient's extremities are cold, or if the patient is severely dehydrated. A skin puncture is not recommended when the patient is edematous, when laboratory tests require more blood than can be gotten through a skin puncture, if the patient has poor circulation, if the patient is in shock, or if the patient refuses the procedure.

The clinical laboratory assistant/phlebotomist must be thoroughly familiar and confident with all equipment used for both the finger and heelstick. The laboratory assistant must perform the finger and heelstick with full attention to the procedure stated in the procedural manual in the clinical laboratory.

Name _____

Date _____

Student Enrichment Activities

Complete the following exercises.

1. Give five reasons why you would choose to do a skin puncture instead of a venipuncture.

   A. _____

   B. _____

   C. _____

   D. _____

   E. _____

2. Give four reasons why a skin puncture might not be possible.

   A. _____

   B. _____

   C. _____

   D. _____

3. What is the composition of blood taken from a skin puncture?

   _____

4. Why is interstitial fluid a potential problem when performing a skin puncture?

   _____

5. Why are the index and fifth fingers not recommended for finger punctures?

   _____

   _____

   _____

Circle T for true, or F for false.

6. T F   Blood for the PKU test on a newborn is taken from a vein.

7. T F   Puncture the finger perpendicular to the fingerprint.

8. T F   Puncturing the finger of an infant can cause damage to the bone.

9. T F   Capillary tubes are used when larger amounts of blood are needed to be drawn by a skin puncture.

10. T F   Microcontainers for drawing blood can have anticoagulants in them.

Match the terms in Column A with the appropriate description in Column B.

Column A

11. ____ osteochondritis

12. ____ osteomyelitis

13. ____ phenylketonuria

14. ____ cyanotic

15. ____ interstitial fluid

16. ____ lancet

17. ____ capillary tubes

18. ____ Unopette®

19. ____ capillary action

20. ____ skin puncture

Column B

A. substance from injured tissue

B. sterile blade

C. bluish

D. inflammation of bone and cartilage

E. hereditary disease

F. bone infection

G. devices that hold a small amount of blood

H. capillary puncture

I. device that automatically dilutes a blood sample

J. blood drawn up into a small tube

Chapter Eleven
Special Blood Collection Procedures

Objectives

After completing this chapter, you should be able to
do the following:

1. Define and correctly spell each of the key terms.

2. Describe how to properly prepare a peripheral blood smear for a complete blood count.

3. Explain how to approach a child before you draw blood.

4. Discuss two methods of restraining a child before drawing blood.

5. Identify the reason for drawing an arterial blood gas.

6. Explain which site a clinical laboratory assistant might use to perform an arterial puncture.

7. Discuss why a bleeding time test might be ordered.

8. Explain the responsibility of the clinical laboratory assistant during the glucose tolerance test.

9. Identify the reason for drawing a blood culture.

10. Discuss special precautions taken when drawing a blood culture.

11. Explain what is meant by therapeutic drug monitoring and the clinical laboratory assistant's responsibility for TDM.

12. Define a vascular access device.

Key Terms

- aerobic
- Allen Test
- anaerobic
- bleeding time test
- blood culture
- brachial artery
- diabetes mellitus
- differential cell count
- femoral artery
- fever of unknown origin
- forensic
- glucose tolerance test

- peak level
- peripheral blood smear
- point-of-care testing
- radial artery
- septicemia
- therapeutic drug monitoring
- toxicology
- trough level
- 2-hour post prandial
- ulnar artery
- vascular access device

peripheral blood smear: a blood smear made from EDTA-anticoagulated blood or capillary blood that is stained for the purpose of microscopic viewing of blood elements.

differential cell count: the counting of 100 white blood cells to obtain the percentage of each type of white blood cells in a blood sample; also includes evaluation of platelet and red blood cell morphology.

Introduction

Blood specimens for most laboratory tests can be collected using routine venipuncture or skin puncture procedures. However, many special procedures are performed by clinical laboratory assistants/phlebotomists. These tests may require special preparation, equipment, handling, or timing. Some can be performed at the patient's bedside, and the results can be reported immediately.

As a clinical laboratory assistant/phlebotomist, you should adopt the attitude of wanting to learn any and all new testing procedures. Your goal should be to become as versatile as possible by learning to draw as many tests as you can. The more skills you master, the more invaluable you are as an employee!

The Peripheral Blood Smear

The **peripheral blood smear** is a commonly performed procedure that enables the laboratory professional to view through the microscope the blood cellular elements in as natural a state as possible, a procedure known as the **differential cell count**. A total of 100 white blood cells are counted and the percentage present of each of the five white blood cells in the circulation are determined. Platelets and red blood cells are also viewed to observe size, structure, and maturity. The blood smear is a routine component of the **complete blood count** order. Today, most automatic cell counters will do a preliminary calculated differential cell count, and that may be all that the physician requires. However, some physicians, especially **hematologists** who specialize in blood disorders, will want a blood smear made for what is now called the **manual differential cell count**.

The peripheral blood smear is made by smearing a drop of EDTA anticoagulated blood (purple stopper) across a microscope slide. The smear must be made within two hours of collection of blood in an EDTA tube. A slide can also be made with a drop of capillary blood without anticoagulant, which is not often an option although this method makes the best slides. The smear is then dried and stained to bring out the different cellular elements.

To make the smear, choose clean microscope slides free from dust and grease. One side of the slide should be frosted, and the patient's identification is written with pencil on the frosted end. Figure 11-1 illustrates a method for preparing blood smears. Wearing gloves, the laboratory assistant places a drop of blood about 1/2 inch to 3/4 inch from the end of a slide, which has been placed on a flat surface. The end of a second "spreader" slide is brought to rest at a 30-35° angle. The spreader is then brought back into the drop of blood until the drop spreads along 3/4 of the edge of the spreader slide. This is performed in a smooth, quick sliding motion.

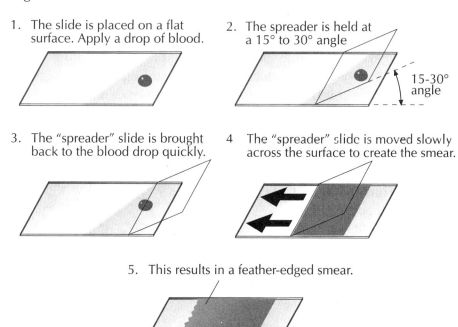

1. The slide is placed on a flat surface. Apply a drop of blood.

2. The spreader is held at a 15° to 30° angle

15-30° angle

3. The "spreader" slide is brought back to the blood drop quickly.

4 The "spreader" slide is moved slowly across the surface to create the smear.

5. This results in a feather-edged smear.

Figure 11-1: A Properly Made Peripheral Blood Smear

The smear should show a gradual transition from thick to thin. It should have a smooth appearance with no ridges or holes in the smear, and it should have a feathered edge. The length and thickness of the smear are influenced by the size of the drop of blood and by the angle in which the spreader slide is held. Slides that are too thin are a result of a blood drop that is too small or the angle of the spreader being too low. Making an excellent blood smear requires practice. In today's sophisticated laboratories, many hematology departments have automatic slide makers to lessen the exposure of employees to bloodborne pathogens. Every bloodborne pathogen precaution must be taken when making slides manually.

The Pediatric Phlebotomy

Chapter Ten discussed the fine points of the technique of performing a skin puncture on small children and a heel puncture on infants. However, there are several challenges associated with drawing blood from children that need to be considered in order to get a sample from children as painlessly and as non-traumatically as possible. Children are less emotionally and psychologically developed than adults. Therefore, a successful outcome requires the use of good interpersonal skills in dealing with children who may not be feeling well, as well as interacting with their sometimes upset and protective parents.

Preparing the Parent and Child

The first step in obtaining blood from a child is to be warm and friendly as he or she approaches your drawing station or as you approach his or her bedside. Show that you are concerned about the child, instilling a sense of trust and confidence in both the child and the parents. A calm, confident approach works with most patients.

Identification can be a bit more difficult with a child. An infant usually has an identification bracelet on the ankle, as the wrist will be too small. Newborns are usually referred to as "Baby Boy Maxwell" or "Baby Girl Castle." The mother will have a bracelet that is cross-referenced to the baby's bracelet to keep identifications straight.

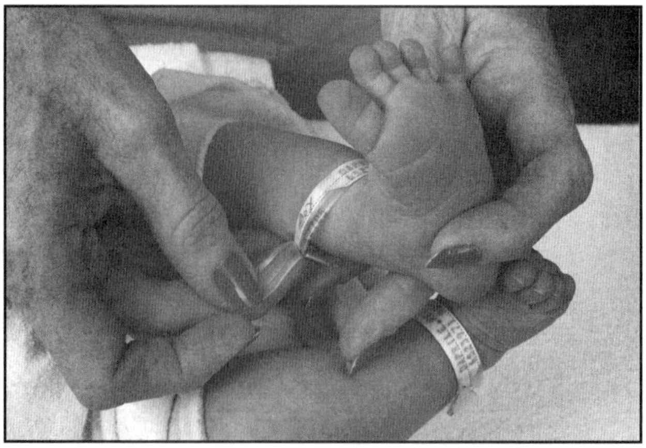

Figure 11-2: Newborns have identification bracelets on their ankles.

It is important to find out about the child's past experience with blood drawing. The child and parent can tell you valuable information about the approaches that have worked effectively. If the child is afraid as a result of a previous bad experience (which is often the case with preschool children), you will need to make a plan as to how to proceed. A plan involves the patient's ability to help you make some choices. If possible, give the child a chance to have some input by asking the child from which arm or finger he or she prefers blood to be taken.

If the child has never had blood drawn, you might explain the procedure while demonstrating what is going to happen. You can use a doll or stuffed animal in the demonstration if possible. If a child wants to hold a favorite blanket or toy during the procedure, it might comfort him or her.

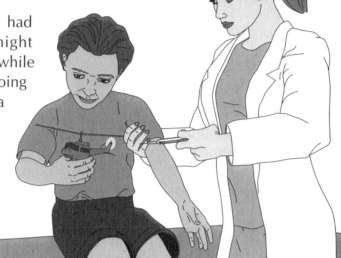

Figure 11-3: A child might want to hold a favorite toy or blanket while you are drawing blood.

Be HONEST with the child. Do not tell a child that the puncture will not hurt at all. As soon as the needle goes into the child, you will lose the child's respect because you had promised that it wouldn't hurt. Instead, tell the child that it will hurt a little bit and that the child should say "Ouch!" or make a big frown. However, the child should be told to make every effort not to move the arm. Reassure the child that you will draw the blood as quickly as possible so that the pain will be over very quickly.

Encourage parental involvement. Most parents will have a beneficial effect in reducing the child's fear. You may find that some parents want to leave because they do not want to see their child in pain. A few parents may actually make the situation worse by being nervous themselves. You must assess each parent's ability to be helpful. Respect a parent's wishes if he or she does not want to be involved.

Just the sight of needles, syringes, and white laboratory coats can frighten a child who has had lots of experience in hospitals. Often people working directly with children wear bright, colorful clothing to create a friendly atmosphere. Equipment can be arranged so that threatening supplies, like needles, are out of sight. It is helpful if the child can be told that there will be a colorful bandage, or perhaps a "hero" badge after the procedure is over.

Restraining the Child

You may have to restrain a child during a venipuncture or skin puncture so that the child's limb is not moved during the procedure. A supportive parent may be asked to assist with the restraining while also providing comfort by speaking continually to the child in a soothing voice.

There are different methods of restraining a child. One method that works well with toddlers is to immobilize the arm with the child in an upright **vertical** position. The parent holds the child on the lap. As the parent hugs the child's body and holds the arm not being used for testing, the clinical laboratory assistant/phlebotomist holds the other arm to perform the procedure.

In the **horizontal** position, the child lies down. The laboratory assistant and the parent stand at opposite sides of the bed. The parent then leans over the child, restraining the child's body and near arm while holding the child's opposite arm extended so that the laboratory assistant can do the procedure. Most infants younger than 3 months do not require assistance for a blood draw.

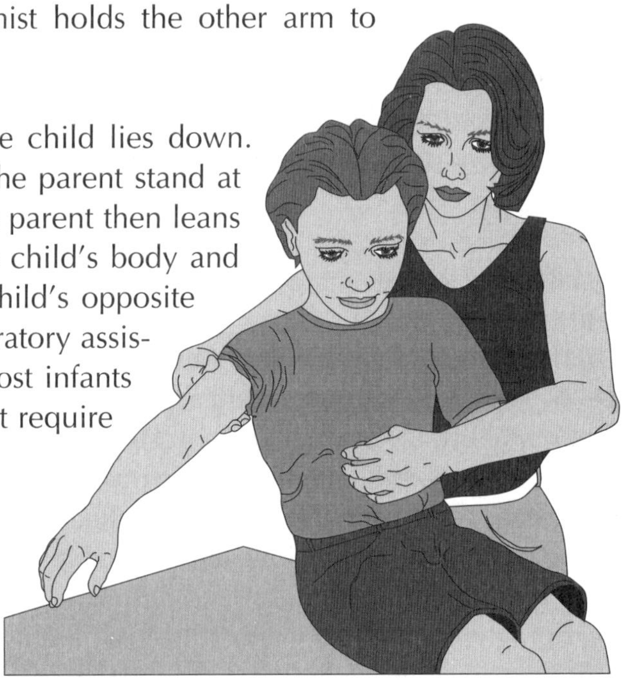

Sometimes children can become uncooperative even after efforts have been made to calm them. Children can kick, scream, and thrash, becoming even more combative when restrained. You then have to decide if there is a risk to the child or to yourself in obtaining the blood

Figure 11-4: Vertical Position for restraining a child during a venipuncture. The parent puts the child in his or her lap while holding the child's body and immobilizing the child's arm that is not being used in the procedure.

sample. You may have to ask more people to help restrain the child. If you still feel that the child will not be restrained properly, you should discontinue the blood collection attempt and notify the nurse (if the child is an inpatient) or the physician (in the case of an outpatient) that you were not able to obtain the sample.

Thinking It Through ...

Annie is a tiny, frail 4-year-old. She comes to the laboratory to have her blood drawn frequently. Most of the time Annie's father brings her, but today Mrs. Clifford, Annie's mother, is with her.

Diane is going to draw Annie's blood. She has performed many successful venipunctures on Annie, and they have a good **rapport**. She has never met Mrs. Clifford.

"Hi, Annie! Remember me, Diane? We're going to ..."

"Hold on a minute," says Mrs. Clifford. "What are you going to do to my Annie? Can't you see she is pale and scared? I don't want you hurting her. Please promise Annie you won't hurt her. Come on, tell her the blood test won't hurt at all!"

Annie and Diane's good relationship has now changed. All of a sudden, Annie is frightened and begins to cry. What should Diane do?

Arterial Blood Gases

The arterial blood gas (ABG) provides useful information about the respiratory status and the acid-base balance of patients with lung disorders as well as other diseases where acid-base balance might need to be measured (as in a diabetic in a coma). Arterial blood is used rather than venous blood because the composition of arterial blood is relatively consistent throughout the body, while the venous blood varies in relation to the metabolic needs of the area of the body it serves.

Some healthcare facilities do not require the clinical laboratory assistant/ phlebotomist to perform the ABG test. The arterial puncture is technically more difficult to perform and potentially more painful and hazardous to the patients than the venipuncture. As a result, many times nurses, clinical laboratory technologists and technicians, respiratory therapists, medical students, emergency medical technicians, and physicians obtain arterial blood gases more often than the clinical laboratory assistant. According to NCCLS, all personnel who perform ABG procedures should be certified by the healthcare institution after successfully completing training involving theory, demonstration of technique, observation of the actual procedure, and performance of arterial puncture under the supervision of qualified persons.

Today, noninvasive monitoring systems, such as the pulse oximeter, attach to the patient's fingertips and continually monitor the arterial blood status of the patient by registering the oxygen saturation in the blood. These systems cut down on the frequency of blood gas draws, although ABGs are still drawn on a regular basis on some patients.

Sites for the Arterial Puncture

The procedure that the clinical laboratory assistant/phlebotomist might be asked to perform after much training would be an arterial puncture of the **radial artery** (Figure 11-6). The best puncture location for the radial artery is on the thumb side of the wrist (Figure 11-5), an artery that is typically close to the surface. Arterial blood flows into the hand from both the radial artery and the **ulnar artery** (Figure 11-6), located on the other side of the wrist. Although the radial artery is smaller than many arteries, it is readily accessible. The ulnar artery is not used for an arterial puncture.

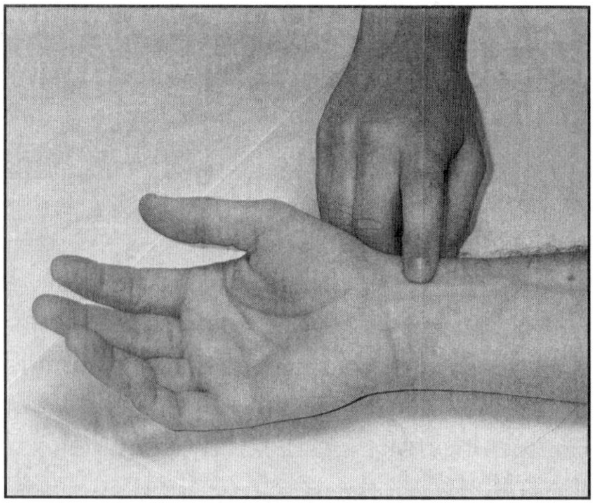

radial artery: the artery located near the radius in the wrist; one of the places suitable for taking a pulse.

ulnar artery: an artery located in the wrist opposite the radial artery; not used for arterial puncture.

Figure 11-5: Palpating the Radial Artery on the Thumb Side of the Wrist

The **brachial artery** is the second choice for an arterial puncture. The easiest access site for this artery is in antecubital space. This artery is deeper than the radial artery, often making the puncture more difficult. The brachial artery is also next to a large vein (the basilic vein) and the median nerve, both of which could be punctured accidentally. Disturbing a vein can cause pain to the patient, and entering a vein instead of an artery will result in incorrect results when arterial blood is required. The clinical laboratory assistant/phlebotomist is often restricted from blood draws on this artery.

brachial artery: the large artery in the arm on the anterior inner aspect of the elbow.

The **femoral artery** is located superficially in the groin. It is the largest artery used for puncture, and is generally punctured only by physicians or specially trained emergency room personnel.

femoral artery: the largest artery used to obtain blood; access in the groin area near the femur.

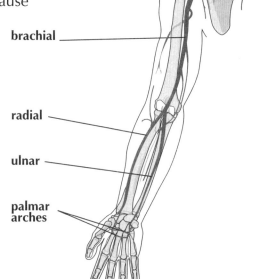

Figure 11-6: Arteries of the Arm

The Allen Test

As the clinical laboratory assistant/phlebotomist is often restricted to puncturing the radial artery, you must be aware of the **Allen Test**. When puncturing the radial artery, it is necessary to check first to see if the ulnar and the radial artery are both supplying blood to the hand. If there is some impediment in either artery, the radial artery must NOT be used.

Allen Test: a test performed to verify blood flow to the hand from the radial and ulnar arteries before performing arterial blood gas testing.

To perform the Allen Test:

1. Have the patient make a fist.

2. Maintain pressure on both the radial and ulnar arteries of the patient at the same time with the middle and index fingers of both hands. (Figure 11-7).

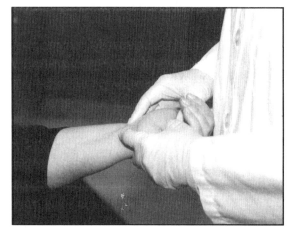

Figure 11-7: When performing the Allen Test, press both the radial and ulnar arteries of the patient at the same time.

3. While maintaining pressure, have the patient open and close the hand slowly several times. The hand should be drained of color.

4. Lower the patient's hand, and release pressure on the ulnar artery.

5. The patient's hand should flush pink within 15 seconds, indicating that both arteries are functioning. If this does not occur, this site must not be used for an arterial draw.

Performing the Arterial Blood Gas Test

The procedure for performing an arterial blood gas test is generally not learned during training as a clinical laboratory assistant/phlebotomist. You will be required to be trained to the specifications of each facility for which you work. A detailed procedure is not included in this textbook, but the following points are important to understand before you learn to draw arterial blood gases.

- Arterial blood gases are generally more painful to draw than venipunctures due to the depth of the artery and the surrounding nerves. The patient may be very tense before you begin the procedure, especially if the patient has already experienced the test. It is important to explain to the patient what you are doing, that the procedure will be over quickly, but that the procedure will be a bit painful, perhaps more so than the venipuncture.

- An artery has a pulse. That is how you can really tell the difference between an artery and a vein. You must never feel for an artery with your thumb, as the thumb has its own pulse. You do not want to mistake your own thumb pulse for the patient's pulse.

- Because of the depth of the artery, the site for puncture must be cleaned with alcohol and then with povidone iodine. Allow the site to dry as you would with a venipuncture.

- The angle of a radial arterial puncture is 45°, unlike the 15° angle of the venipuncture (Figure 11-8).

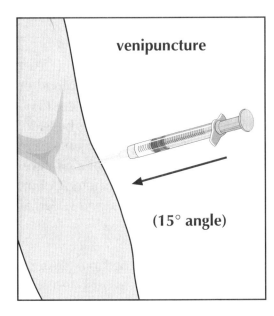 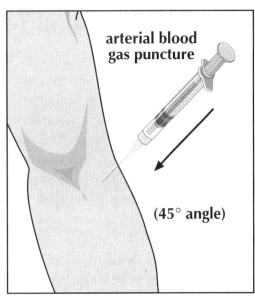

Figure 11-8: Angles of the Venipuncture and of the Arterial Blood Gas Puncture

- A syringe is used to draw arterial blood gases. Generally, you will not have to pull back on the syringe as the pressure on the artery will automatically push the blood into the syringe, another way of telling whether you have penetrated a vein or an artery. Remember that veins have much less pressure than arteries, because the blood from arteries is pumped directly from the heart. Glass syringes are not used often because of the use of disposable blood drawing products.

- You have to be particularly careful never to inject air into the patient's artery (or vein when you are using a syringe). All air must be expelled from the syringe before use.

- After withdrawing from an artery, you must hold pressure on the site for at least 5 minutes. Since the artery is under much more pressure than the vein, the puncture site can bleed longer. If inadequate pressure is applied, the patient could receive a painful hematoma and a great deal of bruising. The site could be tender for days.

Point-of-Care Blood Testing

point-of-care testing: collection of a blood sample and immediate testing at the site of patient care.

In today's healthcare environment, the focus is on rapid results in the least amount of time without sacrificing quality. This involves collecting blood or urine and then performing immediate testing at the patient's site. This could be in an emergency room, operating room, a physician's office, a patient's bedside, or even in a patient's home. The new capabilities of testing instruments have made it possible to provide a very rapid response at the patient's **point-of-care**. This type of testing can include tests for glucose (most commonly), hemoglobin, urine dipstick, sodium, potassium, ionized calcium, blood gases, and coagulation studies.

New instruments developed for point-of-care testing are designed to make tests less dependent on the technical skill of the operation; in some cases, tests can be used by the patients themselves. This gives the clinical laboratory assistant/phlebotomist opportunities in new areas of training and expansion of skills. Each institution will make a decision about who is involved in point-of-care testing. Of course, quality control must be integrated into each of these types of tests.

Bleeding Time Testing

[handwritten: pump to No. prep take surgout]

bleeding time test: a procedure designed to evaluate how long it takes a patient to stop bleeding from a standardized tiny incision.

The **bleeding time test** is a useful tool for testing platelet plug formation in the capillaries. It is used with other coagulation tests to detect problems in blood clotting. This test is often used as one of the battery of coagulation tests to check a patient's bleeding status before surgery.

The test is performed by making a minor standardized incision on the forearm. The length of time for bleeding to cease is recorded. The duration of bleeding from a punctured capillary depends on the quantity and quality of the patient's platelets. If the patient bleeds a long time, usually more than 8 minutes, a platelet problem is expected. However, some drugs, especially aspirin, can cause a prolonged bleeding time. Physicians generally require that patients refrain from taking aspirin for at least 7 days prior to surgery.

[handwritten: keep going up to 15 min   norm. 3-7 min]

A device known as the "Simplate" is often used to make uniform incisions for the bleeding time test. In many states, the clinical laboratory assistant/phlebotomist is not allowed to perform this test because of the judgment required to determine the end point of the test.

[handwritten: blot every 15 sec]

Specialized Glucose Testing

Due to the high presence of diabetes in our society today, there are many types of glucose tests. The **glucose tolerance test** (**GTT**) is the most frequently ordered multiple-timed test on the blood. It is effective in helping physicians diagnose carbohydrate metabolic problems such as **diabetes mellitus**.

The clinical laboratory assistant/phlebotomist should ask the patient before the test starts if the patient is currently using any of the following substances: alcohol, blood pressure medications, diuretics, estrogen or birth control pills, corticosteroids, anticonvulsive medications, or salicylates. If any of these drugs are taken by the patent, it should be noted on an order slip.

The patient is given a commercial glucose preparation, frequently 75 to 100 grams for an adult and about 1 gram per kilogram for a child. Then the patient stays in the waiting area near the drawing room, and urine and blood are collected every hour or half-hour for up to 6 hours, but usually not for less than 3 hours. Instructions vary according to procedures developed by the pathologist or laboratory director.

After collection, the several blood specimens are tested and graphed for the physician. (Urine also is tested for the presence of glucose). Figure 11-9 shows how the glucose preparation a patient drinks at the beginning of the test is metabolized in the blood during the next few hours. It illustrates normal patient reaction to the glucose and the reaction of a patient with diabetes mellitus. Notice how the glucose stays in the blood of the diabetic, but starts to be absorbed by the normal patient.

In addition to the glucose tolerance test, there are the fasting and **2-hour post prandial** glucose tests. These tests simply require drawing blood after a patient has fasted for at least 8 hours, or 2 hours after the patient has eaten a prescribed meal.

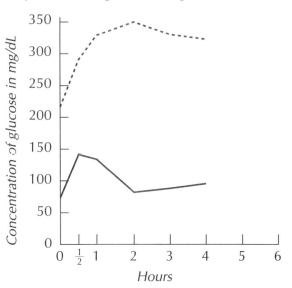

Examples of glucose tolerance over time

――― Normal   ------ Diabetes mellitus

Figure 11-9: Glucose Tolerance Test Values for a Normal Patient and for a Patient with Diabetes Mellitus

glucose tolerance test: GTT; a test for imbalance in glucose metabolism in which a patient follows a special diet and has blood drawn in timed intervals after ingesting a glucose drink. Urine also is tested at timed intervals as part of the test.

diabetes mellitus: a chronic disorder caused by the failure of the pancreas to produce enough insulin or the failure of cells to accept insulin, causing an increase in blood sugar; commonly referred to as diabetes.

2-hour post prandial: a blood test drawn 2 hours after a meal.

Glucose Tolerance Test Procedure

Materials needed:
✓ urine containers
✓ venipuncture equipment
✓ commercial glucose preparation

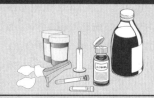

1. Procedure: The client should receive instructions several days before the glucose tolerance test (GTT). Instructions are usually given by the physician ordering the test or the laboratory. Patients should eat well-balanced meals for several days before testing. Then, for 12 hours before the test, patients should not eat, chew gum, exercise rigorously, or drink anything but water.
Reason: Preparation before the testing is critical to the success of the test. The patient should be hydrated to make urine collection easier, and rigorous exercise should be avoided to discourage an overstimulated digestive process.

2. Procedure: Make sure that the patient has followed all dietary preparations, and determine if the patient has ingested any substances that might interfere with the analysis.
Reason: If dietary preparations have not been taken, a decision can be made by a physician or a nurse (if the patient is an inpatient) to terminate and reschedule the procedure.

3. Procedure: Collect a fasting blood sugar and have the patient collect a fasting urine specimen. These specimens should be labeled "Fasting" along with regular identification.
Reason: A glucose baseline level must be determined before the glucose solution is administered. Accurate labeling is critical for this testing, including the timing of each specimen.

4. Procedure: If the fasting blood level is within normal range, the patient is given the adult dose of a commercial glucose preparation (about 100 grams). A child receives about 1 gram per kilogram body weight. If the glucose level is above the normal range, the test may be canceled and the physician notified.
Reason: A GTT may be canceled if the fasting blood sugar is above normal. The patient should not be placed in glucose overload if there is already excess sugar in the blood. The dosage is important to control the conditions of the test for accuracy.

5. Procedure: Record the time of consumption of the glucose solution. Collect both blood and urine specimens every hour for 3-6 hours, depending on the facility's policies. Label each specimen according to the collection time. If the client cannot void, an empty container should be labeled "unable to void."
Reason: The labeling should be accurate in order to interpret the test.

6. Procedure: At the end of the procedure, thank the patient for his or her cooperation.
Reason: The patient generally spends several hours at the laboratory without eating, often spending the time near the laboratory, usually in a waiting room. Having several blood tests drawn can become uncomfortable, and the glucose drink can cause nausea and dizziness. Patients may wish to terminate the test if they are too uncomfortable. If they want to continue, they should be monitored throughout the test period to make sure they are still able to continue.

Blood Cultures

A **blood culture** is often collected from patients who have **fevers of unknown origin** (**FUO**). Blood is normally sterile. However, during a bacterial infection bacteria can get in the blood, causing a condition known as **septicemia**. This condition can lead to the patient's death and must be identified as soon as possible. Infection can be carried all over the body through the blood. When a patient is in the hospital, blood cultures might be drawn before and after a spike in temperature (ordered by the nursing station), when the bacteria might be present in the largest numbers. Often, blood cultures will be ordered in sets of three at different times and from three different sites.

Identifying the Agent Causing Septicemia

In order to see if there are bacteria or other offending pathogens in the blood, a blood collection system must be used for this test. The collection system must be sterile and filled with a medium that will encourage growth of an organism after collection. See Figure 11-10.

Some culture systems are designed to be used with the vacuum tube system. Others require a syringe collection, with the blood culture bottles **inoculated** following the draw. There are two bottles for each blood culture: the **aerobic** and **anaerobic** testing bottles. Some pathogens in the human body require oxygen for life. Those pathogens are called aerobic organisms. Some pathogens, called anaerobic organisms, live best without oxygen. The anaerobic bottles for culture incubate the blood without the presence of air.

Iodine damages blood stopper

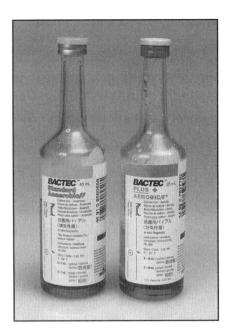

Figure 11-10: A blood culture system is used to encourage the growth of an organism after collection.

blood culture: a liquid broth with a blood sample added to test for possible infection in the blood.

fever of unknown origin: FUO; an illness of at least three weeks duration with a recurrent fever and no diagnosis.

septicemia: the presence in the bloodstream of infectious microorganisms or their toxins.

aerobic: \ requiring oxygen to maintain life.

anaerobic: 2 able to live without oxygen.

Skin Preparation for the Blood Culture Draw

When drawing blood cultures, the site for a puncture must be prepared using special disinfection techniques to avoid any bacterial contamination from the skin. After locating the vein, the area of the puncture is specially prepared for venipuncture. With the tourniquet off, the site is scrubbed thoroughly with an antiseptic agent made with iodine. Scrub a 3 to 4 inch-square area for 2 minutes with the iodine antiseptic. Allow the site to air dry. Do not touch the area after disinfecting.

Culture bottles should also be cleaned off thoroughly before inoculating them with blood. Most culture bottle stoppers should be cleaned with alcohol, not iodine, as iodine can damage the rubber.

Therapeutic Drug Monitoring

therapeutic drug monitoring: TDM; collection and testing of blood to evaluate and manage medication therapy effectively and safely.

The collection of **therapeutic drug monitoring (TDM)** specimens is a very important task often assigned to the clinical laboratory assistant/phlebotomist to aid the physician in the diagnosis and safe management of drug treatment of a patient. Physicians do not want to prescribe a dosage of a medication that is too toxic to a patient. However, at the same time a dosage that is too weak will not treat the patient adequately. When dealing with drugs that can be toxic in overdose, the physician wants to find an optimal effective therapy for the patient until recovery is achieved.

Therapeutic drug monitoring can be ordered for any therapeutic substance being administered to the patient, such as antibiotics, anticoagulants, seizure medications, cardiac medications, and psychiatric medications. Each patient's system breaks down drugs at a different rate, so blood levels of each patient must be checked to see how effective the dosage is for that patient.

The clinical laboratory assistant/phlebotomist is often asked to draw **peak levels** and **trough levels** of drugs. A requisition will be sent to the clinical laboratory specifying the time that the TDM testing should be drawn. The two types of levels are listed below.

Trough Level: A trough level is described as a drug level in the blood collected when the lowest serum concentration is expected, which is usually just before the next drug dose is given.

Peak Level: A peak level is defined as a drug level in the blood collected 15 to 30 minutes after the medication has been given to a patient and when the highest level of the drug is expected in the blood.

Complications of Therapeutic Drug Monitoring Testing

A surprising number of errors can be made during TDM testing that can affect patient results. Some of these errors include the following:

- The clinical laboratory assistant/phlebotomist fails to collect the blood at the time ordered on the requisition. Once the time is missed, another level cannot be drawn again until the next cycle of medication, which could be as much as 12 to 24 hours. This could delay very valuable information for the physician who must know if the patient is being undertreated or overtreated.

- The laboratory assistant fails to document when the blood was drawn, which could result in confusion.

- The drug was not administered on time. The laboratory assistant can draw a peak level on an inpatient and find out later that the drug had not been given to the patient.

- The nursing station or physician fails to document when the next dosage is due and does not order the next TDM testing.

- An inaccurate dosage of the drug is given that is not in the physician's orders, causing confusion when the physician receives results.

The clinical laboratory must be responsible for sending blood drawers at specified times for both the peak and trough testing. It is always a good idea to check at the nurse's station to make sure that the drug was given (or will be given) on time.

peak level: a drug level in the blood collected 15 to 20 minutes after the dosage has been administered or when the highest serum concentration of the drug is expected.

trough level: a drug level in the blood collected when the lowest serum concentration is expected, which is usually immediately before the administration of the next dosage.

Forensic Specimens

toxicology: specimens evaluated for the presence of drugs.

Occasionally, you might be asked to draw blood for a blood alcohol determination or for the presence of other drugs (**toxicology** specimens) for **forensic** purposes. Your healthcare facility will give you specific instructions on how to draw a blood alcohol. In this instance, you will not use any type of alcohol for cleansing because that alcohol could falsely elevate the blood alcohol level. Toxicology specimens may also follow a protocol developed by your laboratory director to ensure accurate and reliable analytical results that will be credible as evidence.

forensic: pertaining to the law.

Intravenous Therapy

Intravenous therapy for inpatients can create a variety of challenges for venipuncture collections. Healthcare facilities have varying policies about drawing blood from below an IV site when there are no other sites available. NCCLS recommends the following steps if it becomes necessary to draw blood below an IV:

- Ask the patient's nurse to turn off the IV for at least 2 minutes.

- Apply the tourniquet below the IV site.

- Discard the first sample of blood taken before collecting test blood. 5 ml is the minimum for regular testing; 10 ml is required before drawing coagulation tests.

- Locate a different suitable vein not being used for the IV.

- Collect the venipuncture, and tell the nurse that the IV needs to be turned on again.

- Document that the blood was taken from an IV arm, describe precautions, and identify the fluid being administered through the IV.

vascular access device: VAD; a device used to automatically remove blood from a patient without having to stick the patient with a needle.

Vascular Access Devices (VAD)

Blood collection from **vascular access devices (VADs)**, which are indwelling lines such as a central venous catheter, heparin lock, or cannula, is beyond the scope of the clinical laboratory assistant/phlebotomist. Collection involves flushing and clearing the lines before blood can be collected. However, you may be asked to pick up specimens drawn from such lines.

Chapter Summary

In addition to routine venipunctures and skin punctures, there are also special procedures that the clinical laboratory assistant/phlebotomist may or may not be required to perform. You will often make blood smears and draw blood from pediatric patients in most facilities. You will be responsible for administering the glucose tolerance test, you will draw blood cultures, and you will be involved in drawing peak and trough levels during therapeutic drug monitoring. You may not be allowed to draw arterial blood gases or perform bleeding time tests. Whether you are routinely assigned to any or all of the special procedures listed in this chapter, you should be knowledgeable about them and be willing to learn any new procedure when given the opportunity.

Name _____

Date _____

Student Enrichment Activities

Circle T for true, or F for false.

1. (T) F   Two methods of restraining a child include using a vertical position and a horizontal position.

2. T (F)   Parents should be encouraged to leave the room while you draw blood from their children.

3. T (F)   Venous blood composition is consistent throughout the body.

4. (T) F   In general for most patients, an arterial puncture is more painful than a venipuncture puncture.

5. (T) F   The Allen Test must be performed before doing the brachial artery puncture procedure.

6. (T) F   Arteries are under greater pressure than veins.

7. (T) F   You must hold pressure on an arterial puncture for at least 5 minutes.

8. T (F)   Veins have their own pulse.

9. (T) F   Your thumb has a pulse.

10. (T) F   Point-of-care testing produces quick results for the patient.

Complete the following exercises.

11. Briefly explain point-of-care testing. Collection of a blood sample
     and immediate testing @ site of pt care. Get results in
     1-2 min

12. Three arteries in the arm are the radial , ulnar , and
     brachial .

13. The bleeding time test is performed for testing how long it takes a pt
     to stop bleeding from a standardized tiny incision & assess vascular
     integrity

14. A physician would order a blood culture on a patient when a bacterial
     infection of the blood is suspected or FUO.

15. Glucose tolerance testing is ordered when a patient is suspected of having a
     Carbohydrate metabolic problems

16. What is the difference from peak and trough levels for therapeutic drug testing?
     Peak is when drug level is suspected to be
     the highest, usually 15-30min after med is given. Trough is when
     Med is expected to be lowest, usually before next dose

     or length of infusion —

17. Describe briefly how to prepare a peripheral blood smear. Smear a drop of
     EDTA blood onto slide, 2H after obtained. Dry smear. Before
     putting blood on slide, make sure name is on frosted
     side & slide is clean, Blood is put 1/2 -3/4 in from side,
     rest spreader @ 35° angle on drop of blood, slowly spread
     across surface.

     not on final

18. Why is a peripheral blood smear made? Manual blood count,
     certain diseases

Name _____

Date _____

19. Why wouldn't you use alcohol to cleanse the puncture site when drawing a blood alcohol level? _It would give false results_____

20. Give two examples of a VAD. _central venous catheter, fistulas_____

Match the terms in Column A with appropriate description in Column B.

Column A

21. _D_ point-of-care testing

22. _C_ GTT

23. _E_ FUO

24. _B_ TDM

25. _A_ blood cultures

Column B

A. drawn to rule out septicemia

B. tests to see if a patient is responding well to drug therapy

C. test to rule out diabetes

D. testing that is done at the patient site

E. a fever without a known cause

Chapter Twelve
Hazards and Complications of Blood Drawing

Objectives

After completing this chapter, you should be able to
do the following:

1. Define and correctly spell each of the key terms.

2. Discuss the legal and physical risks an employee might encounter while drawing blood.

3. Explain why a clinical laboratory assistant could be the object of litigation as a result of a blood draw.

4. Identify several complications related to the patient that could affect a venipuncture or a skin puncture.

Key Terms

- burden of proof
- hemorrhage
- litigation

- petechiae
- syncope
- thrombi

Introduction

This chapter discusses risks to the clinical laboratory assistant/phlebotomist that are related to the blood draw as well as complications that can occur during the act of drawing blood. It would be simple if every blood draw was uneventful, with patients having large, full veins. However, that is not reality. Patients are often in poor health and have had many venipunctures in tired veins, posing real challenges to the blood drawer.

As a clinical laboratory assistant/phlebotomist, you must be prepared for a variety of complications and have the knowledge and confidence to approach each problem with a calm, professional attitude. At the same time, you must minimize any risk to yourself and must also keep the patient's welfare foremost in mind.

The Risk of Bloodborne Pathogen Exposure

Chapter Five of this text discusses the risk posed to the clinical laboratory assistant/phlebotomist by bloodborne pathogens. The potential exposure to HIV and hepatitis must be a consideration at all times. Protective practices must be in place at the workplace to minimize all risks to those collecting blood specimens. This information must be maintained within a procedure manual or in a separate safety manual developed by each facility. These procedures are set forth by OSHA, JCAHO, CLIA, CDC, and NCCLS, to name several organizations who are dedicated to employee safety.

NCCLS Guidelines

Of particular interest to the clinical laboratory are the NCCLS guidelines (National Committee for Clinical Laboratory Standards) for performing laboratory procedures accurately and safely. The NCCLS standard M29-A is particularly important because it was developed by experts in laboratory medicine including physicians and members of the CDC. This standard addresses laboratory procedures and practices of laboratory personnel who are at risk of exposure continuously. The standard incorporates the OSHA and CDC guidelines.

Review of Safety Precautions Taken During Blood Draws

The following points are summaries of suggestions taken from NCCLS documents.

1. Venipuncture is considered a risky procedure for a number of reasons. The employee is manipulating a sharp needle, the employee can accidentally puncture an artery instead of a vein, and the process of transferring blood from a syringe to vacuum tubes presents a risk to the employee. Blood can contaminate your gloves, clothing, or mucous membranes. A patient can move suddenly during the procedure, leading to potential exposure to bloodborne pathogens. NCCLS recommends clean, fresh gloves, a nonpermeable protective gown or laboratory coat, and eye protection.

2. Gloves should cover the cuffs of the protective garment. If gloves are loose, blood could flow inside the gloves.

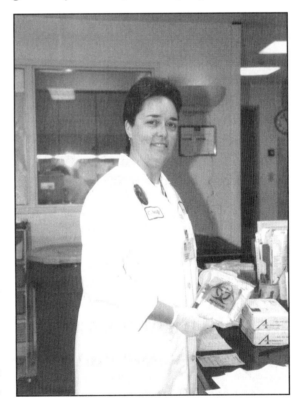

Figure 12-1: A Clinical Laboratory Assistant/ Phlebotomist Dressed for a Blood Draw in Accordance with NCCLS Standards

3. Sharps containers must be in reach for immediate disposal of the needles. NEVER recap, cover, bend, or set down a used needle.

4. NCCLS recommends that a fresh solution of 10% household bleach or a comparable product that is effective against the HIV and hepatitis B virus be available where blood collection takes place in case of an accident or contamination. The bleach must be poured over the blood and allowed to sit for at least 15 minutes. An employee, wearing fresh gloves, then wipes up the area. The contaminated material is then put in a biohazard container. If the spill is spread over a large area, bleach should be poured over the spill and allowed to cover the spill for 15 minutes. Then a substance to solidify the spill should be added so that clean up can be done with a pan or similar device.

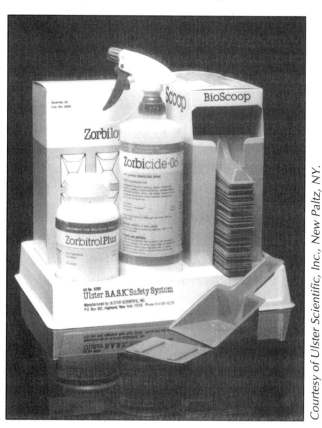

Courtesy of Ulster Scientific, Inc., New Paltz, NY.

Figure 12-2: A safety system such as this is used to clean up contaminated spills.

5. NCCLS recommends regular decontamination of blood drawing equipment such as tourniquets and vacuum tube holders.

Risk of Litigation for the Clinical Laboratory Assistant/Phlebotomist

As discussed in Chapter Four , phlebotomy is an invasive procedure. Therefore, if a patient has an injury that he or she feels is directly caused by the blood drawer, a claim of malpractice or negligence can result in **litigation**.

litigation:
a lawsuit.

Providing the **burden of proof** is the patient's responsibility. A significant injury from venipuncture is difficult to prove. For a suit to be proved against a phlebotomist, four conditions must occur.

1. A standard of care must exist.

2. This standard must be breached.

3. An injury must be sustained.

4. The injury was caused by a breach of the standard of care.

NCCLS has developed a standard of care involving professional standards in the practice of collecting blood. It must be proven that the clinical laboratory assistant was not trained to a standard of care that includes competency in all areas of phlebotomy.

Errors That Can Lead to Litigation

Several mistakes that can be made through negligence will increase the risk of litigation. They include the following:

- misidentification of a patient
- mislabeling or failing to label a patient specimen
- patient infection caused by failure to use sterile technique during the blood draw
- reusing needles with resulting infection
- injury to patient veins or nerves
- scarring as a result of a blood drawing procedure
- failure to inform a patient of risks associated with fainting and injuring his or her self
- drawing blood without patient's consent
- breach of confidentiality on such matters as AIDS, HIV screening, abortion, paternity, pregnancy, patient diagnosis, drug or alcohol abuse
- equipment breakage causing patient injury

The key is to FOLLOW POLICY AND PROCEDURES IN THE PROCEDURE MANUAL EXACTLY!

burden of proof: the obligation to prove the facts of a dispute by evidence presented.

Complications of Blood Drawing

As mentioned in the introduction of this chapter, it would be wonderful to have every blood draw proceed with no complications. However, when you are working with human beings (some being very ill), there will be problems that come up periodically. You as a clinical laboratory assistant/phlebotomist must be aware of the potential for complication and be ready to solve any problem resulting from a blood draw.

Hematoma

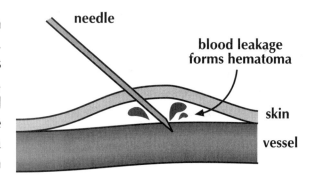

The most common complication from phlebotomy is a **hematoma**. This occurs when the needle is placed improperly in the vein, allowing blood to escape and collect under the skin (Figure 12-3). The first indication that a hematoma is forming comes with a swelling around the venipuncture site while the needle is in the vein. The needle can be adjusted to stop the formation, but in most

Figure 12-3: A hematoma occurs when an improperly placed needle results in blood escaping from a vein.

cases it is best to remove the needle and apply firm pressure to the site. The patient will be bruised, but the bruising should go away in a few days. Applying firm pressure to a hematoma is mandatory to prevent complications.

Failure to Obtain Blood

Several factors can cause the clinical laboratory assistant to fail to get blood during a blood draw. The needle may not be inserted deeply enough (a common problem with nonaggressive beginners), the needle is inserted clear through the vein, the bevel of the needle is against the vein wall, or the vacuum is lost in the tube. Figure 12-4 illustrates some needle positions that will result in failure to obtain an adequate specimen.

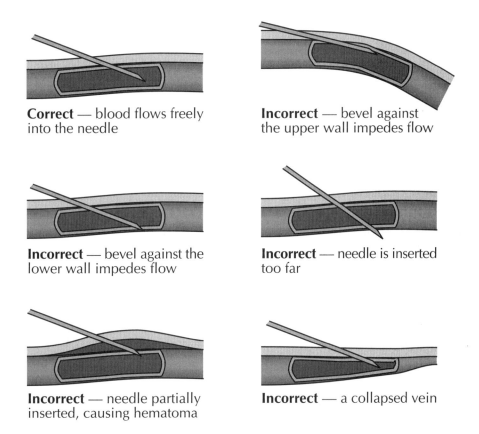

Correct — blood flows freely into the needle

Incorrect — bevel against the upper wall impedes flow

Incorrect — bevel against the lower wall impedes flow

Incorrect — needle is inserted too far

Incorrect — needle partially inserted, causing hematoma

Incorrect — a collapsed vein

Figure 12-4: Needle Positions That May Result in Failure to Draw Blood

Occasionally a tube may not have adequate vacuum pressure. The tube is placed in the vacuum tube adapter, but no blood comes out. Sometimes a tube will be punctured before the procedure is performed. This will result in no blood entering the tube after it is in place. For these reasons it is always good to have extra tubes on hand in case there is a tube problem.

Another problem that can occur when the needle is not screwed properly into the adapter during a vacuum tube draw is that the needle can become unscrewed. In that case, the phlebotomy must be stopped immediately as there is no other way to correct this problem. Make sure that the needle is always seated properly in the adapter.

Veins can also collapse because the vacuum draw of a tube is too strong for a fragile vein. You can tell if this happens because the vein will disappear as soon as the needle penetrates it. Blood flow may be reestablished by tightening the tourniquet. If the blood flow doesn't increase immediately, withdraw the needle and attempt a second venipuncture at another site.

If blood is not forthcoming immediately, sometimes the needle can be readjusted gently. DO NOT PROBE! If the blood is not flowing after a few readjustments, discontinue the venipuncture. Clinical laboratories have a maximum amount of times that you may stick a patient to get blood, usually two or three times. After attempts fail, you must ask another laboratory assistant to attempt the venipuncture.

Fainting

Many patients become dizzy and faint at the thought or sight of blood, especially their own blood. The clinical laboratory assistant/phlebotomist should respect a patient's comment that "I often faint when my blood is taken." Immediately have the patient moved to a reclining position.

syncope: fainting; sudden, brief, and temporary loss of consciousness; passing out.

Even when the patient has no history of fainting (**syncope**), consider fainting as a possibility that could occur with all patients. However, patients seated in the blood collection chair with the locked arm rest will avoid the possibility of falling during a faint. If you find that a patient is becoming faint, the tourniquet should be immediately released and the needle removed from the patient's arm. Attempt to keep pressure on the venipuncture site with gauze. Place the patient's head between his or her legs, and tell the patient to breathe deeply.

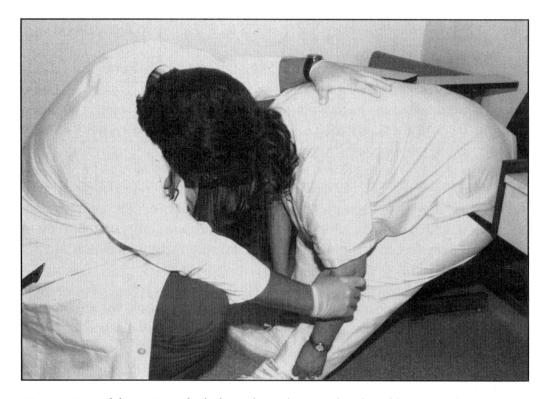

Figure 12-5: If the patient feels faint, have her put her head between her legs.

Since it is always a possibility that a patient may faint during a blood draw procedure, it is helpful reassure him or her and distract his or her attention from the collection procedure. If a patient does completely faint, carefully help the patient to the floor, and ask for help if possible. The patient should eventually be placed on a bed if he or she isn't already on one, and the laboratory assistant should stay with the patient for at least 15 minutes. A wet towel gently applied to the forehead and a glass of juice may help the patient recover faster. The patient can experience nausea, as well, and may refuse any drink but water.

Patients who do not admit to fainting problems can display symptoms even before you begin a blood draw. Their skin color can change (becoming pale), and their skin can become clammy with signs of perspiration on their face. If a patient does faint, an incident report must be filed. Many healthcare facilities require that the patient see an emergency room physician before he or she is released.

Allergies

Some patients are allergic to iodine or other solutions used to disinfect a puncture site. They can also be allergic to adhesive tape. Always respect their request for a different type of disinfectant or tape.

Seizures

A rare complication that can occur during a blood draw is a seizure. If a patient begins to have a seizure, the healthcare worker should immediately remove the tourniquet and needle from the patient's arm, trying to maintain pressure on the venipuncture site. Call for help while making sure the patient does not hurt himself or herself. Move anything that could harm the patient and try to protect the patient's head from striking an object that could cause harm. Never leave the patient alone. DO NOT ATTEMPT TO PUT ANYTHING IN THE PATIENT'S MOUTH.

Excessive Bleeding/Petechiae

A patient usually stops bleeding at the site of the venipuncture within a few minutes. However, patients on anticoagulant therapy (heparin, coumadin) or other medications such as arthritis medication can bleed for a longer period of time. Patients may tell you that they are on such therapy, or it may be noted on a laboratory order form. Pressure must be applied to the venipuncture site until the bleeding stops. The clinical laboratory assistant/phlebotomist should not leave the patient until the bleeding stops.

petechiae: red spots seen on skin, associated with a decrease in platelet function.

Petechiae are small red dots that appear on the skin because of capillary **hemorrhage**. Capillaries can bleed excessively as a result of a coagulation problem, generally one related to platelets. If you see petechiae on a patient's arm or elsewhere, you must assume that this patient may take a little longer than normal to stop bleeding from a puncture site. Petechiae can also be caused by tying the tourniquet too tightly and leaving it on too long.

hemorrhage: the severe, abnormal internal or external discharge of blood.

Edema

Edema results when excessive fluids collect in the tissues of a patient, resulting in swelling of the tissues. Venipunctures usually are not successful in such areas because it is difficult to feel a vein in the swollen area. Additionally, the specimen can become diluted by the fluid surrounding the tissues.

Damaged, Scarred Veins

Some patients have had many venipunctures, often related to a chronic illness that has required many medical procedures. Sometimes veins will build up scar tissue as a result of numerous phlebotomies. Intravenous drug users can have much scar tissue.

thrombi: blood clots.

Veins can also be blocked by other diseases and disorders, and only a small amount of blood might come from a blocked vein. Veins can have **thrombi** inside them as well, solid masses derived from blood constituents that reside in blood vessels. A thrombus can completely or partially block a vessel. An alternative site must be located.

Burns

Burned areas cannot be sites for blood drawing, as they are very susceptible to infection. Careful attention to sterility must be maintained when drawing a burn patient, because he or she is very susceptible to contracting infection from any source. An alternate site should be found.

Too Much Pain

Occasionally patients, especially those already in pain, will complain about the pain associated with the needle entering the skin. They may also complain about the tourniquet being painfully tight. Warn the patient before the venipuncture that there will be a small amount of pain associated with a routine venipuncture or skin puncture. The stinging sensation of the alcohol can be avoided by allowing the alcohol to dry before needle penetration. Probing with the needle should always be avoided, especially with a pain-sensitive patient.

Thinking It Through ...

Mrs. Jackson has been chronically ill for years. Several laboratory assistants can't even remember a time when Mrs. Jackson wasn't having some procedure performed at their healthcare facility.

Mrs. Jackson hates having her blood drawn. She complains from the time she comes into the drawing area until the time she leaves. Today she is not feeling well and faces surgery. She is coming in to have her pre-surgery blood testing, which is very important.

Jennifer seats Mrs. Jackson in the blood drawing chair. Mrs. Jackson immediately says she is going to faint. She also says that she doesn't want a tourniquet, that she has no good veins, and that she wants to go home. She is not about to let anyone put any more needles in her veins.

1. What should Jennifer do?

2. Should Jennifer send Mrs. Jackson home immediately?

3. What could be done to help Mrs. Jackson feel more comfortable?

Nerve Damage

Excessive or blind probing while performing a blood draw can lead to injury of a main nerve, most commonly the median cutaneous nerve. This injury could cause permanent damage to the patient, who might then institute a lawsuit.

Accidental Arterial Puncture

If the accidental puncture of an artery takes place during a venipuncture procedure, it is important to hold pressure over an arterial puncture for AT LEAST 5 MINUTES. You can recognize arterial blood by the bright red color or by the fact that arterial blood spurts into the tube. You should notate "possible arterial blood" on the sample because arterial blood can have different values for some tests.

Obesity

Occasionally, obese (extremely fat) patients will have veins that are not able to be felt at all. With practice, you should be able to palpate a vein even though it appears very deep. Generally, hand veins are more visible.

Intravenous Lines

Whenever a patient has an intravenous line, the arm with the IV line should not be used for venipuncture because the specimen will be diluted with IV fluid. Instead, the other arm or another site should be considered. Sometimes nurses or physicians can discontinue the IV line and draw blood from the needle that is already inserted. In this instance, the first few milliliters of the specimen should be discarded to remove IV fluid. Notes should be made on the laboratory requisition that this step was performed. IV therapy can also cause vein damage.

Mastectomy

A female patient who has had a mastectomy may have reduced lymph flow (or none at all) on the side of the body where the breast was removed. This happens because the lymph nodes next to the breast have also been removed. Without lymph flow on a particular side, the patient is highly susceptible to infection. Pressure from a tourniquet can also lead to injury. Perform the blood draw on the side unaffected by the mastectomy. If the patient has had both breasts removed, consult the physician about what course to follow.

Chapter Summary

The great majority of blood draws are carried out without complication. The clinical laboratory assistant/phlebotomist must continually be aware of the precautions that must be taken to avoid infection by bloodborne pathogens. Drawing blood can also present complications to the patient, and if serious, can result in litigation. Remember that adherence to prescribed venipuncture and skin puncture procedures will minimize the risk to you and to the patient. Have patience and compassion. Listen to the patient's instructions as well as fears about the venipuncture; this attention will help greatly in avoiding undue complications for you and the patient.

Name _____

Date _____

Student Enrichment Activities

Define the following terms.

1. bloodborne pathogens: <u>pathogens in blood</u>

2. syncope: <u>fainting; sudden, brief, & temporary loc,</u>
<u>passing out</u>

3. NCCLS: <u>National Committe for Clinical Laboratory</u>
<u>Standards. Guidelines for procedures & practices</u>

4. legal liability: <u>Proof of liability and responsible</u>

5. petechiae: <u>red spots seen on skin, associated c̄ ↓</u>
<u>platelet function</u>

Circle T for true, or F for false.

6. T (F) When a hematoma starts to form while drawing blood, ignore it until you are able to safely get the blood specimen.

7. T (F) In a lawsuit against a laboratory assistant, providing the burden of proof is the responsibility of the laboratory assistant.

8. (T) F Petechiae are a result of capillary hemorrhage.

9. T ~~F~~ ~~Try to put something into the mouth of a seizure patient to prevent~~
    him or her from swallowing his or her tongue.

10. (T) F Making sure the alcohol on the arm is completely dry before a skin or vein
    puncture will reduce the pain for the patient.

Complete the following statements.

11. In the course of the venipuncture, some patients can be allergic to the _iodine_
    and/or the _adhesive tape_.

12. Another word for fainting is _syncope_.

13. Excessive bleeding after a venipuncture could be related to the patient
    being on _anticoagulants_.

14. A drug addict can have _scarring_ of the veins.

15. A clinical laboratory assistant can puncture an _artery_ instead
    of a vein during a venipuncture.

Circle the correct answer.

16. The following conditions can cause venipuncture complications, except:
    A. thrombi.
    B. hematomas.
    C. obesity.
    (**D.**) patience.

Name _____

Date _____

17. A woman who has had a mastectomy:

   A. poses no complication for the venipuncture.

   B. can have an increased risk of infection on the mastectomy side.

   C. will never have problems from tourniquet use.

   D. should never have blood drawn anywhere.

18. Edema:

   A. can cause swelling in a venipuncture site.

   B. can cause dilution of the blood sample.

   C. can make it hard to feel veins.

   D. all of the above.

19. When a patient is becoming faint, symptoms might include:

   A. perspiration.

   B. pale skin.

   C. clammy skin.

   D. all of the above.

20. NCCLS recommends that a blood spill should be disinfected with a fresh solution of
     10% household bleach or a comparable product for at least:

   A. 5 minutes.

   B. 10 minutes.

   C. 15 minutes.

   D. 20 minutes.

12-16

Chapter Thirteen
Obtaining Blood Samples from Animals

Objectives

After completing this chapter, you should be able to
do the following:

1.   Define and correctly spell each of the key terms.

2.   Identify job situations in which a clinical laboratory
     assistant/phlebotomist might be asked to draw blood
     from animals.

3.   Discuss some general guidelines for drawing blood
     from animals.

4.   List venipuncture sites from which to draw blood from cats,
     dogs, guinea pigs, rats, mice, and rabbits.

5.   Discuss how to handle blood specimens from animals
     correctly in order to avoid inaccurate test results.

Key Terms

- canine
- cephalic vein
- feline
- femoral vein
- jugular vein
- lateral saphenous vein
- medial saphenous vein

Introduction

Employment opportunities also exist for clinical laboratory assistants/phlebotomists in research facilities. Some of these facilities do work with animals, and the same venipuncture skills used on humans can be used when drawing blood from animals. For example, in some areas where veterinary technicians and veterinary assistants are in short supply, the clinical laboratory assistant may be employed by a veterinarian to run simple tests and to perform venipunctures. Chapter Nine of this textbook goes into detail about venipuncture procedures. Since most of the mechanical considerations for performing a human venipuncture are the same as those for performing an animal venipuncture, this chapter is a quick overview of the techniques used when drawing and handling blood from certain animals, such as cats, dogs, guinea pigs, rats, mice, and rabbits. These animals are used often in research and also are found in households as pets.

General Venipuncture Techniques for Animals

When a human patient is frightened of an impending venipuncture, it is often possible to reason with the patient to convince him or her that a blood test is necessary. Obviously, this technique does not work with an animal. Although venipuncture sites differ with various animals, they all respond to several techniques that help make the venipuncture as painless and quick as possible:

- Animals should be treated with kindness and respect. They may be in pain, frightened, and confused. Just as you would do with a small child or frightened adult, speak in soothing, quiet tones to the animal. Handle the animal gently, and avoid creating undue stress to the animal. As with humans, an animal that is upset can lead to changes in the blood that may not be reflective of its true blood picture.

Thinking It Through . . .

Judy works as a clinical laboratory assistant in a veterinary clinic that is also a research facility. Today, Judy is drawing blood from a dog, Bucky, who is having a blood test to assess thyroid function.

Bucky is a hyperactive spaniel who is adored by his owners. Mrs. Black insists on being present for Bucky's blood test and also wants to bring her 6 year-old twin boys with her into the room while the blood is being drawn. Bucky is nervous about being in the clinic. Mrs. Black has definite opinions about how to get Bucky's blood sample. One of the twins is standing on the examination chair.

1. Is this the best atmosphere for drawing blood on an anxious dog?

2. How do you improve the situation?

3. How is this situation similar to drawing blood from a child with a protective parent?

- Veterinarians often wish to take blood when the animal is under anesthesia to avoid having the animal struggle and to avoid putting it through the fear and discomfort of a procedure. If the animal only needs a blood test and no other procedures, help is almost always needed, especially with larger animals, to accomplish a successful venipuncture.

- Unlike human skin, animal skin is typically covered in fur. Some assistants clip the fur over a venipuncture site before attempting to feel for the vein.

- When a vein is found, stabilization is as necessary in this situation as it is with a human because veins can shift if not held down.

- With larger animals, such as medium-sized dogs, a Vacutainer™ system can be used. However, in small animals, a needle and syringe may be used to avoid undue pressure to a small, fragile vein. The needle and syringe selected are determined by the size and location of the vein to be used, much the same as in humans of different sizes and ages.

- Some facilities do not require the use of gloves during a venipuncture. In the interest of measures taken to keep the venipuncture site free from infection and because of the small chance that an assistant could contract a disease from an animal, gloves are generally recommended.

- The position and angle of entry of the needle is the same in animals as it is in humans. When using a syringe, the removal of blood should be slow and continuous, just as in a human venipuncture to prevent hemolysis of the blood.

- The area to be punctured should be cleaned with a suitable antiseptic, depending on the study or test to be obtained. Just as it is with humans, infection of the site is to be carefully avoided in animals.

- If an anticoagulant is used in a blood collection tube, the correct ratio of anticoagulant and blood must be considered as it is in human draws.

- Animals should be placed on a fasting diet, similar to that given to humans if fats from a diet will interfere with testing.

- After a blood draw, the wound of the stick should be watched for clotting just as a human's puncture is watched. Applying pressure to the area for a few minutes is generally enough to ensure a clot.

The Animal Venipuncture

Obtaining blood samples from various animals requires some knowledge of unique animal anatomy and of ways to restrain individual species so that the blood test can be gotten as rapidly and as safely as possible.

The Cat

It is not surprising that cats (**felines**) require special handling in the event of a venipuncture. Cats are very independent and are not enthusiastic about any veterinary procedure. The environment in which to draw blood should be quiet and unhurried. Most commonly, the **cephalic**, **jugular**, and **medial saphenous veins** are used to draw blood (see Figure 13-1).

---

feline:
of or pertaining to a cat.

cephalic vein:
a superficial vein of the arm and forearm that winds anteriorly up the arm; a common venipuncture site in the antecubital area (in front of the elbow at the bend of the elbow).

jugular vein:
the major vein that runs on either side of the trachea; a major venipuncture site in animals.

medial saphenous vein:
a superficial vein that travels along the medial surface of the ankle (tibiotarsal joint) and the distal tibia; a common venipuncture site for cats.

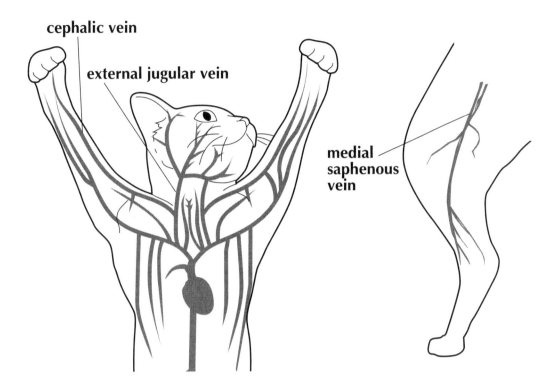

Figure 13-1: Common Venipuncture Sites for Felines

Cephalic Vein Venipuncture: After wrapping the animal in a heavy towel, an assistant holds the cat on a table and places an arm under the chin and neck of the cat. The laboratory assistant/phlebotomist grasps the foreleg at the level of the carpus, gently extends the leg, and rolls it outward slightly prior to starting the venipuncture. Holding the foreleg firmly extended, the venipuncture is started. It may be necessary to muzzle the cat with a soft cloth muzzle if restraining techniques do not control the cat's head completely.

Jugular Vein Venipuncture: After wrapping the cat in a heavy towel with the head and neck exposed, an assistant extends the cat's head and neck with one hand, giving the laboratory assistant/phlebotomist a view of the jugular vein. The thumb can hold the jugular vein in place. Putting a soft cloth muzzle on the cat may also be helpful.

Medial Saphenous Vein Venipuncture: Many animal experts recommend the medial saphenous vein as an excellent vein to use to obtain cat blood because the site is away from the animal's mouth and front claws, and because it is easily accessible, being close to the skin's surface. The cat is put snugly in a heavy towel with one hind leg exposed. The fur may have to be clipped on the inner thigh. An assistant applies pressure above the vein while the phlebotomist uses a thumb to anchor the vein, completing the venipuncture.

Because of the cat's habit of scratching and biting anyone who presents a threat, these animals require firm restraining. A cat's body should be wrapped tightly in a heavy towel. The cat is then placed on its side.

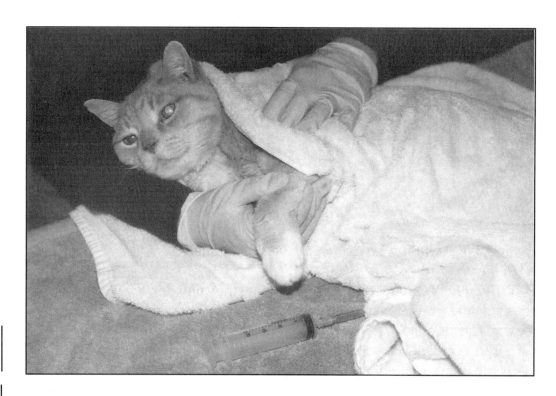

Figure 13-2: A heavy towel may be used to restrain a cat effectively.

canine: of or pertaining to dogs.

lateral saphenous vein: a superficial vessel that obliquely crosses the lateral surface of the distal tibia; a common venipuncture site for dogs.

femoral vein: a large vein located in the groin area.

The Dog

In general, it is easier to obtain blood from **canines** (dogs) than from other small animals. This is due to most dogs' need to please, their calmer nature, and their larger size. The most common sites for venipuncture are the **lateral saphenous**, **jugular**, cephalic, and **femoral veins**.

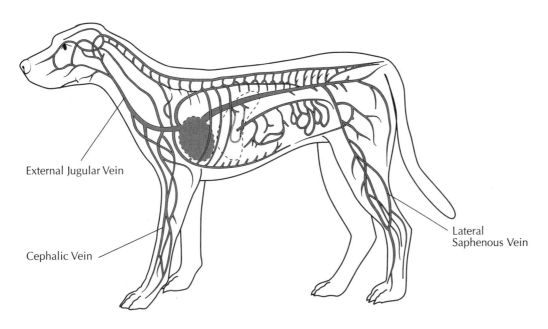

External Jugular Vein

Cephalic Vein

Lateral Saphenous Vein

Figure 13-3: Common Venipuncture Sites for Canines

Lateral Saphenous Vein Venipuncture: The lateral saphenous vein is located on the outside lower hind leg. It can be a good site for a difficult dog as the person drawing the blood is positioned away from the head. The animal is placed on its side, with the assistant holding the leg under the dog. Pressure is applied to the dog's neck to keep the head and neck on the examining table. The laboratory assistant/phlebotomist extends the upper rear leg.

Jugular Vein Venipuncture: The fur over the jugular area of a dog is usually clipped in order for the vein to be visible. An assistant extends the dog's head and neck with the left hand, and with the right hand and arm controls the dog's front feet and legs. The clinical laboratory assistant/phlebotomist puts a thumb on the jugular vein to distend the vein.

Cephalic Vein Venipuncture: Clipping the fur on the top of the foreleg helps the laboratory assistant to see the cephalic vein of the dog. An assistant holds the dog on a table, placing a restraining arm under the chin and neck of the dog. The laboratory assistant/phlebotomist holds the cephalic vein at the level of the dog's elbow and rolls it outward with the thumb. Holding the foreleg firmly extended, the venipuncture is completed.

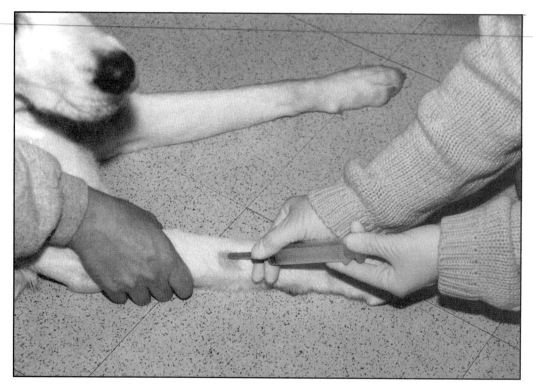

Figure 13-4: A Cephalic Vein Venipuncture of a Dog

Femoral Vein Venipuncture: Like the lateral saphenous vein, the femoral vein is a good vein to use to obtain dog blood because the site is away from the animal's mouth. However, because it lies deeper in the tissue, it is less accessible than the lateral saphenous vein. The dog is held on its side with one hind leg exposed. The fur may have to be clipped on the inner thigh. An assistant applies pressure above the vein while the phlebotomist uses a thumb to anchor the vein, completing the venipuncture.

The Guinea Pig

The guinea pig is often considered a fine animal for laboratory research due to its docile nature and cleanliness. Blood is often taken from the ear vein, heart, or jugular vein.

As with other animals, the guinea pig's ear vein will yield a small amount of blood. The ear should be warmed before attempting blood collection. Generally the blood in this area will be obtained by taking a scalpel and penetrating the vein, draining some blood in a glass capillary tube or a pipette. This is best done under anesthesia.

As with the guinea pig's ear vein, blood can be collected in a heart puncture and through the jugular vein, but should be done under anesthesia. Drawing blood from the jugular vein requires surgical exposure. The heart puncture is made with the anesthetized guinea pig placed on its side, and its heart is entered through the chest wall. A 1-inch, 23-gauge needle is generally recommended. This procedure is performed ONLY as a terminal procedure. In other words, rodents and rabbits are not expected to recover from the anesthesia and will be **euthanized** at the completion of the procedure.

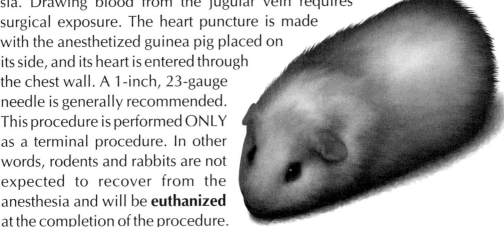

Figure 13-5: The guinea pig is a common laboratory animal.

The Rat and Mouse

Traditionally, rats and mice are the most common laboratory animals. They are inexpensive, breed frequently, and are easy to handle. However, obtaining blood does require general anesthesia.

A puncture of the retro-orbital sinus often is performed to obtain blood from anesthetized rats and mice. To do this, the assistant secures the rodent's head using his or her thumb and forefinger. Then the puncture is performed by inserting a capillary tube or blunted needle at the medial edge of the eye socket, and directing it toward the back of the eye socket. The tube is rotated carefully to puncture the blood sinus. Pasteur pipettes may work better than capillary tubes when drawing retro-orbital blood from rats.

A heart puncture is done by placing the animal on the side and feeling its chest wall for the area of maximum heart beat. A 25-gauge needle, generally on a 3-ml syringe, is advanced into the chest wall. In order to avoid heart injury, the needle should not be moved once the heart chamber is entered. Again, as with the guinea pig, this is procedure is performed ONLY as a terminal procedure.

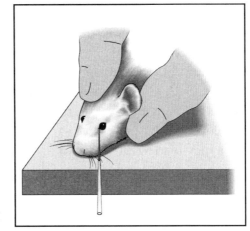

Figure 13-6: Retro-orbital bleeding often is performed to obtain blood from anesthetized rats and mice.

The jugular vein can be used in rats, but not in mice. Again, the animal is put under anesthesia, and the neck is shaved. A small gauge needle is used. A tail vein may also be used, especially when the animal must survive. The lateral tail veins are easy to see if the tail is warmed before the procedure.

A new technique has recently been developed that makes it possible to draw blood from rats or mice using the lateral saphenous vein. This is noteworthy because the procedure can be performed without general anesthesia. However, perhaps because the procedure is so new, the method is not used commonly.

The Rabbit

As with the cat, a heavy towel can be used with the rabbit to restrain it effectively. Although docile, the rabbit's hind feet and claws can cause injury to the restrainer and to the blood drawer. The most common sites for drawing rabbit blood are in the ear and the heart.

The central ear artery of a rabbit runs down the center of the ear. The fur may have to be clipped for easy visibility. The rabbit is restrained, and the artery is stabilized with pressure from the finger and thumb on each side of the ear. A 20 to 23 gauge, 1-inch needle will yield good results.

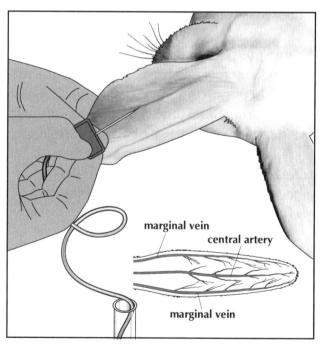

A heart puncture on a rabbit requires anesthesia and is done ONLY as a terminal procedure. The left chest wall is palpated for the area of maximum heart beat. An 18 to 21 gauge, 1½ inch needle is used to puncture the heart. However, since this procedure may lead to the death of the animal, the ear artery generally is most recommended.

Figure 13-7: The central ear artery is a common site for drawing blood from a rabbit.

Handling the Animal Blood Specimen

Not surprisingly, the animal blood specimen requires the same type of care that the human blood specimen requires. As with humans, if the animal has had a fatty meal before the blood is drawn, the fats in the blood (lipemia) will interfere with many tests. A 12-hour fast is recommended before sampling animal blood. Specimens should be processed as rapidly as possible after being drawn.

Additionally, animal blood can be disturbed by placing too much pressure on a syringe during drawing, rough handling (such as forcing blood through a needle into a collection tube too rapidly), vigorous mixing of the sample after drawing, temperature extremes, and wet equipment coming into contact with blood. This kind of treatment can easily break red blood cells in the sample, causing hemolysis and resulting in incorrect results.

Always keep in mind that correct labeling is as necessary for accuracy in handling animal specimens as it is in human specimens. When animal blood testing is being done in a veterinary environment, the tests are expensive and animal owners are depending on you to be as careful and accurate as possible. In a research setting, accuracy of drawing and testing of blood is also mandatory, as incorrect results can impede the process of research projects.

Chapter Summary

Drawing blood from animals is very similar to drawing blood from humans. Animals require compassion, calmness and efficiency from blood drawers just as humans do. Although the sites may be different and restraining animals can present specific challenges, blood must be drawn accurately with attention being given to avoidance of lipemia and hemolysis. In both the research laboratory and veterinary clinic, results of animal blood tests need to be accurate. This requires careful labeling and handling of specimens.

Appendix F in the back of this textbook gives an overview of normal laboratory values for selected animal blood tests.

Name _____

Date _____

Student Enrichment Activities

Complete the following statements.

1. Restraining a cat in a _____ _____ can help protect the blood drawer from being injured.

2. Talking to animals in a _____ voice helps to calm the animal.

3. The medial saphenous vein is located on the medial surface of the ankle (_____ _____) and the _____ _____.

4. Feline is word that refers to _____.

Circle T for true, or F for false.

5. T F   The word canine refers to rabbits.

6. T F   Animal blood is not subject to hemolysis.

7. T F   Fasting is required for some animal blood tests.

8. T F   The retro-orbital plexus is an area used for venipuncture in the dog.

9. T F   When an animal is under anesthesia, it is a good policy to obtain blood while the animal is anesthetized.

Circle the correct answers.

10. The jugular vein is often used for obtaining blood in the following animals except:
    A. the dog.
    B. the mouse.
    C. the cat.
    D. the rat.

11. The easiest and most docile animal to keep as a laboratory animal is the:
    A. rat.
    B. cat.
    C. dog.
    D. guinea pig.

12. Two major reasons why laboratory results can be incorrect in animals include:
    A. animal pain and distress.
    B. lipemia and stress.
    C. hemolysis and bad technique.
    D. small veins and incorrect venipuncture technique.

13. Reasons for hemolysis of animal blood specimens include:
    A. chilled glassware.
    B. too vigorous mixing of the blood sample.
    C. too much pressure on the syringe while drawing the blood.
    D. all of the above.

14. Blood can be obtained in small amounts from the ear vein in the following animals except:
    A. rats.
    B. rabbits.
    C. guinea pigs.
    D. none of the above.

Chapter Fourteen
Urine Specimen Collection

Objectives

After completing this chapter, you should be able to do the following:

1. Define and correctly spell each of the key terms.

2. Explain what kind of urine specimen is collected for urinalysis.

3. Identify the importance of clean-catch urines and why they are necessary for the urine culture and sensitivity.

4. Explain why a 24-hour urine collection might be ordered by a physician.

5. Describe general instructions given to a patient about a 24-hour urine collection.

6. Explain why urine might be used to test for pregnancy.

7. Describe steps that might be required to collect a urine drug screen.

Key Terms

- aliquot
- clean-catch urine specimen
- human chorionic gonadotropin
- midstream urine specimen

- random urine specimen
- 24-hour urine specimen
- urinary tract infection
- urine culture and sensitivity
- void

Introduction

urinary tract infection:
UTI; a cluster of symptoms characterized by dysuria, frequent urination, urgency, and white blood cells in the urine.

Urine is the second most often analyzed body fluid. It is second only to blood. Analysis of urine can help the physician diagnose and treat **urinary tract infections** (UTIs), and it can also be an aid to diagnosis for many other diseases. Although often the floor nurse is responsible for instructing inpatients about obtaining a urine specimen, usually the clinical laboratory assistant/phlebotomist is responsible for instructing outpatients about collecting specimens. There are many different types of urine specimens. The clinical laboratory assistant must understand the differences and must be able to instruct the patient about how to collect several types of urine specimens.

The clinical laboratory assistant/phlebotomist needs to be aware that the same precautions that are taken with blood MUST be taken with urine. Urine is capable of transmitting diseases, so urine specimens are always handled with gloves.

The Urinalysis

void:
to urinate.

random urine specimen:
a urine specimen collected at any time of the day or night.

The **urinalysis** is the most common test performed on urine. The type of specimen preferred for most urine studies, including the urinalysis, is the first urine **voided** in the morning because this urine is the most concentrated. However, urine collected at any time of day, called **random urine specimens**, can be used for the urinalysis as well as for chemistry studies such as sodium, potassium, and uric acid testing. Many physicians prefer 24-hour urine collections for chemistry studies, as explained later in this chapter.

The urinalysis consists of a physical, chemical, and microscopic examination. The clinical laboratory assistant/phlebotomist may be required to set up urine specimens for testing, as well as to perform the physical and chemical examinations.

Urine is treated with as much caution as any other body fluid, including blood. Urine containers for urinalysis testing should be clear and clean containers with tight-fitting lids (Figure 14-1). Formerly, urine was often collected with paper lids that were not secure. **Standard Precautions** dictate that all body fluid containers should be secured tightly to minimize the potential for contamination.

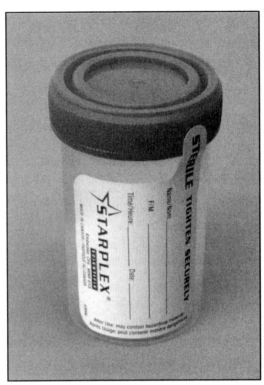

When obtaining the specimen for urinalysis, the patient should be instructed to obtain the specimen in a manner that prevents contamination of the specimen by genital secretions, pubic hair, and bacteria around the urinary opening. This can be accomplished using a procedure known as the midstream urine collection. The patient is often given WRITTEN instructions along with the container

Figure 14-1: A container used for collecting urine for urinalysis testing must have a lid that can be secured tightly.

and a label for the **midstream urine specimen**. This label should contain the patient's name and healthcare facility identification number. Labeling the specimen IS ALWAYS A PRIORITY for all body fluid specimens as soon as the specimen is collected.

midstream urine specimen: a urine sample collected in the middle of the urine flow.

Obtaining a Midstream Urine Specimen

Materials needed:
✓ gloves
✓ cleansing solution and/or wipes
✓ sterile specimen container
✓ bedpan or urinal (if needed)

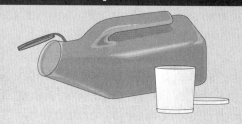

1. Procedural Step: Complete the laboratory requisition form.
   Reason: This is sent with the specimen to the laboratory.

2. Procedural Step: Wash your hands.
   Reason: Standard Precaution.

3. Procedural Step: Put on gloves.
   Reason: Standard Precaution.

4. Procedural Step: Identify the patient by his or her identification bracelet.
   Reason: To make sure you obtain the correct patient's specimen.

5. Procedural Step: Explain the procedure to the patient in terms he or she can understand.
   Reason: The patient will assist with the procedure.

6. Procedural Step: Instruct the patient to clean the urinary **meatus** with the antiseptic solution you provide.

Reason: This ensures a clean specimen.

7. Procedural Step: Instruct the patient to clean from front to back.
   Reason: This avoids contamination.

8. Procedural Step: If the patient is an uncircumcised male, instruct him to retract his foreskin before cleansing.
   Reason: This allows a thorough cleaning.

9. Procedural Step: Instruct the patient to begin urinating and capture only the midstream urine in the specimen container. Explain that the midstream urine is that which comes out after the flow has begun and before the flow ends.
   Reason: Only midstream urine is desired.

10. Procedural Step: If the patient cannot obtain the specimen unassisted, you will need to capture the midstream urine in a clean urinal or bedpan.
    Reason: The urine must not be contaminated.

Obtaining a Midstream Urine Specimen (Cont.)

11. Procedural Step: If a urinal or bedpan was used, cover it and take it and the specimen container to the bathroom, and pour the urine from the bedpan or urinal into the specimen container. Do not touch the inside of the container.
Reason: To avoid contamination.

12. Procedural Step: When the specimen has been collected, replace the cap on the container.
Reason: To secure the contents.

13. Procedural Step: Label the specimen container with the patient's name, the date, and the time.
Reason: To ensure correct identification.

14. Procedural Step: Remove your gloves.
Reason: Universal precaution.

15. Procedural Step: Wash your hands.
Reason: Standard Precaution.

16. Procedural Step: Document the procedure as appropriate.
Reason: To provide documentation.

Thinking It Through ...

Elizabeth is a new clinical laboratory assistant/phlebotomist. She has just given Mrs. Castle a urine container and instructions to collect a midstream specimen. Mrs. Castle seems a bit confused, so Elizabeth carefully goes over the procedure with Mrs. Castle.

When Mrs. Castle finishes collecting the specimen in a nearby bathroom, she does not leave her specimen in a collection box. She comes out of the bathroom and hands the urine specimen to Elizabeth. The lid is not on the urine, and it is evident that Mrs. Castle has urinated on the outside of the container.

1. How should Elizabeth handle this situation?

2. Should Elizabeth just take the specimen and put the lid on it herself?

3. Should Elizabeth instruct Mrs. Castle to throw this urine away and get another specimen?

The Urine Culture and Sensitivity

urine culture and sensitivity: a test where a urine specimen is placed on special growth media to grow an organism for identification and also for testing with antibiotics to ascertain the best antibiotic to use to kill the infectious organism.

Another test ordered frequently on a urine specimen is the **urine culture and sensitivity**. A culture and sensitivity is a test that is performed in the microbiology department to determine if there is bacterial growth in the urine. The "culture" includes growing the potential bacteria on media in the microbiology department. The "sensitivity" involves finding out what antibiotics will kill the bacteria found in the urine. This test requires a sterile urine container so that the bacteria recovered are from the patient's body and not from the container itself.

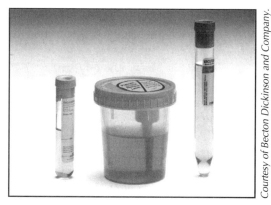

Figure 14-2: A urine container used for a urine culture and sensitivity must be sterile.

clean-catch urine specimen: a method of obtaining a urine specimen so that it is free of contaminating matter from external genital areas.

To obtain a urine specimen in a sterile container that is also not contaminated during the collection process, a procedure called the **clean-catch urine specimen** collection is used. The patient is instructed to collect the urine midstream as in the urinalysis collection. The clinical laboratory assistant/phlebotomist must be able to explain this procedure to both males and females.

Clean-Catch Urine Collection Procedure

Materials needed:
- ✓ Patient identification label
- ✓ Clean-catch urine specimen written instructions
- ✓ Clean-catch specimen container
- ✓ Sterile towelettes

Males:
1. <u>Procedural Step:</u> Wash hands thoroughly. <u>Reason:</u> *This is a "hands on" procedure for males so hands need to be clean.*

2. <u>Procedural Step:</u> Clean the end of the penis (pulling back foreskin if needed) with sterile towelettes

provided with the sterile container (prelabeled with patient information), beginning at the urethral opening and working in a circular fashion away from it. <u>Reason:</u> *Cleaning the urethral opening reduces or eliminates contamination of the urine stream from microorganisms on the genitalia.*

Clean-Catch Urine Collection Procedure (Cont.)

3. Procedural Step: Repeat the above procedure using two successive sterile towelettes.
   Reason: To assure a contamination-free specimen.

4. Procedural Step: Void the first portion of urine in the toilet, collect a portion into the container, then void the rest of the collection into the toilet, being careful not to touch the inside or lip of the container with hands or other body parts.
   Reason: The midstream collection of urine cuts down upon or eliminates contamination of the urine, as well as not touching the lip or inside of the container.

5. Procedural Step: Cover the container with the sterile lid, touching only the outside surfaces of the lid and the container.
   Reason: The specimen is covered to prevent any contamination of the specimen and to keep the urine contained to prevent contact with the skin of others.

6. Procedural Step: The patient leaves the specimen in a designated area, washes his hands, and leaves the collection area.
   Reason: The patient must be instructed as to where to leave the specimen so the specimen is not misplaced and/or lost. Handwashing is a sanitary precaution.

Females

1. Procedural Step: Assume a squatting position just above the toilet seat.
   Reason: This position gives the patient much more room in which to collect the specimen.

2. Procedural Step: Separate the folds of skin around the urinary opening, cleansing the area with special towelettes provided with the container.
   Reason: Cleansing around the folds of skin near the urinary opening reduces the risk of contaminating the specimen.

3. Procedural Step: Cleanse the area again with clean towelettes, wiping from front to back.
   Reason: To further reduce the risk of contamination.

4. Procedural Step: Void the first portion of the urine into the toilet, collect a portion of urine into the container, and void the remainder of urine in the toilet, being careful not to touch the lip or inside of the container.
   Reason: To reduce possibility of contamination to the specimen.

5. Procedural Step: Cover the specimen with the lid provided, touching only the outside of the container.
   Reason: To prevent contamination of the specimen and to keep the urine contained to prevent contact with the skin of others.

6. Procedural Step: The patient leaves the specimen in a designated area, washes her hands, and leaves the collection area.
   Reason: The patient must be instructed as to where to leave the specimen so the specimen is not misplaced and/or lost. Handwashing is a sanitary precaution.

Specimens for culture and sensitivity testing should be transported to the laboratory and processed immediately. Refrigerate the specimen if a delay is unavoidable. If a culture and sensitivity and a urinalysis are ordered on the same specimen, the specimen should be processed first in the microbiology department and then given to the urinalysis department. In some cases, a sterile **aliquot** is poured off immediately for microbiology before the specimen is taken to the laboratory.

aliquot:
a portion of a sample used for testing.

Timed Urine Studies

For some clinical laboratory urine tests, a 24-hour (or other timed period) specimen must be obtained. Sometimes a physician will order a **24-hour urine specimen** collection to evaluate kidney function accurately. In order to diagnose certain diseases and conditions, it is important to see how the kidney functions over a longer period than just one collection. Substances excreted by the kidney may not appear in urine all of the time and may vary from day to night.

24-hour urine specimen:
urine collected in a container over a period of 24 hours.

The 24-hour collection involves collecting a specimen in a suitable container (Figure 14-3), often with a preservative. Refrigeration is required during the collection process. Two of the most frequent errors made in collecting 24-hour urine specimens are incorrect collection and improper preservation of the urine collected. There are several steps that should be taken for this type of collection. The patient MUST receive written instructions as the procedure is too complicated to be committed to memory.

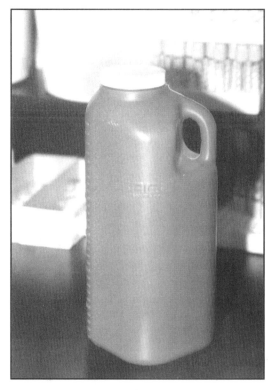

Figure 14-3: A 24-hour Urine Collection Container

1. The patient is given a clean, 3 to 4 liter container with a tight-fitting lid. The laboratory assistant should have an up-to-date list of preservatives (or no preservatives) required for specific 24-hour testing. The preservative and any precautions related to the preservative (some are acid) should be written on the collection container label. Some laboratories have separate warning stickers to be placed on the container. Other information on the label should include the following:

    - patient's name and identification number
    - starting collection date and time
    - ending collection date and time
    - laboratory test to be performed on the urine
    - optional: physician's name, patient location (inpatient, outpatient)

2. The patient should be instructed by the clinical laboratory assistant that the collection of a 24-hour urine specimen begins with EMPTYING THE BLADDER AND DISCARDING THE FIRST URINE. Collections usually start between 6 and 8 am, with the exact time noted on the label.

3. After the first urine is discarded, ALL urine should be collected during the next 24 hours. The last specimen should be included in the collection.

4. Instructions to the patient should include telling the patient to collect the urine specimen before having a bowel movement to prevent contamination with fecal material.

5. The ENTIRE collection should be refrigerated each time a new specimen is collected. Urine is an ideal culture medium for bacteria. Preservatives do not necessarily protect the specimen from bacterial contamination.

6. Some preservatives are potentially dangerous if spilled and can burn the patient's skin. Make sure that the patient is aware of any corrosive preservatives.

7. The patient must not add anything except urine to the container and must not take anything out of the container throughout the entire collection.

8. In general, normal intake of fluids is required. There may be some special dietary considerations for some tests, and these restrictions should be given to the patient.

9. Physicians often ask their patients to refrain from taking medications for up to 72 hours prior to the collection as a precaution against interference with the testing.

10. The specimen must be brought to the laboratory as soon as possible after collection. It is best to bring the specimen in a portable cooler to maintain a cooler temperature.

11. If the patient does not speak English, he or she should receive written instructions in the language the patient speaks. If that is not possible, a translator should be given written directions to help the patient.

Commonly ordered 24-hour urine specimen tests include the following:

- sodium, potassium, and chloride (electrolytes)
- magnesium
- creatinine clearance
- uric acid
- calcium

Other timed tests include a glucose tolerance test in which blood and urine are collected hourly for up to six hours. The blood and urine are both checked for the presence of glucose at regular intervals.

Pregnancy Testing

human chorionic gonadotropin: HCG; a hormone found in the blood and urine of a pregnant human female.

Human chorionic gonadotropin (HCG) is the first detectable substance in blood and urine that is produced in pregnancy. Its determination in blood and urine is the basis for pregnancy tests. Normally called HCG, this substance is produced by placental cells approximately 10 days after conception.

Excretion of HCG into the urine peaks during the first trimester of pregnancy, up until about 10 weeks. There are several pregnancy tests used to determine urinary HCG levels. A **first morning specimen** (first voiding after the patient arises) is preferred for testing because of its concentration.

Pregnancy tests can be performed not only to confirm a pregnancy, but also to eliminate the threat to an unknown pregnancy by a procedure. Some surgical and diagnostic procedures are postponed or reconsidered if a patient is pregnant. HCG levels are also elevated in the urine of persons with various types of tumors (for instance, a certain kind of lung cancer).

Urine Drug Screens

Urine testing remains the most economical method of screening people for drugs. Many potential employees use urine testing for screening large number of employees. Common drug tests that can be performed on urine include the following:

- alcohol
- amphetamines
- barbiturates
- cocaine
- opiates
- marijuana
- LSD
- sedatives
- tranquilizers

You may be asked to receive urine specimens from patients who are being screened for drugs. Strict procedures may be put in place by your facility for this process. Typical precautions that you would be required to take might include the following:

1. Properly identify the patient by asking for photo identification before the urine is collected, because some patients may send other people in their place to be tested.

2. After the urine is collected, you may be asked to take the temperature of the urine to make sure that the specimen was just produced. Some patients may take another specimen into the bathroom and put that precollected specimen into the container. To avoid this kind of tampering, some employers ask that you be present during the urine collection (females accompany females, males accompany males).

3. As in all samples, the urine should be labeled carefully with a numeric code that matches the paperwork. Confusing specimens can have especially complicated results in this case.

4. A sample may be specially sealed after it is collected. The patient signs the seal after collection. This will avoid tampering with the specimen after collection.

5. A document may have to be signed by the patient after producing the specimen in which the patient swears that the urine has been collected properly.

6. Specimens that will be saved for 30 or more days often have special requirements.

Chapter Summary

Urinalysis is the most common test performed to look for urinary tract infections. Several other tests are also performed on urine, including cultures and sensitivities to identify the bacteria involved in a urinary tract infection and to find out which antibiotic will kill the bacteria. Single urine tests and 24-hour collections are also ordered to get a more accurate picture of urine production over a time range. Urine can also be used for pregnancy testing and drug screening.

Often the clinical laboratory assistant/phlebotomist is charged with the responsibility of explaining the specifics of urine testing by making sure the patient receives verbal and written instructions. The laboratory assistant must also continually remember that urine is treated as a biohazardous substance.

Name _____

Date _____

Student Enrichment Activities

Complete the following exercises.

1. The preferred type of urine specimen for most urine studies is the _____ urine collected in the _____.

2. Briefly describe each of these types of urine specimens.
   random urine specimen: _____
   _____
   _____
   clean-catch urine specimen: _____
   _____
   _____
   midstream urine specimen: _____
   _____
   _____
   24-hour urine specimen: _____
   _____
   _____

3. A routine urinalysis includes a _____, _____, and _____ examination.

4. A urine _____ _____ _____ may be ordered on a patient suspected of having a urinary tract infection.

5. _____ _____ dictate that urine containers should have tight fitting lids to prevent contamination of the urine specimen and of the person who will handle the urine after the specimen is collected.

Circle T for true, or F for false.

6. T   F   A patient should obtain a midstream urine collection for urinalysis testing.

7. T   F   UTI stands for urinary tract infection.

8. T   F   Males collect urine in the exact same manner as females during the clean-catch collection.

9. T   F   Sterile containers are not necessary for routine urinalysis testing.

10. T   F   It is approved procedure to perform a urinalysis on a specimen first, before sending the specimen to the microbiology department for culture and sensitivity testing.

Circle the correct answer.

11. A urine specimen collected for a culture and sensitivity should be:
    A. collected midstream.
    B. a clean-catch specimen.
    C. collected after wiping the urethral area with sterile towelette.
    D. all of the above.

12. The two most common mistakes made with 24-hour urine collections are:
    A. incorrect collection and improper preservation.
    B. mislabeling and contaminating the container.
    C. collecting the urine for less than 24 hours and not refrigerating the specimen.
    D. forgetting to return the urine and not labeling the specimen correctly.

13. The 24-hour specimen collection begins by:

    A. collecting the first specimen and discarding the last.

    B. partially emptying the bladder and voiding the rest into the toilet.

    C. collecting a separate specimen and not adding it to the 24-hour container.

    D. emptying the bladder and discarding the first urine of the collection.

14. Pregnancy tests on urine are based on the presence of:

    A. white blood cells.

    B. excess urine.

    C. human chorionic gonadotropin.

    D. HDG.

15. Urine drug screens may require the following precautions taken during collection:

    A. the temperature of the urine should be taken after collection.

    B. the specimen may have to be specially sealed after collection to avoid tampering.

    C. a photo identification may have to be seen by the laboratory assistant to verify the patient's name.

    D. all of the above.

Chapter Fifteen

Collection of Other Non-Blood Specimens

Objectives

After completing this chapter, you should be able to do the following:

1. Define and correctly spell each of the key terms.

2. Explain why it is so important to follow Standard Precautions when handling any specimens collected for testing in the clinical laboratory.

3. Explain why stool, cerebrospinal fluid, sputum, semen, various body fluids, gastric secretions, throat and nasopharyngeal specimens are tested in the clinical laboratory.

4. Describe the importance of transport media when collecting specimens for microbiological testing.

Key Terms

- cerebrospinal fluid
- gastric secretions
- lumbar puncture
- meningitis
- nasopharyngeal
- occult blood testing

- ova and parasite testing
- pericardial fluid
- peritoneal fluid
- pleural fluid
- semen
- synovial fluid

gastric secretions: fluid collected from the stomach.

cerebrospinal fluid: CSF; the clear, watery fluid that flows through the brain and spinal column, protecting the brain and spinal cord.

occult blood testing: an examination for blood, usually found in the stool, that is present in such minute quantities that it cannot be visually detected.

ova and parasite testing: a microbiology test performed on stool to determine whether a patient has parasite eggs and/or parasites themselves in the stool.

Introduction

Blood and urine are not the only specimens that the clinical laboratory assistant/phlebotomist will need to handle during a routine workday. Many other body fluids and other specimens are tested in all departments of the clinical laboratory including stool, sputum, **gastric secretions**, **cerebrospinal fluid**, body cavity fluids, joint fluids, tissue specimens, and throat and nose secretions. Special attention must be paid to the manner in which such fluids are transported to the clinical laboratory. In particular, specimens for the microbiology department must be delivered to the department in containers that keep specimens from being contaminated and allow potential pathogens to stay alive for identification.

The clinical laboratory assistant/phlebotomist must always practice Standard Precautions in the handling of all body fluids and other body substances.

Stool Specimens

Stool (fecal) specimens are sent to the clinical laboratory for a variety of tests, including an examination for blood (**occult blood testing**), and **ova and parasite testing**. Stool should be collected in clean containers made of plastic-covered cardboard or in glass jars with screw covers. Some stool testing is done in special containers with preservative to ensure the best specimen possible. The patient should make every effort not to contaminate the collection with urine. The patient is given written instructions before making a stool collection because some testing requires special dietary considerations. The clinical laboratory assistant/phlebotomist may be called upon to give special containers and instructions to the patient who is going to be collecting stool.

Ova and Parasite Testing

Stool samples are collected regularly to screen for parasites (ova and parasites or O & P). Figure 15-1 illustrates two containers that are used routinely by patients to collect stool samples for parasitic infections. There are two containers for every O & P test, and each container holds a different preservative. Patients must receive written instructions enclosed with the two containers to collect the specimens correctly. Often a physician will order "ova and parasites X 3," which means that the patient will collect stool specimens on three different occasions, filling a total of six vials.

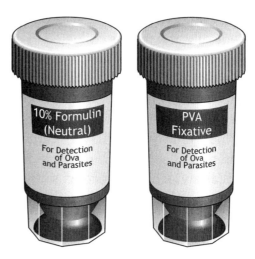

Stool for Occult Blood

Another common test for stool is the occult blood test, which is a test to detect invisible (occult) quantities of blood in the stool, often used as a

Figure 15-1: Ova and parasite collection containers are used to retain stool samples.

screening test for **gastrointestinal lesions** and **colorectal cancer**. This test is collected on special test cards. Cards can be mailed in or brought to the clinical laboratory by the patient.

Stool Culture

A stool specimen also can be collected for culture by the microbiology department. The container for this test is not critical, but should be a wide-mouthed plastic or waxed cardboard container with a tight fitting lid. The patient should bring the specimen to the laboratory as quickly as possible after the collection. The microbiology department is looking for pathogens such as Salmonella, Shigella, and other organisms.

Stool also can be tested for fat and fibers. Stools can also be ordered as a 72-hour collection, which requires that the patient be given a large container and written instructions as to how to collect this specimen.

Cerebrospinal Fluid

lumbar puncture:
a diagnostic test in which a specimen of cerebrospinal fluid is removed and analyzed for diseases such as meningitis; a spinal tap.

Cerebrospinal fluid (CSF) is a clear, colorless liquid that circulates within the cavities around the brain and spinal cord. CSF has many of the same contents as blood plasma. It is obtained through a **lumbar puncture** (also called a **spinal tap**, a procedure in which spinal fluid is removed and analyzed for disease). Generally, the fluid is collected in three sterile containers (Figure 15-2), and it is numbered in the order in which it was collected. The first tube is usually contaminated with blood due to the needle puncture. The second and third tube are used for analysis. Tests commonly performed on CSF include total protein level, glucose, cell count, a culture and sensitivity, chloride levels, and crypto-coccal antigen (cryptococcus is a fungus that can appear in the CSF of AIDS patients).

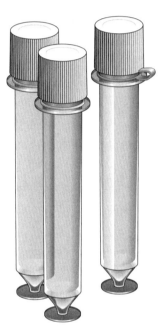

Frequently, cerebrospinal fluid testing is ordered STAT. The clinical laboratory assistant/phlebotomist often handles the specimens for distribution to various departments in the clinical laboratory. The physician is often anxious about the results because the patient could be running a high fever and therefore could be suspected of having **meningitis** (an inflammation of the membranes covering the brain and spinal cord), which can be particularly serious in children if not treated rapidly.

meningitis:
inflammation of the membranes covering the spinal cord and brain; marked by severe headache, vomiting, fever, and a stiff neck, and usually caused by infection.

Figure 15-2: Three Containers Used to Collect CSF

Sputum

Sputum is fluid from the lungs that is collected from patients, usually for microbiology testing. Sputum must be collected in a sterile container and transported as soon as possible after the patient collects the specimen. Patients must be instructed to cough deeply to bring up lung fluid rather than to simply spit into the cup. Saliva is not an acceptable specimen for culture.

A physician usually orders tests on sputum to determine what organism(s) might be growing in a patient's lungs. There are also a few other tests that can be run on sputum, but the culture and sensitivity testing is the most common.

The clinical laboratory assistant must wear gloves when handling all specimens brought to the clinical laboratory. Often a specimen will be handed to you by a patient. Some patients may partially miss the container, and specimen can be clinging to the outside of the container. Some laboratories will require that you refuse to accept such a specimen. Always treat all specimens as if they are contaminated with pathogenic organisms!

Semen

Semen (also referred to as **seminal fluid**) is the thick, white secretion discharged by the male sex organs that carries sperm. Semen specimens can be examined in the clinical laboratory to do the following:

- determine the effectiveness of a vasectomy

- assess fertility

- investigate possible sexual criminal activity

The clinical laboratory assistant may be responsible for giving written instructions to a male patient for obtaining a proper specimen. Semen must be collected in containers that are clean and free of detergents. Condoms can be used to collect the semen, initially, if the condoms do not contain spermicidal substances. Specimens must not be exposed to extremes of light or temperature and should be transported within 2 hours of collection. It is important to emphasize to the patient that the specimen should be brought to the laboratory AS SOON AS POSSIBLE after collection for the most accurate results.

Body Fluids

Body fluids that are collected routinely for laboratory testing include **synovial fluid** collected by aspiration from joint cavities, **pleural fluid** obtained from the lung cavity, **pericardial fluid** extracted from the heart cavity, and **peritoneal fluid** collected from the abdominal cavity. All such collections are made by an invasive procedure performed by a physician using sterile technique with special needles and other equipment. These specimens should be handled carefully and taken to the testing site as soon as possible. It is very difficult to obtain more of these specimens if you accidentally drop and break the container containing the fluids.

semen:
the thick, white secretion discharged by the male sex organs that carries sperm.

synovial fluid:
the clear fluid surrounding a joint.

pleural fluid:
fluid in and around the lungs.

pericardial fluid:
fluid surrounding the heart.

peritoneal fluid:
the clear fluid secreted by the tissue in the peritoneum.

Several different types of testing can be done on fluids, including cell counts and cultures and sensitivities. Upon receiving any of these specimens, it is important to ALWAYS verify that the container is labeled properly with the patient's name, identification number, the date, the time of collection, and the type of specimen collected.

Gastric Secretions

Gastric secretions (fluids from the stomach) are collected by a physician by use of a tube inserted into the stomach through the mouth and sent to the laboratory for testing to determine stomach function by analyzing stomach acid production. Often, this test is performed in the clinical chemistry laboratory. Gastric secretions are usually sent in a clean container that must be delivered promptly to the testing site.

Throat and Nasopharyngeal Culture Collections

Throat cultures are ordered by a physician most commonly to determine whether or not the patient has a **streptococcus** infection. This specimen is often collected by a clinical laboratory assistant/phlebotomist when the patient is an outpatient, and the specimen has not been collected by the physician's office.

In order to collect a throat specimen, the patient's tongue is pressed down with a tongue depressor, and the patient is instructed to say "ah." The culture is obtained by swabbing the back of the throat and the surfaces of the tonsils (if they are present) with a special sterile disposable swab. (See Figure 15-3.) The clinical laboratory assistant must try to avoid letting the swab touch the mouth surfaces or the tongue, which are filled with bacteria normally residing in the mouth (mouth **flora**) that can contaminate the swab.

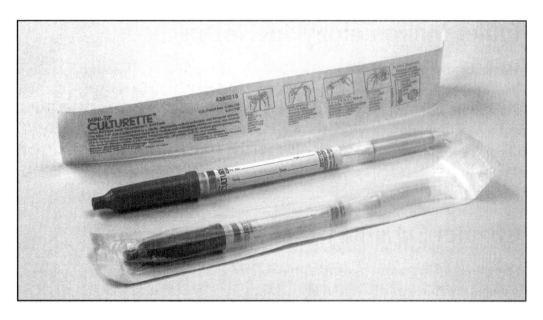

Figure 15-3: Nose and Throat Culture Transport Media

Nasopharyngeal cultures are taken from the nose to detect different organisms that might reside in the nose. Sometimes the patient can be a carrier, someone who is not infected by an organism but carries the organism in the nose. The organism can shed from the nose and infect other individuals. Occasionally nurses who work in a nursery in a healthcare facility will be tested by nasopharyngeal cultures to make sure they are not carrying organisms in their noses that can infect newborns.

nasopharyngeal: of or relating to the nose and throat.

Transport Media

As with other specimens that are collected for microbiological testing, throat and sputum cultures are placed in transport media that assure that organisms are not allowed to die before they can be cultured in the microbiology department. Some organisms such as gonorrhea (caused by a bacterium) can die without proper transport material. Some organisms cannot survive at all with oxygen and must be put in special containers.

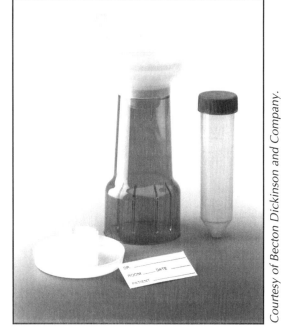

Courtesy of Becton Dickinson and Company.

Figure 15-4: Sputum Culture Transport Media

Other Microbiology Specimens

Sterile swabs are adequate for specimens collected from infected body openings such as the throat, nose, ears, vagina, cervix, penis, infected wounds, body fluids, and blood. The swabs are placed on the infection site and then placed in holding medium, depending on what organisms are suspected. Generally, this medium is a broth or a gel. All transport media are disposable, and none are reused.

Chapter Summary

The clinical laboratory assistant/phlebotomist is often given the task of giving patients containers and written instructions for non-blood specimen collection. As an important part of customer service in the healthcare facility, the clinical laboratory assistant plays an important part in making sure that the specimen received for testing in the clinical laboratory has been collected correctly.

The clinical laboratory assistant/phlebotomist should be familiar with most commonly collected specimens for testing in the laboratory, including stool, sputum, cerebrospinal fluid, gastric secretions, body fluid collections, and the various specimens collected for culturing in the microbiology department. The clinical laboratory assistant must be familiar with transport media and dedicated to transporting specimens into the laboratory for testing as soon as possible.

As with all specimens collected from the human body, every precaution must be taken to protect the employee from being contaminated by potentially pathogenic materials. The laboratory assistant must also take great care to see that the specimens themselves are not contaminated after collection as well.

Name _____

Date _____

Student Enrichment Activities

Complete the following statements.

1. Another term for a stool specimen is a _____ specimen.

2. A test performed on stool is _____ _____ _____.

3. CSF stands for _____ _____.

4. Three tests that might be performed on CSF are _____,
    _____, and _____.

5. Sputum comes from the _____.

6. Three body fluids that are tested in the clinical laboratory are _____,
    _____, and _____.

7. Semen is often tested in the clinical laboratory to _____
    _____
    _____.

8. A nasopharyngeal culture is taken from the _____ _____.

9. Ova and parasite testing is performed on _____ _____.

10. Semen is also known as _____ _____.

Circle T for true, or F for false.

11. T   F   Cerebrospinal fluid orders are usually routine and are not STAT orders.

12. T   F   Cerebrospinal fluid is located in the intestines.

13. T   F   Gastric secretions come from the stomach.

14. T   F   Synovial fluid comes from joints.

15. T   F   A lumbar puncture is done on the lungs.

Match the terms in Column A with the appropriate description in Column B.

Column A

16. ___ semen

17. ___ pericardial fluid

18. ___ CSF

19. ___ gastric

20. ___ peritoneal fluid

21. ___ throat

22. ___ nose culture

23. ___ stool

24. ___ sputum

25. ___ Standard Precautions

Column B

A. used when handling all kinds of specimens

B. from the stomach

C. from the lungs

D. nasopharyngeal

E. seminal fluid

F. around the heart

G. specimen used to screen for streptococcus

H. specimen used for O & P test

I. from the abdominal cavity

J. gotten through a lumbar puncture

Chapter Sixteen

Quality Assurance and the Clinical Laboratory Assistant/Phlebotomist

Objectives

After completing this chapter, you should be able to do the following:

1. Define and correctly spell each of the key terms.

2. Explain the significance of Total Quality Management in the healthcare facility.

3. Describe the difference between the concepts of quality assurance and quality control.

4. Identify several quality control measures that must be taken by clinical laboratory assistants/phlebotomists to ensure quality service for the patient.

Key Terms

- accuracy
- Clinical Laboratory Improvement Act of 1988
- controls
- floor book

- quality assurance
- quality control
- standards
- Total Quality Management

Introduction

quality assurance: QA; a process of policies, principles, and procedures that provides accurate, reproducible, and reliable test results.

Total Quality Management: TQM; an overall institutional process to assess quality and constantly improve patient care.

One of the most important practices throughout the healthcare facility is the continual adherence to a **quality assurance (QA)** program. In many facilities, the quality assurance program is part of an institutional ten-step process designed by the Joint Committee for Accrediting Healthcare Organizations, (JCAHO), and is known as **Total Quality Management (TQM).** The goal of TQM is to assess the quality of care in a healthcare facility and to constantly improve patient care by involving every employee in achieving customer satisfaction.

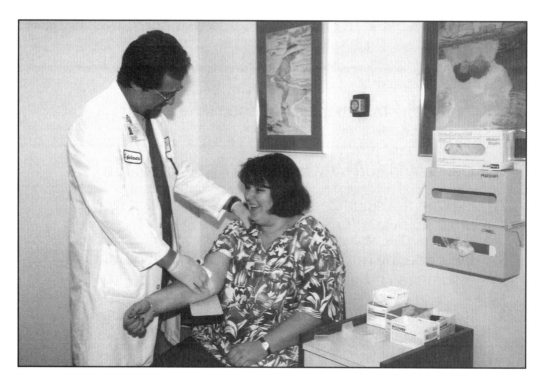

Figure 16-1: A clinical laboratory assistant completes a venipuncture for a satisfied patient.

Policies, principles, and procedures that promote accurate, reproducible, and reliable test results are the aspects of quality assurance programs that most directly affect the clinical laboratory assistant/phlebotomist. These test results help the healthcare team make accurate and reliable diagnoses for the patient. Therefore, the clinical laboratory assistant/phlebotomist must assess his or her job performance continually to make sure that each procedure reflects the best possible quality of service for the patient.

Quality control (QC) is a critical component of any quality assurance program. A quality control program is achieved by following specific steps. In the clinical laboratory, for example, a step in the coagulation studies procedure is to fill the sodium citrate vacuum tube completely, thus avoiding a dilution effect that takes place with less than a full tube. Another rule that must be complied with while drawing blood is that a tourniquet must not remain on a patient's arm for more than one minute. In both instances, specific steps are followed by the clinical laboratory assistant/phlebotomist; this conformance to quality control directives assures that the patient receives accurate, reliable results and quality service.

Clinical Laboratory Improvements Act of 1988

The **Clinical Laboratory Improvement Act of 1988 (CLIA '88)** emphasized the need for clinical laboratories to have regulations placed on all laboratory procedures, regardless of where such procedures are performed. The same regulations apply to small laboratories in doctors' offices as well as large university medical centers. Implemented in 1992, CLIA sets stringent requirements and standards that must be met for every procedure used in the testing of human specimens. The consequences of not adhering to such standards of quality assurance can be application of fines; revocation of the certificate of performance so that a procedure can no longer be performed in a facility; and termination of reimbursements from government medical programs such as Medicare and Medicaid.

Under CLIA, all laboratory procedures are categorized as "waived tests," "moderately complex tests," and "highly complex tests." These categories are based on the difficulty of the procedure, as well as the training and competency level needed for the employee to perform the procedure accurately.

quality control: QC; also called quality assurance; a program throughout the healthcare facility that contains specific policies and procedures that help ensure patient safety and accurate testing results; the program includes maintaining procedure manuals, monitoring equipment, maintaining records, and hospital inspections.

Clinical Laboratory Improvement Act of 1988: CLIA '88; an act signed into federal law in 1988, which mandates that all laboratories be regulated using the same standards regardless of location, type, or size.

Total Quality Management

Total Quality Management (TQM) is designed to be a continuous effort to seek opportunities for improving services to the patient. The following are the four principles involved in TQM:

1. Customer satisfaction

2. Constant improvement of services

3. Employee participation

4. Procedure orientation

The TQM program stresses constant monitoring to find opportunities to improve service with innovations. In order to make these improvements, every employee participates in a quality assurance program.

Quality Assurance/Quality Control for the Clinical Laboratory Assistant

accuracy: the closeness of a result compared with the true or actual value.

For the clinical laboratory assistant, components of quality assurance and quality control are frequently the same process. While Total Quality Management dictates general directives about a procedure, for example, when performing venipunctures, **accuracy** should be achieved on the first attempt 95% of the time; quality assurance further dictates that a worker can attempt a venipuncture on a patient only two times. A quality control procedure might be further detailed by dictating the specific angle of the arm when drawing the blood specimen. Often these concepts do overlap. Also, some people may not understand the difference between quality assurance and quality control, so they use the terms interchangeably.

The following sections deal with specific procedures that come under the category of clinical laboratory quality control. All of the procedures are a part of a quality assurance program, which in turn may be a part of TQM.

Quality Control Procedures

Patient Preparation

When interacting with patients, quality control measures begin by making sure that the patient is prepared properly before a test specimen is collected. In today's healthcare facility, many nursing stations have a book of instruction called the **floor book** (user manual) that is provided by the clinical laboratory. The nursing staff can then look at a blood test order from a physician and find out in the floor book whether the patient needs special preparation before the blood is drawn. For instance, if a fasting blood glucose is ordered for the following morning, the nurse wants to make sure that the patient is not served breakfast before the clinical laboratory assistant is able to draw the patient's blood.

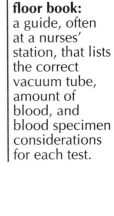

floor book: a guide, often at a nurses' station, that lists the correct vacuum tube, amount of blood, and blood specimen considerations for each test.

In an outpatient setting, the clinical laboratory assistant/phlebotomist must ask the patient questions about his or her preparation before certain tests. For instance, some tests may require a 12-hour fast, others a 16-hour fast. Sometimes patients are given containers to take home to collect other specimens for later testing. The clinical laboratory assistant may see that the patient receives proper written instructions on how to collect, for example, a 24-hour urine sample or a 72-hour stool sample. If a sample is obtained from a patient who has not been prepared properly, the results can be worthless. This means that the specimen will be collected again, unnecessary costs will be incurred, and the patient will be inconvenienced. That is not quality service!

Patient Identification

One of the most critical aspects of quality control in the clinical laboratory is the proper identification and labeling of a patient sample. If the patient is an inpatient, he or she will be wearing proper identification in the form of a wrist band. Before drawing blood, the wrist band must be checked for the proper name of the patient (checked with the blood draw requisition) as well as the patient's identification number. Two patients may have the same name, but no two patients should have the same identification number.

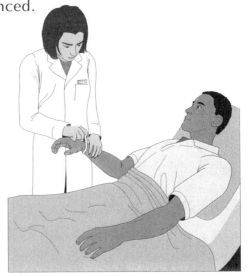

Figure 16-2: A clinical laboratory assistant must always check the identification band of the inpatient before obtaining a blood specimen.

In the outpatient setting, the patient's name must be verified. Some facilities actually band the patient for outpatient work as well. So, do not merely ask the patient, "Are you Mr. George?" Confused people or people who speak limited English may agree with you regardless of their name. "Please tell me your name" is a much better way to obtain an outpatient's name. If the patient is confused, ask someone with the patient to verify the patient's name.

Labeling is a critical part of patient identification. Most healthcare facilities will have computerized labels that can be put on the specimen as soon as it is drawn or collected from a patient. Mislabeling a specimen can have drastic consequences for a patient and can result in termination of employment for the laboratory assistant/phlebotomist.

Figure 16-3: A Computer-generated Identification Label for a Blood Specimen

Collection Technique

The technique of phlebotomy must be taught carefully and clearly to the clinical laboratory assistant/phlebotomist. This technique must be followed by every employee and must be stated clearly in writing in a procedure manual in the clinical laboratory for clinical laboratory assistants/phlebotomists.

A proper quality assurance program in the clinical laboratory should also detail the procedure of what to do if the clinical laboratory assistant/phlebotomist is unable to collect a blood specimen. Most laboratories put a limit on how many times one blood drawer can attempt unsuccessful venipunctures on a patient. Periodic review of phlebotomy technique is an important part of an excellent quality assurance program.

Collection Priorities

The clinical laboratory assistant must have a clear understanding of which requests have priority when several requests on different patients appear in a short period of time. For example, when staffing is short, a clinical laboratory assistant/phlebotomist could conceivably get requests for an immediate (STAT) blood draw in the emergency room, the nursery, and in intensive care. Knowing what to do in this situation comes from experience and from guidelines already set in the clinical laboratory for such an occasion.

Priority should always be given to a life-threatening emergency (a patient needs blood drawn in order to receive an immediate transfusion, a newborn is in dire distress, a patient is having a massive heart attack in the emergency room, and so on). Timed specimens should always take priority over routine draws. Physicians are often interested in how much drug is in a patient's system after a dosage has been given and before the next dose is taken. It is important to time the draws carefully to measure the amount of a drug in the patient's system accurately.

Thinking It Through ...

Jared is a clinical laboratory assistant/phlebotomist who works the PM shift in a small healthcare facility. He is the only laboratory assistant in the clinical laboratory in the evenings.

On a very busy night, Jared suddenly has four requisitions in front of him for drawing blood. All of the specimens must be drawn STAT.

- Specimen #1 is for a patient in the emergency room with a bleeding ulcer.

- Specimen #2 is on a child in pediatrics who has a 105° fever.

- Specimen #3 is on an elderly lady who had abdominal surgery earlier in the day and is experiencing terrible pain in the lower abdomen.

- Specimen #4 is on a male inpatient who is overdue to go home and cannot be released until his blood is drawn. A nurse forgot to send down the orders to the laboratory.

1. In what order would you place these blood draws?

2. If two orders are equally urgent, what would you do?

3. What if you are not able to find a vein on one of these patients who urgently needs blood drawn?

4. Can being in a hurry make it harder for a blood drawer to find a vein?

Equipment and Supplies

Clinical laboratory assistants are often put in charge of a blood drawing area that can contain various pieces of equipment. Such areas usually have refrigerators to store specimens until the specimens can be taken back to the clinical laboratory itself for testing. Recording the temperature of laboratory refrigerators is an important part of a quality assurance program in the clinical laboratory.

Centrifuges are also used by clinical laboratory assistants. Centrifuges have to have frequent control checks to make sure the speed of the centrifuge is correct for spinning down blood. A centrifuge that is too fast may damage the blood cells. A centrifuge that is too slow may not recover an adequate amount of plasma or serum. Centrifuges and refrigerators must also have routine maintenance, which is to be recorded each time the maintenance is done. The clinical laboratory assistant/phlebotomist may also have to record temperatures elsewhere in the laboratory, as well as perform a variety of other daily checks on equipment.

Clinical laboratory assistants are asked periodically to be a part of a quality control program regarding supplies that are ordered for the laboratory. In some laboratories, there are quality control procedures for evaluating evacuated test tubes, stoppers on tubes, and additives in blood collection tubes. Expiration dates on all supplies are checked periodically.

Documentation

Recording quality control measures is an integral part of the quality assurance program in the clinical laboratory. Every time the clinical laboratory assistant reads a temperature, it must be recorded neatly next to the correct date. A floor book must be kept up-to-date with all information necessary to draw a blood specimen, ie, the minimum amount needed, special handling, normal values for the test, testing days available, and turnaround time.

Further, some tests that are ordered are not run in the clinical laboratory of that facility. Some are sent to another laboratory. All of these samples must be logged carefully in a reference log book, which includes the patient's name and identification number, the date sent out, and the date the results were received.

Laboratory procedure manuals must be made available to all employees. The manual must be updated annually, as there are always changes that are made to procedures, new tests introduced, new equipment installed, and so on.

Incident reports, discussed in Chapter Five, are an integral part of any quality assurance program. As the TQM program emphasizes, the healthcare facility must always work for improvement in all phases of customer service. When incidents occur, they must be documented. Examples of incidents include an employee sticking his or her self with a needle, a patient fainting during a blood draw, and a patient receiving a serious hematoma after a blood draw. Incident reports always require the employee to describe the incident in detail. Most reports also include a section in which the employee explains how the incident could have been prevented and what measures can be taken to avoid similar incidents.

Continuing education also must be documented. To maintain proficiency and consistency in their workplace and to obtain recertification in their profession, laboratory assistants/phlebotomists must participate in continuing education. For example, they may be asked to read literature about new job-related practices. Generally, supervisors document and maintain the records on these requirements.

Operating Automated Instruments

In some states, clinical laboratory assistants/phlebotomists are allowed to use certain automated instruments. For example, some laboratory assistants operate cell counting instruments. When running tests in the clinical laboratory, there must be **controls** performed on the instrument before patient specimens can be tested. Controls are done to check reagents, technique, and equipment. They are substances that have preset values that must be reproduced by the laboratory worker. Often controls are classified as "low," "medium," and "high." They are performed at least once a shift, sometimes with each test. Before a test result is reported, the control results must be within the range listed on the manufacturer's directions. If the control is not in the proper range, the result can not be reported. Adjustments must be made, usually by a supervisor, and the test redone. Controls are carefully recorded, either by computer or by hand. Control charts are prepared so that trends can be easily seen. Commercially prepared controls are generally made from human blood, with the same safety precautions used with them as used with regular specimens.

controls: comparisons of known values that are run with patient tests to check equipment, reagents, and technique.

standards: substances having a known value used in quality control testing.

Standards are solutions of known concentrations of a pure substance. Standards are not run with all types of tests. However, when they are required, they must be within certain guidelines or results cannot be reported. Records must be kept of all standard testing.

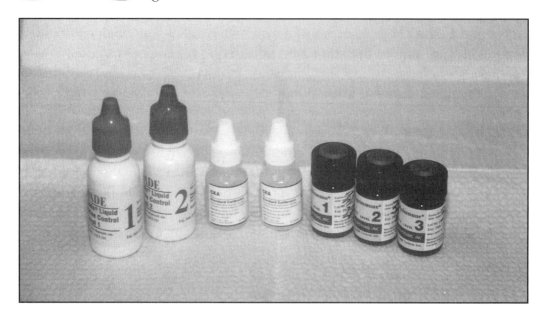

Figure 16-4: Controls are available on the commercial market.

Clinical Laboratory Inspections

The "honor system" method of quality assurance does not apply to clinical laboratories. Rather, each clinical laboratory, as well as all healthcare facilities, are subject to inspections from county, state, and federal agencies at any time. Inspectors can recommend closures of facilities if certain standards are not met.

Inspections are very detailed and always include the inspection of all quality assurance documentation, which must always be up-to-date or laboratories can receive penalties.

Chapter Summary

There is nothing more important in a clinical laboratory assistant/phlebotomist's routine workday than working continually to improve service to the patient. Total Quality Management programs in healthcare facilities assure the existence of quality assurance programs. These quality assurance programs are a combination of policies, principles, and procedures that assure accurate, reproducible, and reliable laboratory results.

Specific quality assurance tasks that the clinical laboratory assistant/phlebotomist can accomplish include the following:

- correctly preparing a patient for testing
- accurately identifying patients and properly labeling specimens
- consistently performing venipunctures according to a specific protocol
- thoroughly understanding collection priorities
- consistently performing quality control procedures on equipment and supplies
- carefully documenting all quality control measures performed
- competently running controls and standards (when mandated) whenever performing tests.

16-12

Name _____

Date _____

Student Enrichment Activities

Complete the following exercises.

1. Explain the goals of Total Quality Management.

   _____

   _____

   _____

   _____

2. Define both quality assurance and quality control.

   _____

   _____

   _____

   _____

   _____

   _____

3. Name three types of quality control documentation in the clinical laboratory.

   A. _____

   B. _____

   C. _____

4. What is the purpose of a floor book?

   _____

   _____

   _____

   _____

5. Why is an incident report part of a quality assurance program?

_____

_____

_____

_____

Circle T for true, or F for false.

6. T F   Refrigerator thermometers in the clinical laboratory must be read on a
regular basis.

7. T F   Blood drawing technique should always be consistent and vary little.

8. T F   A procedure manual must be updated every month.

9. T F   All outpatients have identification bands on their wrists.

10. T F   CLIA is a regulatory agency that makes sure quality assurance is performed
in the clinical laboratory.

Complete the following statements.

11. Quality control is the responsibility of _____ _____.

12. TQM stands for _____ _____ _____.

13. _____ and sometimes _____ must be performed before patient tests
can be run on instruments.

14. _____ _____ is necessary for all employees to keep up with
new developments in their fields.

15. There is usually a prescribed limit on how many times a clinical laboratory
assistant can attempt to perform a _____ on a patient.

Chapter Seventeen

Transporting, Processing, and Distributing Clinical Specimens

Objectives

After completing this chapter, you should be able to
do the following:

1. Define and correctly spell each of the key terms.

2. Identify several specimens that might have to be specially
    handled during transport.

3. Discuss the time constraints imposed on certain specimens
    for delivery to the clinical laboratory.

4. Explain how specimens for testing are centrifuged.

5. Describe how specimens are processed after centrifugation.

6. Discuss how specimens are distributed throughout the
    clinical laboratory.

7. Explain how some clinical laboratory specimens for testing
    are prepared for shipment to other laboratories.

Key Terms

- ASAP
- bilirubin
- central processing
- centrifuge

- icteric
- jaundice
- QNS

Introduction

To make sure a sample is adequate for testing purposes, the clinical laboratory assistant/phlebotomist must be very careful when drawing a blood specimen and when giving a patient instructions for collecting other body fluid specimens. However, the responsibility for the specimen does not end after the sample has been produced. What happens to the specimen after it is collected is very important for maintaining specimen quality.

A specimen must be transported to the clinical laboratory as quickly as possible, and processed with speed and accuracy. Also, this must be done with consideration for preventing accidental exposure to a potentially infectious body fluid. Then the specimen must be distributed to the correct department for testing, whether in your immediate facility or to a laboratory in another location. All of these steps require a commitment on the part of the clinical laboratory assistant to make sure that the specimen tested is the best quality specimen that can be delivered.

Transportation of Specimens to the Clinical Laboratory

ALL specimens should be transported to the clinical laboratory as soon as possible and with the safety of the specimen utmost in the laboratory assistant's mind. Agitation and unnecessary shaking should be avoided because such movement can damage the specimen. Specimens transported within the same healthcare facility should be placed in resealable biohazard bags or in leakproof biohazard containers with securely fitting lids to prevent accidental spillage. Specimens that are to be shipped to another facility will be discussed later in this chapter.

Blood tubes should be transported with the stopper up, which aids in clot formation of the serum tubes. This position also reduces agitation that can cause hemolysis. The stopper can be a source of contamination to the specimen, releasing contaminants into the air during stopper removal.

When handling additive tubes, the clinical laboratory assistant must always remember that these tubes need to be gently inverted as soon as they are drawn. Inadequate mixing may cause anticoagulant tubes to form clots that can lead to incorrect results, especially for hematology testing. These tubes should be gently inverted ten times immediately after drawing. If you remember later that you did not initially invert the tubes, gently invert the tubes before transporting them. It may not be too late.

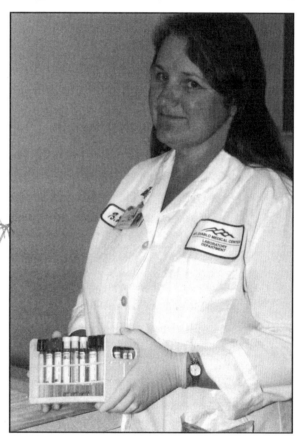

clotting—not mix
Inverted
*   appropiately*

Figure 17-1: A laboratory assistant/ phlebotomist transports blood tubes in a rack.

Specimens That Require Special Handling

Some specimens require special conditions soon after they are collected from the patient. Special considerations include the following:

bilirubin:
a product
produced from
the breakdown
of red blood
cells; excessive
blood levels
may indicate
liver disease.

• Some blood components are broken down when exposed to light, causing false readings. So, these specimens must be protected from the light after they are collected from a patient (Figure 17-2). The most common component requiring protection from light is **bilirubin**. Other components that need protection from light include vitamin B12, carotene, folate, and urine specimens for porphyrins. Specimens can be protected from light by wrapping them in aluminum foil. Amber-colored collection containers are available for collecting bilirubin specimens from infants.

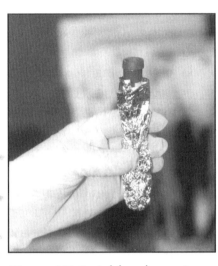

Figure 17-2: A blood specimen for bilirubin testing can be wrapped in aluminum foil to protect the blood from the light.

• Metabolic processes continue even after a specimen has been collected from a patient. Chilling a specimen can slow down this process. Specimens requiring cooling can be immersed in a combination of crushed ice and water. Specimens should be cooled when components such as arterial blood gases, ammonia, lactic acid, acetone, catecholamines, corticotropin, fibrinogen, ketones, and serum gastrin are to be tested.

• A few specimens have to be transported at or near body temperature (37° C). Specimens should be kept at this temperature when testing components such as cold agglutinins, and cryofibrinogen. A 37°C heat block can be used in these cases.

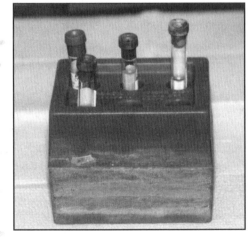

Figure 17-3: A 37° C heat block can be used to transport specimens that need to be kept warm.

- If you draw blood or receive another type of specimen from a patient whose skin, whites of the eyes, and mucous membranes are obviously **jaundiced** (yellowed), it is possible that this patient has hepatitis, which is highly infectious. You might also notice that as the blood settles before you transport the specimen, the plasma or serum is bright yellow or gold in color. When it looks like this, it is called **icteric**. Although all members of the laboratory team are supposed to treat ALL specimens as potentially biohazardous (Standard Precautions), many laboratories go a step further and place a biohazard label or other precautionary label on certain blood tubes that look potentially hazardous to alert fellow workers to a possible biohazard.

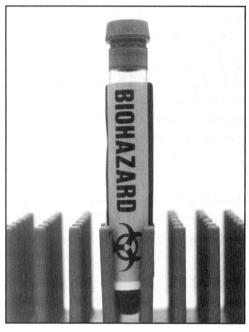

Figure 17-4: A biohazard label may be placed on a potentially biohazardous blood tube.

jaundice: yellow discolorization of skin and eyeballs caused by excess bilirubin in the blood.

icteric: referring to jaundice; yellow discolorization of skin and eyeballs caused by excess bilirubin in the blood.

milky-whitish increase lipids
turbid-cloudy-contaminated

Time Constraints for Delivering Specimens

ALL specimens should be transported to the clinical laboratory immediately after being drawn. Ideally, routine blood specimens should arrive at the laboratory within 45 minutes and be centrifuged within 1 hour. Guidelines recommended by the National Committee for Clinical Laboratory Standards (NCCLS) document H18-A set the maximum time limit to separate serum and plasma from cells at 2 hours from the time of collection. Less time may be recommended for certain specimens.

STAT - now within the hour
ASAP - now but not rushed for it.
routine - no hurry

Specimens that cannot reach the clinical laboratory within these allotted time periods should be allowed to clot (if applicable), should be centrifuged, and the resulting serum or plasma should be separated and transferred to a suitable container for transport. If blood is drawn in **serum separator tubes** (**SST**), the separator gel should prevent metabolic changes up to 24 hours after centrifugation.

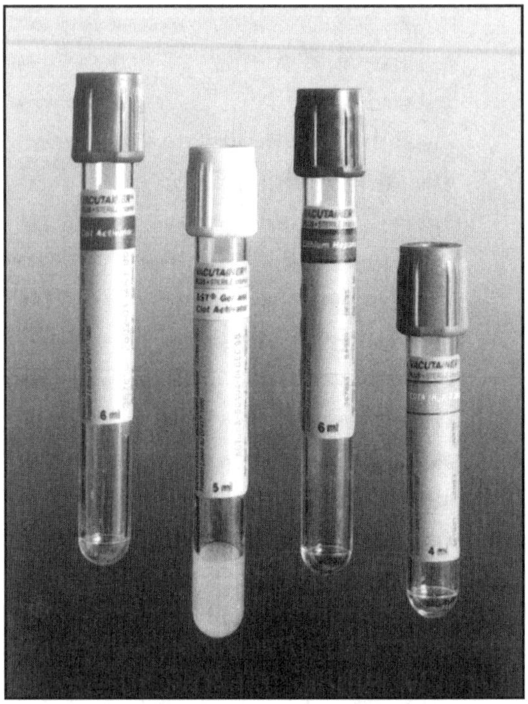

Exceptions to the above time constraints include "STAT" or "medical emergency" orders. In these cases, specimens should be transported and processed immediately. Physicians

ASAP:
as soon as possible.

may also order a test **ASAP** (as soon as possible), which means that the physician really would like the test

Figure 17-5: Serum Separator Tubes

Courtesy of Becton Dickinson and Company.

run immediately if possible. Some anticoagulated tubes such as **sodium fluoride** tubes (for glucose determinations) and EDTA (ethylenediamine tetraacetic acid) tubes keep blood stable for up to 24 hours at room temperature.

Processing Specimens

Central Processing

central processing: also known as specimen processing, the area of the clinical laboratory where specimens are processed for testing in various departments of the clinical laboratory as well as for preparing specimens for transport to other facilities.

Most laboratories have a specific area often called **central processing** (also called specimen processing) where all specimens are received and processed for testing. In many laboratories, one or more clinical laboratory assistants may work at this position, usually in a rotating capacity. For example, a clinical laboratory assistant/phlebotomist might work in central processing one week, draw outpatients one week, draw inpatients one week, and work in laboratory departments one week.

In central processing, specimens are identified, logged, and sorted by department and type of handling required. Many specimens, such as urine and certain hematology specimens that require the entire blood specimen (whole blood), are distributed to the proper department immediately.

Specimens requiring processing, such as those that need serum or plasma to be removed, must be centrifuged. Many tests require only the liquid portion of the blood. After centrifuging the specimen, the liquid portion rises to the top of the blood tube. The blood cells remain at the bottom of the tube. Remember: the liquid portion of the blood without cells is called plasma. If a chemical agent such as an anticoagulant is added to prevent clotting, the plasma and cells can be separated by means of centrifugation. If a blood specimen without any additives is allowed to clot, the result is serum on the top plus blood cells meshed in a clot on the bottom of the tube. Serum contains essentially the same chemical constituents as plasma, except that the clotting factors and the blood cells are contained within the fibrin clot.

Special Considerations for Serum Processing

Serum specimens must be completely clotted before centrifugation. A complete clotting typically takes 30 to 45 minutes at room temperature. Serum specimens from patients on anticoagulant medication may take longer to clot, as do chilled specimens. Specimens in serum separator tubes (SSTs) and other tubes containing clot-activating particles usually clot within 15 minutes.

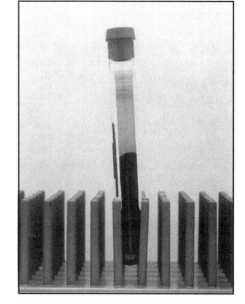

Centrifugation

The **centrifuge** is a machine that spins the blood at high revolutions per minute (rpms). This high speed spinning motion creates

Figure 17-6: Complete clotting takes from 30 to 45 minutes in a nonadditive blood tube.

centrifuge: a device used to separate substances of different densities through spinning.

centrifugal force, which separates cells from plasma or from serum. Once blood specimens that contain serum have fully clotted, they can be centrifuged. The liquid portion of the blood rises to the top. The red cells, white cells, and platelets move toward the bottom. Stoppers should remain on all tubes awaiting centrifugation. Removing stoppers from a blood specimen can cause a loss of CO_2 and an increase in pH, leading to inaccurate test results for certain tests such as pH, CO_2, and acid phosphatase. Leaving tubes unstoppered also increases the risk of specimen contamination and evaporation. Furthermore, it is safer to leave the blood specimens stoppered as long as possible.

The following procedure describes the steps taken to safely centrifuge blood specimens.

Centrifuging a Blood Specimen

Materials needed:

✓ a pair of new gloves
✓ a laboratory centrifuge, properly checked for safety
✓ stoppered blood specimens
✓ balance tubes

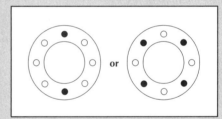

1. Procedural Step: Wearing gloves, open the centrifuge and determine how many holders are available in the centrifuge. Count the blood specimens to be centrifuged.
   Reason: To assess how much room is available in the centrifuge, and determine how many specimens can be spun at one time.

2. Procedural Step: You must make sure that tubes of equal volume of specimen are placed opposite one another. This is known as "balancing" the centrifuge (Figure 17-8). Tubes must be approximately equal in weight and size. They must be filled to near equal volumes of liquid. Tubes that are half full must be balanced across from an equal volume tube. If you have an uneven number of tubes, a balance tube containing water must be placed opposite the extra tube.

Reason: An unbalanced centrifuge may break specimen tubes, ruin the specimen, and create aerosols (escaping contaminants that become airborne) that can be dangerous to the clinical laboratory assistant.

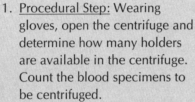

Figure 17-7: Some balancing configurations in a centrifuge.

3. Procedural Step: Make sure that all tubes are stoppered tightly. You may have the opportunity to centrifuge microbiological specimens, some of which can be extremely hazardous. In these cases, you may be required to put the specimen inside a special sealed vial.
   Reason: Specimens should not be allowed to create aerosols inside a centrifuge that can be harmful to laboratory employees when the centrifuge lid is

Centrifuging a Blood Specimen (Cont.)

opened. Special vials for extremely hazardous materials protect you and others if the specimen container breaks by containing the specimen in the special vial, preventing contamination of the centrifuge.

4. Procedure: The lid of the centrifuge is closed, and the centrifuge is not opened again until the machine has come to a complete stop without using the brake.
Reason: The lid must be closed securely before the centrifuge is started. An open, running centrifuge can pose many dangers, such as releasing harmful aerosols. Therefore, the machine must stop on its own. In fact, trying to stop a centrifuge manually can lead to personal injury; for example, body parts can get caught in the centrifuge. Further, using a brake before the centrifuge stops is not recommended (unless you hear breakage occurring or unless there is something wrong with the motor) because the sudden stop can disrupt cells in the sample and interfere with the testing.

5. Procedure: The specimens should be centrifuged for 10 minutes. Speeds will vary according to individual laboratory specifications and machine specifications.

Reason: It is important to follow instructions on the exact speed recommended for specific centrifuges in order to recover the greatest amount of serum or plasma without damaging any contents of the blood tubes.

6. Procedure: If, when opening the centrifuge, you find that tubes have broken, you must extract the spilled blood and glass and decontaminate the interior of the centrifuge, according to OSHA and NCCLS guidelines posted in the laboratory. Care must be taken to wear heavy gloves that glass cannot penetrate. Goggles and a mask must be worn also. Periodic cleanings must be scheduled for the centrifuge.
Reason: Contamination must be removed as soon as possible from the centrifuge to protect employees. Heavy gloves keep the hands safe from cuts by broken glass, and goggles and a mask help protect the eyes and the lungs from contamination from the broken glass and any aerosols from the specimen. A strong disinfectant is applied to the inside of the centrifuge to decontaminate the centrifuge surfaces, another reason to wear heavy gloves to protect the skin. Periodic cleanings help keep the centrifuge free from contamination.

Preparing the Specimens for Testing

After centrifugation, specimen tubes should be removed CAREFULLY from the centrifuge and placed in a test tube rack.

Stopper Removal

The stopper of a blood tube has to be removed to obtain the serum or plasma that is needed for testing. Stoppers can be removed by commercially available stopper removal devices. If such a device is not available, stoppers should be removed with a gloved hand and first covered with a 4 X 4 piece of gauze or tissue to catch any aerosol that might be released. The stopper should be slowly twisted off away from the laboratory assistant's face. Sometimes face shields are used for this process to avoid a possible spray of blood or the formation of an aerosol.

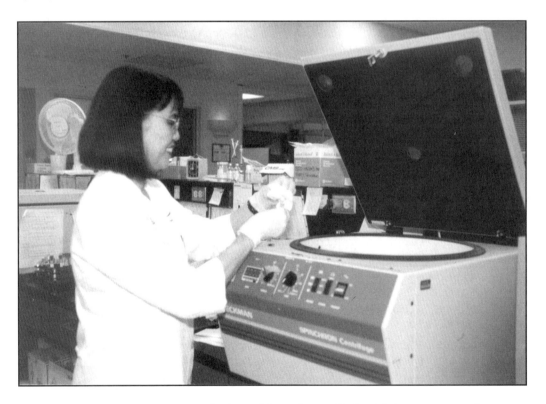

Figure 17-8: Using gauze and gloved hands, a clinical laboratory assistant opens a centrifuged blood tube.

Separating Serum or Plasma for Testing

Using a disposable plastic Pasteur pipette (Figure 17-10), and wearing gloves and a face shield, the clinical laboratory assistant/phlebotomist separates the liquid portion of the blood from the cells. The liquid is then placed in another aliquot tube that is used for transporting or storing the specimen. The aliquot tube must be labeled with the same identification information as the collection tube.

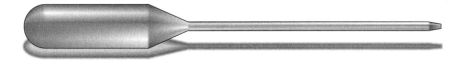

Figure 17-9: A Disposable Pasteur Pipette

The liquid is removed down to the gel separation material (if present) or to the formed elements. BE CAREFUL NOT TO DISTURB THE CELLULAR PORTION OF THE TUBE. If this should occur, reapply the stopper and recentrifuge the entire tube. Serum and plasma must not contain cells. After a specimen is transferred into the aliquot tube, the tube is covered or capped and taken to the proper department for testing.

Evaluating Specimen Integrity

When working in the central processing area of the clinical laboratory, you may be responsible for screening blood specimens for their integrity. There are certain situations in which you might have to reject specimens for testing. Of course, in cases when you have a question, you must consult your supervisor. A rejected specimen often means that a patient will have to be recalled, and the patient's blood will have to be drawn again for a new sample.

Reasons to reject specimens include the following:

- **QNS** means "quantity not sufficient." An anticoagulated tube must have an acceptable volume of blood for testing accuracy. Many tubes must be filled to the top in order to balance the blood and the anticoagulant volume. Too little blood means that the anticoagulant could dilute the specimen.

- A clotted additive tube is not an acceptable specimen. This occurs when a laboratory employee does not gently mix the blood in an additive tube IMMEDIATELY after collection.

- Visible hemolysis in serum or plasma (cherry red color) is not acceptable for many tests. Plasma or serum should be golden-colored.

- Specimens that require protection (such as bilirubin tests) are not protected properly after the draw and will yield inaccurate results.

- Specimens for a specific test may be drawn in an additive tube or nonadditive tube that is not recommended for the test.

- Unlabeled specimens are NOT accepted, even if you have a good idea of where the specimens came from.

Distributing Clinical Specimens

After processing, specimens are delivered to your healthcare facility's clinical laboratory, or the specimens are sent elsewhere for testing.

Distributing Specimens to Various Departments

Every clinical laboratory has a specific protocol for receiving specimens in each department of the clinical laboratory, including hematology, clinical chemistry, blood bank, clinical microbiology, immunology/serology, as well as in the coagulation and urinalysis sections of the laboratory. STAT tests must be delivered as soon as possible after collection. Employees in each department should be informed each time you deliver specimens.

Each department and section in the clinical laboratory will have specific areas where it wishes the specimens to be placed. Always remember to place the specimens where they can be seen and tested as soon as possible.

Thinking It Through ...

> Larry has just drawn a STAT blood test from an outpatient. He takes the specimen back to the laboratory immediately and processes the specimen at once. He then takes the specimen into the chemistry department for immediate testing.
>
> As he approaches the chemistry department, he sees no one anywhere in the department. As stated, he has a test that must be run immediately. He calls out, but no one answers. The physician has already called the laboratory for the test results.
>
> What should Larry do?

Preparing Specimens for Shipment

Today's healthcare environment is very concerned with keeping close watch on the budgets of all healthcare facility departments. It has been found that sharing services with other healthcare agencies in the same area is of fiscal benefit to all facilities involved. For example, if one local clinical laboratory purchases an expensive instrument for a highly complex test, other clinical laboratories may send all their tests to be done on this machine rather than buying their own equipment. Therefore, specimens are often sent daily from one laboratory to another in a metropolitan area. Also, some tests are so specialized that they may be sent across the country to one of a few centers that can run such a test.

The transportation of human specimens is closely regulated by the **Department of Commerce**. Policies for transporting specimens vary within and between states. However, the CDC (Centers for Disease Control and Prevention) clearly describe labeling policies for all containers sent through the mail or by courier. Containers must be leakproof as required by law. Accurate labeling of containers and packages is required for the protection of all workers. Labels must include the following information:

1. The package is labeled as biohazardous.

2. The type of tissue, organ, or body fluid is identified clearly.

3. A contact person must be included in case of breakage or loss.

4. The full address of the CDC must be affixed in case of breakage or loss.

Recordkeeping

Accurate records MUST be kept on specimens sent out from the facility. At such times, physicians are informed that test results will not be available as quickly as when the tests are performed in-house. As a result, physicians often will inquire about the status and availability of those test results. Therefore, the path of these specimens must be traceable.

A record of which tests have been sent out is often kept in the area of central processing where "send-outs" are processed. This log might be stored as a data file in a computer or it might be recorded in a book. The laboratory assistant may be charged with the task of recording when a test is sent out and when the results are received. Additionally, a procedure manual should also be available for the clinical laboratory assistant/phlebotomist to refer to when sending out a specimen. The information should be updated frequently and should answer the following questions:

1. Where is the test sent?

2. What are the regulations involved in sending the specimen to a different area? There are stringent federal and varying state regulations for packaging and transporting all body fluids.

3. Are there special considerations for transporting this specimen? Is it sent frozen? At room temperature? Are there special transport media to ensure that an organism to be tested does not die (microbiology specimens in particular)?

4. What is the turnaround time for a test sent to another laboratory? Will the laboratory run tests on weekends? Will they run STAT tests, and if so, is there an additional charge?

5. What days of the week is the test performed?

Other Transport Considerations

When a test is ordered that must be sent a long distance for testing, the specimen should be sent by the most rapid transportation available. Be sure to consult with the physician about the urgency of the specimen results. For instance, some physicians might want to send a specimen in a hurry and do not care about the cost. Others may not want the patients to pay the extra charge of immediate transport. Customer service considerations also require finding the most cost-effective way to send the specimen without compromising the quality of the service.

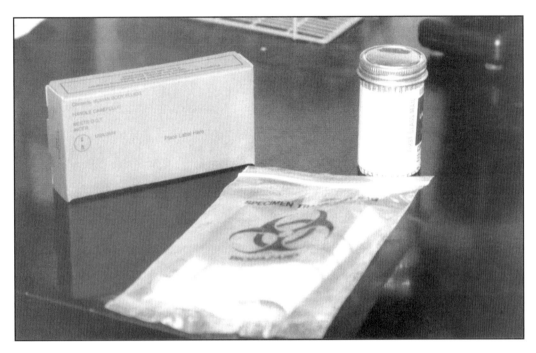

Figure 17-10: A clinical laboratory assistant may be in charge of properly mailing specimens to other laboratories for testing.

Chapter Summary

As in most other tasks routinely performed by the clinical laboratory assistant/ phlebotomist, attention to detail is required of the laboratory professional when transporting, processing, and distributing clinical laboratory specimens for testing. Orders from physicians must be followed as to the urgency of testing (STAT, ASAP, or routine). The specimens must be logged in and processed carefully so that the specimens are not contaminated and do not expose the laboratory employees to bloodborne pathogens. Also, the labeling and relabeling of processed specimens requires that same careful attention. Specimens sent to other laboratories for testing must be recorded properly and packaged carefully following state and federal regulations for hazardous substances.

Name _____

Date _____

Student Enrichment Activities

Complete the following statements.

1. When transporting vacuum blood tubes, the specimens should be positioned with the stopper placed _____.

2. Unnecessary agitation of a blood tube can cause _____.

3. An example of a blood component in a test specimen that must be protected from light when being transported is _____ .

4. An example of a component that must be chilled for specimen testing is a/an _____.

5. Routine blood tests should be centrifuged within _____ of collection.

6. Blood collection tubes without additives generally take _____ to _____ minutes to clot before they can be centrifuged.

7. SST collection tubes can take only _____ to clot.

8. _____ should remain on tubes awaiting centrifugation.

9. Specimens in a centrifuge should be _____ carefully before the centrifuge is turned on.

10. The centrifuge _____ should not be opened until the centrifuge is completely stopped.

Circle T for true, or F for false.

11.   T   F   After blood tubes have undergone centrifugation, stoppers should be removed with caution and with the aid of gauze.

12.   T   F   If you are in a hurry to get a specimen processed, you can use the brake to turn off the centrifuge.

13.   T   F   If a patient is jaundiced, it means that the patient may have hepatitis.

14.   T   F   Aerosols are not a problem when centrifuging specimens.

15.   T   F   The clinical laboratory assistant/phlebotomist is often assigned on a rotating basis to the central processing area of the laboratory.

Circle the correct answer.

16.   It is important to separate the liquid portion of blood from the blood clot in a timely manner. Ideally, for accurate results, this should occur:
   A. within 15 minutes of collection.
   B. within 30 minutes of collection.
   C. within 1 hour of collection.
   D. within 2 hours of collection.

17.   The greatest concern with an icteric specimen is that:
   A. it must be warmed
   B. it must be chilled
   C. the patient could have hepatitis
   D. the results are inaccurate

Name _____

Date _____

18. To balance a centrifuge when five specimens must be processed, you should:

   A. fill five more tubes with water.

   B. use blood previously centrifuged.

   C. fill a balance tube with water.

   D. run the five and hope the centrifuge doesn't unbalance.

19. A blood specimen is not acceptable:

   A. when the specimen tube does not have an acceptable volume of blood.

   B. when hemolysis is visible in the plasma or serum.

   C. when the specimen for testing is collected in the wrong tube.

   D. all of the above.

20. The transportation of human specimens is regulated closely by the:

   A. FBI.

   B. Department of Transportation.

   C. Department of Health Services.

   D. Department of Commerce.

Chapter Eighteen

Operating Laboratory Equipment

Objectives

After completing this chapter, you should be able to
do the following:

1. Define and correctly spell each of the key terms.

2. Explain the difference between general containers and volumetric glassware.

3. List the parts and explain the operation of the compound microscope.

4. Explain how to operate a centrifuge in a safe manner.

5. Explain why a balance might be used in the laboratory by the clinical laboratory assistant/phlebotomist.

6. Discuss the potential role that the clinical laboratory assistant/phlebotomist may play in operating automated equipment in the laboratory.

Key Terms

- analytical balance
- beaker
- calibration
- chemistry autoanalyzer
- compound microscope
- critical measurements
- electronic cell counter
- flask

- general containers
- meniscus
- pipette
- reagent
- TC
- TD
- volumetric glassware

Introduction

One of the interesting aspects of the clinical laboratory assistant/phlebotomist position is the variety of tasks that can be assigned to this job title. It should be noted, though, that in some states, such as California, the laboratory assistant has many task-related restrictions regarding the operating of laboratory instruments and on the performing of any tests that require a specific measurement or "judgment call." However, in other states, clinical laboratory assistants/phlebotomists can do many procedures. Overall, the trend in healthcare is that unlicensed employees are being given more and more responsibility, and the clinical laboratory reflects this trend.

This chapter will concentrate on basic equipment in the clinical laboratory that you might work with in most clinical laboratory assistant/phlebotomist positions throughout the country. For more detail, consult more advanced clinical laboratory textbooks, some of which are named in the bibliography of this textbook.

Clinical Laboratory Glassware

In some clinical laboratories today, the use of glassware is being reduced by the advances of laboratory automation. Glassware is still necessary for many functions in the laboratory, and many pieces are now disposable, designed for one use. Glassware can be made of glass or several types of plastics, including polyethylene, polypropylene, and polycarbonate. (For our purposes, plastics will be called "glassware" in this chapter.) The advantages of plastics include a greater survivability because of greater strength. Also, plastics can resist corrosion better than glass. However, plastics have certain disadvantages too. They may absorb dyes, become stained, allow substances contained in them to evaporate, and so on.

Glassware can be divided into two categories: **general containers** and **volumetric glassware**.

General Containers

General containers are numerous in the clinical laboratory, with many made of plastic. These containers are adequate for storing many substances. General containers are not **calibrated** to hold a particular or exact volume and are not recommended for **critical measurements**. They are not as expensive as glassware requiring more exact volume calibrations (volumetric glassware).

Test tubes are manufactured from either glass or plastic. Most test tubes are disposable and are used for many purposes. They can be containers for liquid samples such as urine, serum, or whole blood. Sometimes the test tube can contain a test reaction.

Test tubes should always be handled with care. They should be examined for any chips and cracks before use. Chips and cracks can cause cuts in the hand, even through gloves, and can introduce infectious materials into the body. Therefore, gloves should always be worn when using test tubes.

Centrifuge tubes look much like test tubes but are designed to withstand the stress of centrifugation. They are used to separate liquid from solids during centrifugation. Centrifuge tubes generally have volumetric marks on them (usually up to 10 ml). Usually, they have a pointed bottom; whereas a test tube has a rounded bottom.

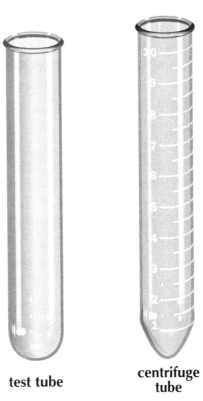

test tube   centrifuge tube

Figure 18-1: A Test Tube and a Centrifuge Tube

general containers: containers such as beakers, graduated cylinders, and certain flasks designed to hold and measure inexact volumes.

volumetric glassware: carefully manufactured glassware to contain, transfer, or deliver exact amounts of substances.

calibration: a determination of the accuracy of an instrument by comparing a measurement with a known standard.

critical measurements: measures that must be made in an exacting manner.

beaker:
a wide-mouthed, straight-sided piece of glassware with a pouring spout in the rim; glassware not critically calibrated.

Beakers have a wide mouth, straight sides, and a pouring spout as part of the rim (Figure 18-2). They are used to estimate liquid amounts, as well as to mix and heat solutions. They can also be used for storage. There may or may not be measurement marks on a beaker; such marks are not critically calibrated, but are marked for estimating volumes. Beakers often are required to be heat and chemical resistant.

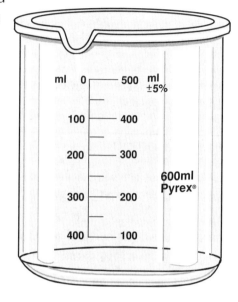

Figure 18-2: A Beaker

flask:
common clinical laboratory glassware that comes in a variety of sizes, usually with rounded sides, a flat bottom, and a long cylindrical neck.

Typically, a general container **flask** (Figure 18-3) is used in the laboratory for holding and mixing liquids. These containers can also have measurement marks for noncritical volumes. For example, Erlenmeyer flasks are designed with a flat bottom and sides that slope up to the neck, with sizes from 1 ml to 2,000 ml. Other flasks, such as the Florence flask, can have rounded sides, a flat bottom, and a long cylindrical neck.

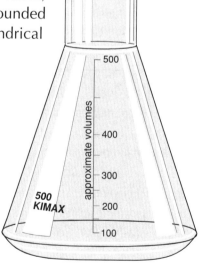

Figure 18-3: An Erlenmeyer Flask

Graduated cylinders are cylindrical pieces of glassware with several calibrated markings, available in many sizes. Precise volumes are not measured with cylinders, but approximate measures can be made (Figure 18-4).

Other pieces of glassware/plastics may be used in the laboratory that are considered general containers. For example, **reagent** bottles hold various reagents used in laboratory testing. Most reagent bottles are made of polypropylene, a plastic that is resistant to most reagents. Some bottles may be clear, and some may be brown to protect the reagents from light.

Volumetric Glassware

Manufactured with a rigorous calibration process to ensure measurement accuracy, volumetric glassware (including flasks and **pipettes**) is used in much of the laboratory's testing. The calibration process is time-consuming; therefore, volumetric glassware is much more expensive than general container glassware.

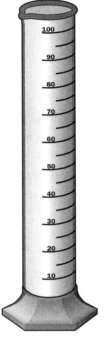

Figure 18-4: A Graduated Cylinder

reagent:
a substance used in laboratory testing procedures to detect and measure other substances.

pipette:
a narrow glass or plastic tube with both ends open; used for transferring and measuring liquids by bringing liquids into the tube with a pipetting device.

Only glass of the finest quality is used in the manufacture of volumetric glassware. Care is taken to make sure the glass is transparent and free of distortions. The temperature of calibration may be etched on volumetric glassware (usually 20° C), as well as the volume, manufacturer, and designated usage. Some volumetric glassware may be marked with a **TD** "to deliver," meaning that the piece of glassware is designed to deliver a designated volume into a receiving vessel. If the glassware is marked **TC** "to contain," that glassware is designed to contain a given volume of liquid at the calibrated mark. If the contents of a TC vessel is poured into another vessel, there is no guarantee that the correct volume would be delivered into another vessel.

Volumetric flasks have a rounded bottom with a long neck on which a calibration mark is found. The National Bureau of Standards sets specifications for the manufacture of volumetric glassware of all kinds. Volumetric flasks come in many sizes.

TD:
initials meaning *to deliver;* glassware has been calibrated to deliver a specific volume of liquid into another vessel.

TC:
initials meaning *to contain;* glassware calibrated to contain the measurement specified.

Volumetric flasks are used to prepare solutions when the accuracy of the concentration is critical. When liquid is placed in this type of flask, it must come up exactly to the calibrated mark on the flask; therefore, the last portion is added slowly. The surface of the liquid will curve when placed in a container. This curvature is called the **meniscus**. To measure the correct volume, hold the flask at eye level and make sure the bottom of the meniscus is right on the calibration mark.

meniscus: the curvature of a liquid's upper surface when the liquid is placed in a container.

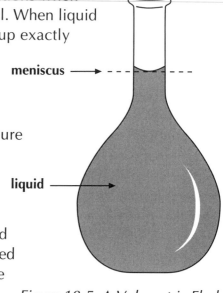

Figure 18-5: A Volumetric Flask

Pipettes are available in both volumetric and nonvolumetric sizes. All pipettes are designed for measuring and transferring liquids. There are different pipettes for specific tasks. These pipetting techniques are common to most pipettes:

- YOU MUST NEVER PIPETTE ANYTHING BY MOUTH! A pipette aid should be attached to the mouthpiece of the pipette (Figure 18-6).

- Pipettes should be examined for cracks, chips, and breaks. If the measurement is critical, any defects can affect the volume that is delivered by the pipette.

- Use a pipette closest to the volume needed to be measured. In other words, if you want to measure 10 ml, do not choose a pipette that measures up to 100 ml.

- Volumetric pipettes must be used for critical volume measurements. Nonvolumetric pipettes are used when measurements are approximate.

- A pipette tip must be placed completely below the surface of a liquid to avoid drawing air in the pipette.

- A pipette must be held in a vertical position while drawing the liquid level to the calibration line and during delivery of the liquid.

- The pipette tip is left in contact with the container surface a few seconds to drain the pipette completely. Some pipettes have a frosted band around the top indicating that the last drop of liquid is not left in the tip but is "blown out" by forcing the last drop out with the **pipette aid**. TD pipettes are not forced out, but TC pipettes must have the last drop forced out.

There are various types of pipettes, including the following:

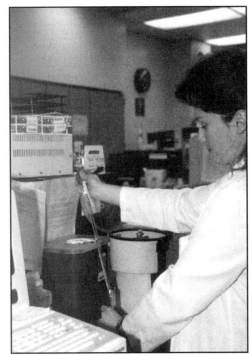

- VOLUMETRIC PIPETTES: Pipettes that consist of a long, narrow tube with an elongated, rounded bulb near the middle. Used when the greatest accuracy and precision is required.

- OSWALD-FOLIN PIPETTES: Specialized volumetric pipettes that are shorter than the regular volumetric pipettes. The bulb is near the delivery tip and the opening is larger for faster drainage.

- GRADUATED PIPETTES: Pipettes that consist of a long straight tube with graduated markings to indicate volume delivered. These pipettes are not accurate enough for critical measurements and are often used to measure reagents.

Figure 18-6: A pipette aid is being used by a laboratory assistant.

- SEROLOGIC PIPETTES: Pipettes that are graduated at the tip and are not used for exact measurements.

- MICROPIPETTES: Pipettes that are used to measure small volumes of a sample, as small as 5 microliters. Generally, these pipettes are used to add a liquid medium to another substance (either liquid or solid). They are rarely used to add a solid because, unlike liquids which can be completely expelled from the pipette, some of the solid can remain in the pipette.

- AUTOMATIC PIPETTES: Pipettes that are designed to pick up and dispense a preset volume of solution when a plunger is smoothly released and then depressed. In some models, disposable plastic tips are used to eliminate carryover from sample to sample.

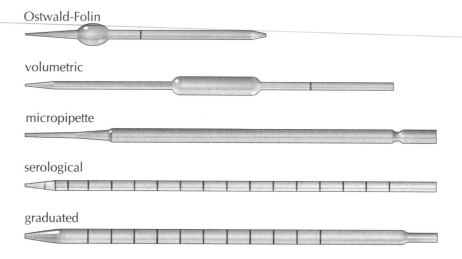

Figure 18-7: Some Examples of Pipettes

The Microscope in the Clinical Laboratory

Microscopes are often used in the clinical laboratory. Although most microscope work will be done by clinical laboratory technicians and technologists, the medical laboratory assistant could, in some situations, use the microscope on a limited basis. Some tasks performed in the clinical laboratory using the microscope include the following:

- evaluating stained blood smears (differential testing)
- examining urine sediment (microscopic portion of the urinalysis)
- evaluating tissue sections
- performing cell counts
- examining different specimens for microorganisms

The microscope allows the operator to see cells, entire organisms, and other structures that cannot be seen with the naked eye. The microscope is a delicate instrument. It can be damaged by improper use, cleaning, or storage.

The Compound Microscope

The **compound microscope** (Figure 18-8) is the microscope used most frequently in the clinical laboratory. It has a two-lens system with one lens next to the eye in the eyepiece and the other set in the objective, located closer to the specimen being viewed.

compound microscope: a microscope that utilizes two lens systems; the most commonly used microscope in the clinical laboratory.

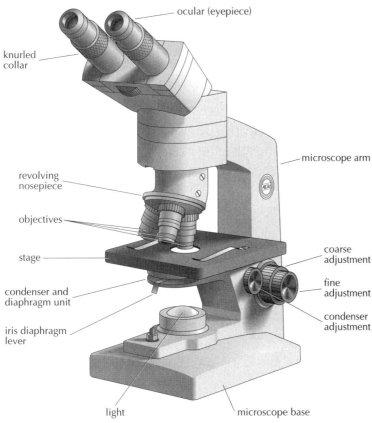

Figure 18-8: Parts of the Compound Microscope

Most compound microscopes offer three or four different magnifications. Magnification is determined by multiplying the magnification of the ocular lens (in the eyepieces of the microscope — usually 10X) by the magnification of the objective lens (near the specimen). If the ocular lens is 10X and the objective lens is 40X, the object is magnified 400 times its normal size.

The objective lenses (low, high, and oil are often used) are held in place by the nosepiece. The low-power lens (an objective lens) is used by the laboratory professional to locate an object in a field. The specimen is generally put on a slide and placed on the microscope stage for observation under the low-power lens. This gets the object in focus before rotating to the higher powered lenses.

The high-power lens is usually a 40X to 43X lens, giving the magnification with the ocular lens of 400X to 430X. After focusing on low power, the high power lens is rotated into place to view the specimen at closer range for better viewing.

The oil immersion lens is used frequently in the laboratory to view blood cells, microorganisms, and sections of tissues. After the object has been found on low power, the lens is rotated to the side. Then a drop of immersion oil is placed on the side, and the oil immersion lens is rotated into place. This has 100X magnification, making the object magnified 1000X. In this situation, the high-power lens is not used.

The microscope is focused by the coarse and fine adjustment knobs. The coarse adjustment is used to focus the low-power lens, and the fine adjustment is used to achieve a clearer picture after the coarse adjustment has been used. The coarse adjustment moves the lenses up and down, and must NEVER BE USED WHEN THE HIGHER POWER OBJECTIVE LENSES ARE IN PLACE. These lenses are too close to the object and can be damaged by contacting the slide and specimen itself.

A light source is located in the base of the microscope, and has a condenser to focus and direct light into the objective lens. The iris diaphragm controls the amount of light that hits the object being viewed.

Care of the Microscope

To function properly, the microscope must be free of dust and must be cleaned after use. Carry the microscope with one hand supporting the base and the other hand holding the microscope arm (Figure 18-9). The following instructions will help you use a microscope efficiently, without causing damage to the scope itself.

1. Use the coarse adjustment only when you are focusing on low power.

2. Keep the microscope clean, using a cover between uses or storing the microscope in a cabinet. Clean the lenses and condenser with a lens-cleaning tissue. Clean all oil immersion lenses after use.

3. Refrain from using eye makeup when using the microscope. Makeup can damage the lenses.

4. When the microscope is not in use, put the low objective lenses in place to assure that the high-power lenses are not damaged (the high-power lens is close to the stage and can be damaged if it contacts the stage).

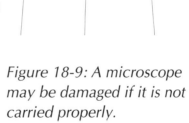

Figure 18-9: A microscope may be damaged if it is not carried properly.

5. Avoid jarring a microscope. Be gentle with its placement.

6. Do not pass the high-power lens through oil. Clean it immediately if this happens. Oil can destroy the lens system. The low-power lens is too short to reach the oil.

7. Never touch the surfaces of the lenses with fingers.

Other Microscopes Used in the Laboratory

If your laboratory is large and complex, there may be several other microscopes in use. The dark-field microscope produces a light object on a dark background, using a special condenser system that prevents light from coming into the objective. The phase-contrast microscope is a specialized microscope, which allows the study of unstained structures such as wet preparations. This microscope can provide give good resolution and detail to such structures.

Often, the fluorescent microscope is used in the microbiology department to view certain organisms (such as those that cause tuberculosis) that absorb fluorescent dyes. When an ultraviolet light is shined through prestained organisms, those that have absorbed the fluorescent dye will be visibly fluorescent. Those organisms that don't absorb the dye will not be visible.

The electron microscope is a very expensive microscope that is used in larger institutions. It uses short wavelength electrons to produce extraordinary resolution. It is much more powerful than the other microscopes discussed here. Operators must have extensive training to use this instrument.

Centrifuges

As discussed in Chapter Seventeen, centrifuges are used in every clinical laboratory department. Centrifuges are an integral part of specimen processing, a task generally assigned to the clinical laboratory assistant/phlebotomist. The main use for the centrifuge is to separate blood cells from plasma and serum. Other body fluids (discussed in Section IV) are also centrifuged, including urine and cerebrospinal fluid. Centrifuges come in various sizes—from tiny centrifuges used to spin capillary tubes of blood to large, refrigerated centrifuges used in the blood bank department to spin down units of blood, that is, if the units received are not already spun down.

Rules for the safe use of the centrifuge are discussed in Chapter Seventeen, including a procedure for operating the centrifuge.

Balances

A clinical laboratory assistant may be asked to help prepare reagents and other chemicals. Most laboratories buy preweighed reagents, but some laboratories on a small budget may do some of their own weighing and reagent preparation using an **analytical balance** (Figure 18-10). It is your responsibility to learn to use the balance or balances used in your facility. Some are easy to operate with digital readouts and very little manipulation on your part. Others are more complex and require some training.

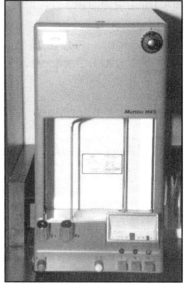

analytical balance: a very sensitive scale used in chemical analyses.

Figure 18-10: An analytical balance may be used to prepare reagents.

Electronic Cell Counters

In the last quarter century, automation has come to the hematology department in the form of **electronic cell counters**. These machines can count red and white blood cells and platelets, determine hemoglobin content, measure and calculate red blood cell size, and determine the approximate numbers of each of the five white blood cells (automated differential count), as well as create graphs, calculate quality control statistics, and make other determinations. In the years before the electronic cell counters, all of these tests had to be done manually (or in some cases, semimanually) with smaller, less sophisticated instruments.

electronic cell counter: an automated system used to count and access formed elements of the blood.

One of the most consistent task-related trends in the modern clinical laboratory is to have the clinical laboratory assistant/phlebotomist run the electronic cell counter (Figure 18-11). This instrument analyzes a tiny sample of EDTA-anticoagulated whole blood (sampled directly from the fully stoppered lavender tube to avoid unnecessary contact with blood by the operator). The blood sample is diluted with saline and is drawn through

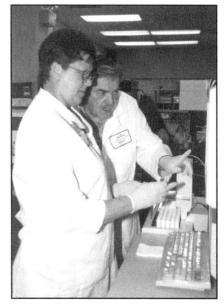

Figure 18-11: An electronic cell counter is used to analyze various aspects of a blood sample.

the machine. These machines are fully computerized and continually report the machine's status to the operator. If a clinical laboratory assistant is allowed to operate these instruments, all results must be reviewed by a clinical laboratory technologist before reporting those results. Operating such a complex machine takes much training and supervision.

Clinical Chemistry Autoanalyzers

Perhaps the most automated department in the clinical laboratory is the clinical chemistry department. Because the clinical chemistry department runs many more tests than the other departments, clinical laboratory assistants/phlebotomists often assist here by preparing specimens for testing.

chemistry autoanalyzer: a general term for highly automated, computerized equipment used to run tests in the chemistry department.

The modern **chemistry autoanalyzer** (Figure 18-12) can analyze many different chemistry tests on the same specimen. In some "discrete analyzers," a sampler probe automatically picks up the needed volume of sample from a specimen cup, dilutes it, and carries the sample into the tubes needed for the requested tests. The employee programs the computer with the patient's identification number and the requested tests. The rest is done by the machine. The machine prints out the review results and automatically sends them to the hospital and laboratory computer systems after being reviewed by a clinical laboratory assistant. Further, the chemistry autoanalyzer calculates its own quality control automatically and monitors itself for any problems within its instrumentation.

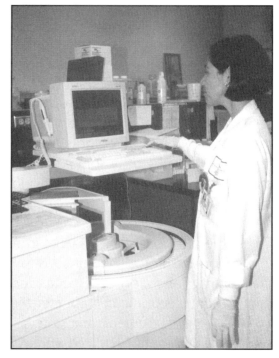

As in all departments, specimens are handled with gloves and often with eye protection. Standard Precautions are practiced continually within the chemistry department, the same as within the other departments.

Figure 18-12: A chemistry auto-analyzer can analyze many different tests on the same specimen.

Additional Laboratory Automation

In addition to the large instruments of hematology and chemistry that run most tests in the clinical laboratory, there are many other machines available that may or may not be operated by a laboratory assistant. For example, coagulation tests are run by a variety of automated instruments. Instrumentation in microbiology can identify organisms and calculate the antibiotic sensitivities of the organisms themselves. Blood types can be determined automatically, and many other tests can be carried out automatically as well. Whether or not state regulations or facility policies allow you to operate these instruments, you may still be called upon to prepare specimens for testing with these instruments.

Chapter Summary

The trend today in the clinical laboratory is to run tests as quickly, efficiently, cheaply, and accurately as possible. The automated instruments in the clinical laboratory can achieve all of these purposes. The clinical laboratory assistant/ phlebotomist is playing an increasingly large role in operating such machinery, with results reviewed by a supervisor before they are reported to nursing stations and physicians' offices.

Understanding how to use basic laboratory glassware and plastics, handling a microscope correctly, running a centrifuge safely, using an analytical balance accurately, and operating automated machinery may fall within your job description. Many of these tasks only can be learned after you are on the job. Each requires attention to detail, a constant vigilance to avoid bloodborne pathogen contact, and a dedication to achieving the best results that can be achieved on the patient's behalf.

Name _____

Date _____

Student Enrichment Activities

Complete the following statements.

1. General containers are not _____, making them less expensive than volumetric glassware.

2. Volumetric flasks have a rounded bottom with a long _____.

3. Three different types of pipettes include _____, _____, and _____.

4. Most microscope work in the laboratory is done by the _____ or by the _____.

5. If an ocular lens is 10X magnification, and an oil immersion lens is 100X, the total magnification is _____X.

6. Three types of microscopes that could be used in the clinical laboratory are _____, _____, and _____.

7. The main use of the centrifuge is to separate _____ from _____ and _____.

8. When a laboratory assistant runs tests on automated equipment, the results must be reviewed by a _____ before they can be reported.

9. The department in the clinical laboratory that produces the most test results is the _____ department.

10. _____ _____ _____ make the job of counting cells much easier for laboratory employees.

Circle T for true, or F for false.

11. T F   A test tube and a centrifuge tube are shaped the same way.

12. T F   Beakers are used for critical measurements.

13. T F   The fluorescent microscope is often used in the microbiology department.

14. T F   Clinical laboratory assistants never run automated equipment.

15. T F   Centrifuges can be refrigerated.

16. T F   A compound microscope has two lens systems that work together.

17. T F   The light source in a compound microscope is generally found in the base of the instrument.

18. T F   Centrifuges can be dangerous to operate if not handled properly.

19. T F   The meniscus refers to the analytical balance.

20. T F   You never pipette anything by mouth.

Match the term in Column A with the appropriate description in Column B.

Column A

21. ___ balance

22. ___ centrifuge

23. ___ electron microscope

24. ___ volumetric flask

25. ___ beaker

Column B

A. measures exact volumes

B. general container

C. weighs substances

D. uses shortwave electrons

E. separates blood from plasma and serum

Chapter Nineteen
Measurements and Calculations

Objectives

After completing this chapter, you should be able to
do the following:

1. Define and correctly spell each of the key terms.

2. Name basic metric units and prefixes.

3. Convert English units to metric units, and metric units into
    English units.

4. Convert Fahrenheit temperatures to Centigrade and
    vice versa.

5. Discuss the difference between the 24-hour clock (military
    time) and Greenwich mean time.

6. Identify how to perform ratio, proportion, and percentage
    solution calculations.

Key Terms

- Celsius
- diluent
- English system
- Fahrenheit
- gram

- liter
- meter
- metric system
- percentage solutions
- ratio

Introduction

The clinical laboratory assistant/phlebotomist does not have to be a mathematics wizard to perform his or her job well. However, a proficiency in addition, subtraction, division, and multiplication is helpful in order to understand the systems of measurement, the terminology used, and the calculations often encountered in the clinical laboratory. The clinical laboratory assistant must also understand temperature measurement and the use of military time in the healthcare setting.

Calculating how much specimen to collect from a patient, measuring how much preservative to put in a collection container, preparing reagents for running tests, and diluting specimens are examples of calculations that a clinical laboratory assistant/phlebotomist might perform.

The Metric System

In the United States when we are asked to measure something, most of us think in terms of the **English system** of measurements. The English system is based on arbitrary body dimensions, with mathematical relationships that are often confusing. However, the **metric system** of measurement is used by over 90% of the world. Science and medicine have consistently used the metric system for measurement.

Clinical laboratory results are always reported in metric units, with all calculations solved using the metric system. In this chapter, the metric units of length (**meter**), weight (**gram**), and volume (**liter**) will be used. There are also metric units for electrical current, intensity of light, and spacial dimension, but they are not used as frequently in the clinical laboratory, and they are not used by the clinical laboratory assistant.

Metric Prefixes

The metric prefixes are added to the front of one of the basic units (meters, grams, liters) to indicate the size of the particular metric unit. The example below uses the liter unit, but meters and grams could be used as well. Examples include kilometer, kilogram, hectometer, hectogram, and so on.

Prefix	Multiple	Example
kilo-	1,000	1 kiloliter = 1000 liters
hecto-	100	1 hectoliter = 100 liters
deca-	10	1 decaliter = 10 liters
deci-	1/10	1 deciliter = 1/10 of a liter
centi-	1/100	1 centiliter = 1/100 of a liter
milli-	1/1000	1 milliliter = 1/1000 of a liter
micro-	1/1,000,000	1 microliter = 1/1,000,000 of a liter

Metric Units

The gram (abbreviated gm) is the metric unit of measurement used to measure weight or mass. **Mass** is the physical measurement of how much an object weighs, regardless of the gravity exerted on the object. **Weight** is the physical measure of an object depending on the physical force of gravity. When measuring within the earth's gravitational field, scientists consider mass and weight the same. Milligrams and grams are used frequently in laboratory calculations. (In the English system, mass or weight is measured in ounces and pounds.)

The liter is a metric measurement of liquid **volume**. Solid volumes are measured as cubic meters. As with mass or weight, milligrams and grams are used frequently in laboratory calculations. (In the English system, volume is measured in cups, pints, quarts, and gallons.)

The meter is the metric unit for linear measurement (length). It is slightly longer than a yard. Millimeters and centimeters are used often in clinical laboratory measurements. Micrometers are used for microscopic measurement. (In the English system, length is measured in inches, feet, yards, and miles.)

The basic metric measures are shown below.

Metric Term	Abbreviation	Measures
gram	g, gm, or Gm	weight or mass
liter	l	volume
meter	m	length

Converting Measurement Systems

In addition to scientific use, the metric system is being used in industry, governmental agencies, education, and many other important areas in the United States. You may be asked to convert the English system of measurements to metric, or possibly even to convert the metric system to the English system. The simplest way is to use a conversion table. The following are two tables with conversion factors for converting the English system to metric and vice versa.

Converting the English System to the Metric System		
English Unit	**Multiply by**	**To Get Metric Unit**
1 pound	0.454	kilograms (kg)
1 pound	454	grams (gr)
1 ounce	28	grams
1 quart	0.95	liters (l)
1 teaspoon	5	milliliters (ml)
1 gallon	3.78	liters
1 inch	2.54	centimeters (cm)
1 foot	0.3048	meters (m)
1 yard	0.9	meters
1 mile	1.6	kilometers (km)

Example: 4 pounds = ? kilograms   4 pounds X 0.454 = 1.816 kilograms

6 ounces = ? grams   6 ounces X 28 = 168 grams

Converting the Metric System to the English System		
Metric Unit	**Multiply by**	**To Get English Unit**
1 gram	0.0022	pounds (lb)
1 kilogram	2.2	pounds
1 milliliter	0.03	fluid ounces (fl oz)
1 liter	1.06	quarts (qt)
1 millimeter	0.04	inches (in)
1 centimeter	0.4	inches
1 meter	39.37	inches
1 meter	3.3	feet (ft)
1 kilometer	0.6	miles

Example: 2 grams = ? pounds   2 grams X 0.002 = .004 pounds

1 liter = ? quarts   1 liter X 1.06 = 1.06 quarts

Measuring Temperature

Two different temperature scales may be used in the healthcare facility. The **Fahrenheit (F)** scale is used to measure body temperature. The **Celsius (C)** scale (also known as the centigrade scale) is also used to measure body temperature as well as temperature ranges of certain equipment in the clinical laboratory.

The freezing point of water in the Celsius system is $0°$, and the boiling point is $100°$. The Fahrenheit scale is based on a system that is less logical and often more cumbersome to use. The freezing point of water on this scale is $32°$, and the boiling point is $212°$.

Most facilities have conversion charts that can be used to change quickly from one scale to another. However, if a conversion chart is not available, it will be helpful for you to know how conversions from one scale to another are done.

Fahrenheit: a temperature scale used in medicine that uses $212°$ as the boiling point of water and $32°$ as the freezing point of water.

Celsius: a temperature scale used in medicine, that uses $100°$ as the boiling point of water and $0°$ as the freezing point of water.

Converting Fahrenheit to Celsius Temperatures

Formula: $C = {}^5/_9 (F - 32)$

Calculation: $F = 98.6°$
$C = {}^5/_9 (98.6 - 32)$
$C = {}^5/_9 (66.6)$
$C = 37°$

Converting Celsius to Fahrenheit Temperatures

Formula: $F = {}^9/_5 (C) + 32$

Calculation: $C = 37°$
$F = {}^9/_5 (37) + 32$
$F = 66.6 + 32$
$F = 98.6°$

The 24-Hour Clock

In the healthcare setting, time is stated in an accurate, concise manner. A time orientation is mandatory for laboratory employees because of the many timed tests that require the laboratory assistant to arrive at a precise time for a blood draw. Physicians will require results by a certain time, especially STAT results.

A clear, concise means of recording time is essential. The **Greenwich system** of time (the one commonly used in homes) has the disadvantage of having twelve of its hours written identically, except for the a.m. and p.m. designations. In contrast, **military time** designates every hour as its own numerical time. For example, the confusion some may have as to whether a noted time is 6:00 a.m. or 6:00 p.m. is nonexistent in military time; those same hours are written as 0600 and 1800 hours. Military time is always expressed in four digits; no colons separate hours from minutes. An "0" is always placed in front of a three-digit number; eg, instead of 200, 2:00 is expressed as 0200. The following table illustrates the conversion from Greenwich to military time.

Conversion of Greenwich Time to Military Time			
Greenwich	**Military**	**Greenwich**	**Military**
1:00 a.m.	0100	1:00 p.m.	1300
2:00 a.m.	0200	2:00 p.m.	1400
3:00 a.m.	0300	3:00 p.m.	1500
4:00 a.m.	0400	4:00 p.m.	1600
5:00 a.m.	0500	5:00 p.m.	1700
6:00 a.m.	0600	6:00 p.m.	1800
7:00 a.m.	0700	7:00 p.m.	1900
8:00 a.m.	0800	8:00 p.m.	2000
9:00 a.m.	0900	9:00 p.m.	2100
10:00 a.m.	1000	10:00 p.m.	2200
11:00 a.m.	1100	11:00 p.m.	2300
12:00 noon	1200	12:00 midnight	2400

Study the clock in Figure 19-1 to make sure you understand the difference between the two times. You will need to become comfortable with using military time.

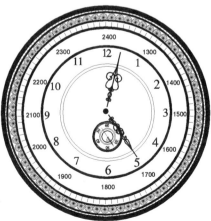

Figure 19-1: A Military Time Clock

Using Basic Mathematics for Clinical Laboratory Procedures

In today's computerized world, you may not have to perform simple mathematical calculations at all in the role of clinical laboratory assistant/phlebotomist. However, some healthcare facilities still require some simple calculations to be performed; therefore it is important for you to have a basic understanding of some simple laboratory calculations, even if it is only to understand what the computer has done automatically for you. Appendix D in the back of this textbook includes some common formulas and calculations used in the clinical laboratory.

Ratios

A **ratio** is the relationship between two substances relating to degree and number. Dilutions are expressed as ratios. For instance, if you dilute blood with a saline solution, the dilution expresses the ratio between the blood and saline. In the clinical laboratory, you might have to dilute a blood specimen if something being tested in the blood is so high that it cannot be read on an instrument. In order to get an accurate reading, you would have to dilute the blood and multiply the result by the dilution to get the final result.

If a procedure requires a dilution of reagent or blood, it will specify the proper ratio to achieve. For example, the problem below requires a 1:50 dilution of serum and saline. The serum is called the specimen and the saline the **diluent**.

Ratio/Dilution Problem

Given: Prepare 50 ml (milliliters) of a 1:50 dilution of serum and saline.
To Solve: A 1:50 dilution has 50 parts total. So you would need 1 part of serum and 49 parts of saline to prepare a 1:50 dilution.

You need 50 ml, so you prepare 1 ml of serum and 49 ml of saline. If you were to prepare 25 ml of a 1:50 ratio, you would take 0.5 ml of serum and 24.5 ml of saline.

ratio:
a relationship between two substances in degree or number.

diluent:
an agent that dilutes a substance or solution to which it is added.

Percentages

A ratio may be expressed as a percentage. Percent means *per 100* and is represented by the symbol %. Two values are involved when a number is expressed as a percent, the number itself and 100. For example, 50% means 50 per 100 or 50 parts in a total of 100 parts.

> **Example:**
> A 50% sale would mean that you would buy everything at $1/2$ of the original price.

To change a fraction to a percent, multiply by 100 and add a percent sign to the result.

> **Example:**
> What percent is 1/5?
> 1/5 X 100/1 = 100/5 = 20%.

percentage solutions: the percentage strength of some clinical laboratory solutions expressed in parts per 100.

Percentage solutions of many reagents are expressed in terms of parts per hundred. When dissolving solids in liquids (usually distilled water for reagent preparation, saline for blood preparations), you use a **weight to volume percentage**. When you mix two liquids together, you use a **volume to volume percentage**. For example, adding acid solution to water is a volume to volume solution.

Weight To Volume Calculation

> Given: Prepare 100 ml of 0.85 percent saline.
> To Solve: A 0.85 percent solution means that for every 100 ml of distilled water, there is 0.85 percent saline.
>
> Therefore, you need to add 0.85 grams of saline to 100 ml of distilled water. You do this by putting about 50 ml of distilled water into a volumetric flask, adding 0.85 grams of salt, mixing gently, and adding distilled water to fill the flask to 100 ml.

Volume to Volume Calculation

Given: Prepare 300 ml of 5 % acetic acid, using concentrated acetic acid.
To Solve: A 5% acetic acid solution contains 5 ml of acid in 100 ml of distilled water.

To prepare 300 ml of 5% acetic acid from a concentrated (100%) acid solution, you must add 15 ml of concentrated acid to 300 ml of distilled water. Remember that YOU MUST ADD ACID TO WATER, AND NOT WATER TO ACID. Adding water to acid can result in acid burns.

Proportions

Proportions are often used when combining reagents. A formula for combining reagents might call for 3 parts of substance A to be combined with 1 part of substance B to produce solution C. Study the following problem and the formula used to solve it.

Proportions Calculation

Given: A reagent is being prepared to do a bilirubin test. You need 3 parts of solution A and 1 part of solution B to make solution C. It is necessary to make 40 ml of solution C. How much of solutions A and B would you need to make solution C?

The formula: $^C/_{A+B} = V$

C = Volume of final solution   B = Total parts of solution B
A = Total parts of solution A   V = Volume of one part

To Solve: $\dfrac{40 \text{ ml of solution}}{3 \text{ parts A and 1 part B}}$ = volume of one part

$^{40}/_4 = 10$ ml = volume of one part

3 parts A = 3 X 10 ml = 30 ml
1 part B = 1 X 10 ml = 10 ml

You would combine 30 ml of solution A and 10 ml of solution B to make 40 ml of solution C.

Chapter Summary

As a clinical laboratory assistant/phlebotomist, you will be required to understand and use the metric system. You may be asked to convert Fahrenheit temperatures to Celsius temperatures. Most temperature measurements are expressed in Celsius units in the clinical laboratory. You must also use military time with ease, as that is the system of timekeeping used in most healthcare facilities.

Some facilities may not require you to do any laboratory math calculations; others may ask you to perform simple calculations. Also, you may have to answer simple ratio, percentage, and proportion problems when taking examinations to qualify for various certifications and sometimes for government jobs.

Careless errors in laboratory calculations can lead to serious consequences for a patient. Care must always be taken to ensure that you are accurate with all calculations.

Name _____

Date _____

Student Enrichment Activities

Complete the following exercises.

1. Define each of the following fundamental units of the metric system:

   A. gram: _____

   B. liter: _____

   C. meter: _____

2. Clinical laboratory results are always reported in _____ units.

3. What is the difference between weight and mass? _____

   _____

   _____

4. The most common measurement conversion in the clinical laboratory is from the

   _____ system to the _____ system of measurement.

5. A yard is _____ (longer, shorter) than a meter.

6. Which measurement is larger?

   A. a foot or a meter? _____

   B. an ounce or a gram? _____

   C. a pound or a kilogram? _____

   D. a quart or a liter? _____

   E. a mile or a kilometer? _____

   F. a liter or a quart? _____

7. What measurement is smaller?

    A. a kilogram or a milligram?_____

    B. a milliliter or a microliter?_____

    C. a milligram or a centigram?_____

    D. a micrometer or a hectometer?_____

    E. a decameter or a decimeter?_____

8. How many meters are in 10 yards?_____

9. How many liters are in 100 quarts?_____

10. How many quarts are in 25 liters?_____

11. You are asked to prepare 20 milliliters of a 1:20 dilution of serum and saline.

    How many parts of serum would you need?_____ml

    How many parts of saline?_____ml

12. In a 1:20 dilution of serum and saline, which one is the diluent?_____

13. Change the following fractions into a percentage.

    A. $^1/_4$ = _____%

    B. $^1/_3$ = _____%

    C. $^2/_5$ = _____%

14. In order to prepare a 400 ml solution of 5% acetic acid, using concentrated acetic acid, how much concentrated acid would you add to 400 ml of distilled water?
    _____ ml

15. Janey is making a reagent. She needs 2 parts of solution A and 3 parts of solution B to make 100 ml of solution C. How many ml of A will be needed? _____ml. How many ml of solution B?_____

Name _____

Date _____

Circle T for true, or F for false.

16.   T   F   The English system is the most commonly used measuring system in
the world.

17.   T   F   The most commonly used temperature scale in the clinical laboratory is
the Celsius scale.

18.   T   F   The Celsius scale is also known as the centigrade scale.

19.   T   F   The Fahrenheit scale is based on an arbitrary scale and is more
cumbersome to use than the Celsius scale.

20.   T   F   1:00 p.m. in Greenwich time is 1300 in military time.

21.   T   F   0300 in military time is 3:00 p.m. in Greenwich time.

22.   T   F   12:00 midnight in Greenwich time is 2400 in military time.

23.   T   F   9:00 p.m. in Greenwich time is 2100 in military time.

24.   T   F   1900 is 8:00 p.m. in Greenwich time.

25.   T   F   4:30 p.m. is 1630 in military time.

Chapter Twenty
Reception and Telephone Technique

Objectives

After completing this chapter, you should be able to
do the following:

1. Define and correctly spell each of the key terms.

2. Explain why a clinical laboratory assistant/phlebotomist
    might use clerical skills while carrying out laboratory
    assistant duties.

3. Discuss how the clinical laboratory assistant can make a
    patient feel comfortable while waiting for a blood test.

4. Identify the proper way to greet a patient.

5. Discuss the role of empathy and listening skills for the clinical
    laboratory assistant.

6. Describe some ways to overcome a language barrier
    with a patient.

7. Explain the importance of registration forms and laboratory test
    requisitions when dealing with patients in an outpatient setting.

8. Describe a pleasant, comfortable reception area in which a
    patient can wait for a blood test.

9. Describe the basics of telephone etiquette in the
    professional setting.

Key Terms

- empathy
- laboratory requisition form

- oncology
- satellite blood drawing station

Introduction

Due to the budget cutbacks that are facing every aspect of the healthcare environment, many patients who formerly would have been admitted to the hospital for procedures are now having the same procedures done on an **outpatient** basis. Most clinical laboratories have had to expand their outpatient blood drawing stations to meet the need for more tests ordered on outpatients. Many larger health facilities have established **satellite blood drawing stations** in physician office complexes, in downtown center locations, and even as separate entities within a healthcare facility (such as dialysis units). This expansion often finds the clinical laboratory assistant/phlebotomist being the only employee in such a station, with many clerical responsibilities in addition to drawing blood.

satellite blood drawing station: an area separate from the clinical laboratory where specimens are collected and transported to the main clinical laboratory for testing.

This chapter focuses on some skills necessary for the clinical laboratory assistant/phlebotomist who may be the only person the patient sees when having blood drawn. Additionally, becoming familiar with some basic medical clerical skills can make you more valuable to the clinical laboratory itself. For instance, what if your facility is making cutbacks, and your job as a laboratory assistant is in jeopardy? At the same time, there could be a shortage of laboratory clerical workers. If you have gotten training that will qualify you to do clerical work, you can work in the laboratory in that capacity until you are needed once again for laboratory assistant duties. In this case, cross-training makes it possible for you to stay employed. You can also impress your laboratory manager and assist the laboratory clerical staff by helping with the telephones during a time when you are not busy, and they are overwhelmed with tasks. To sum up, laboratory employees should work as a team, helping each other whenever possible.

Medical Reception Techniques

The clinical laboratory assistant/phlebotomist is often the only representative of the clinical laboratory that the patient will encounter. If the patient's impression of the laboratory assistant is poor, the chances are that the patient will have some reservations about the laboratory as well. So creating a good first impression is very important. It is equally important to make the patient feel welcomed and relaxed about coming to the facility to have blood drawn. Remember, there is much competition in the healthcare industry. If you do not make the patient feel comfortable, there are other places for the patient to get blood drawn that may be more welcoming.

Receiving the Patient

At certain times of the day, several patients may arrive at the same time; further, they may all want to have their blood drawn as soon as possible. Often, you may open a drawing facility in the morning and be greeted by "early birds" who want their test drawn right away. They want to stop fasting and have breakfast. Around noon, you may find your facility crowded with working people who hope to get their blood drawn on their lunch hour. Late in the day, people may come to have their blood drawn after work.

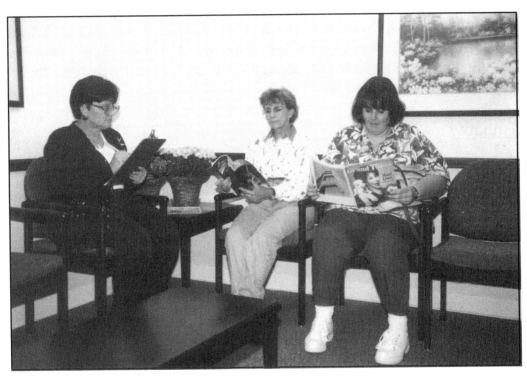

Figure 20-1: Several patients wait in an outpatient facility to have their blood drawn.

So, patients often arrive at the same time, and it is important that every patient be greeted when he or she arrives. Patients may be asked to sign in or put their papers in a certain area. They will be aware of the order in which they arrived and most likely will be vocal if they are not called in that same order.

The Initial Greeting

It is best for patients to be greeted as soon as they arrive. Although you may be in a hurry, your voice should convey warmth and friendliness as you greet patients with a "Good morning, Mrs. Baker. As you can see, I have several patients, but I will make sure you get service as soon as possible." Patients especially appreciate it if you remember their name from your last encounter. It is even better if you can include a personal touch such as "How is that new grandson of yours, Mrs. Jones?" or "How is that garden growing, Mr. Peters?" Address each patient with a title (Mr., Mrs., Miss, or Ms.) except for children or teenagers. If patients asks you to call them by their first name, you can do so. However, many adults resent being greeted by their first name by someone they do not know.

Be alert to the state of mind of your patients. Many people will not be feeling well. They may be in pain and anxious about what their doctor just told them. Some patients may arrive with STAT orders, and they will have to be seen before people who have been waiting longer. Explain to the other patients that this blood draw has been ordered STAT and that you are required to draw the blood right away.

Empathy

empathy:
to understand and relate to the emotional state of another; to show concern.

As you receive patients who are obviously stressed and perhaps in great pain, show them that you have **empathy** for their pain and will be with them as soon as you can. You may think that you are being sympathetic by sounding that way, but your body language may be telling the patient something different. If you are in a hurry, you may not feel like hearing about Mrs. Little's terrible gas pains and her ungrateful daughter. Your facial expression and your hurried manner may tell the patient quite a bit about the way you really feel. Mrs. Little may sense that you are really not interested in her problems at all. Understanding different forms of communication will be discussed further in Chapter Twenty-Three.

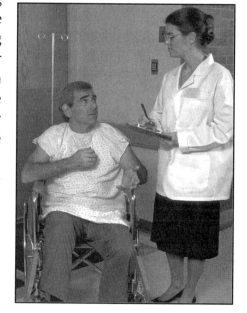

Figure 20-2: A clinical laboratory assistant/phlebotomist listens carefully to a patient in pain.

Thinking It Through ...

Maggie is in charge of a large satellite drawing station connected with General Hospital. On a busy day, Maggie can see more than 100 patients at her station for blood draws. There are two large **oncology** practices near the drawing station, and many cancer patients are sent to Maggie each day for blood draws to monitor their chemotherapy treatments. Mrs. Lyman is a frequent patient whom Maggie knows well.

On Monday, Maggie is swamped with customers. Mrs. Lyman comes in for a blood draw, having just received news from her doctor that her cancer has returned. Of course, Mrs. Lyman is very upset. Her family lives far away, and she lives alone, having been recently widowed. She feels the need to talk to someone about her news. She knows Maggie is a sympathetic listener and wishes to linger to talk with her after the blood draw. Maggie has no time for this interaction.

1. What does Maggie tell Mrs. Lyman when she begins to cry while telling Maggie her news?

2. How does Maggie extend kindness to this woman while serving other patients as well?

oncology: the area of medicine concerned with the diagnosis and treatment of tumors.

Listening Skills

You must develop excellent listening skills when you work as closely with patients as the clinical laboratory assistant/phlebotomist frequently does. Patients often will want to tell you where the last blood was drawn successfully. They may also have a special way they wish to have the tourniquet applied, or they may not want the type of tape you use because it causes a rash. They may just want a little sympathy from you. Listen to and respect their requests.

Because of the hurried nature of the laboratory environment, it is hard to be a good listener, as clearly illustrated in this chapter's *Thinking It Through*. Chapter Twenty-three discusses in more detail how you can improve your listening skills. This will give patients the feeling that they are not being interrupted and that you are truly hearing them.

Language Barriers

As our society becomes more culturally diverse, you will encounter patients who do not speak English. Some facilities have bilingual laboratory assistants who may be asked to draw a patient with whom you cannot communicate. But, in some parts of the country, such as California and New York, there are people of many nationalities. As a result, the chances are that no one at the facility will be able to communicate clearly with some patients. Often the patient will bring a family member who can translate. If not, there are some tips to use if you do not speak a patient's language.

1. Be patient and unhurried.

2. Listen carefully and sympathetically without interrupting.

3. Try to pick up a few words that might give a clue to the total message. With languages similar to English, this is not too hard. However, with languages such as Asian languages, you may not recognize any words.

4. Find out if there are other languages you both might know. Many foreigners, especially Europeans, know several languages. You might get to use your high school French after all!

5. Use body language because the face, voice tone, and hands can express a great deal.

6. Speak slowly and clearly, using short sentences. Do not use technical language.

7. Use drawings and magazine pictures to illustrate key concepts when necessary.

8. Remember not to shout. This does not help communication.

9. Smile as much as possible to help put the patient at ease.

Confused people who may be on medication or who have a form of dementia also present challenges in communication. You may ask the patient to be seated and to wait, but he or she may not understand why waiting is necessary and may become difficult. Hopefully, you can call upon a relative or friend who is accompanying the patient to help explain what is going to happen at this station. Children may also not understand why the wait is necessary. Again, you must communicate carefully and clearly, not being impatient or talking too rapidly.

Registration

Often in an outpatient facility, patient registration is accomplished before the patient comes to you to have blood drawn. However, in smaller blood drawing stations that are removed from the large healthcare facility, you may be in charge of registering the patients. Sometimes during the evening shifts when clerical help is not available, you may also have to register outpatients who are seen after regular hours. Registration techniques vary among facilities. However, some aspects of the process are fairly constant:

- Make sure patients receive registration forms as soon as they enter the facility. You do not want the process delayed by waiting for patients to fill out forms after they have already been waiting. Filling out the forms also gives patients something to do while they are waiting.

- It is ALWAYS necessary for patients to fill out the forms as completely as possible. Minimum acceptable information on such a form usually includes the patient's full name, address, telephone number, birth date, sex, marital status, occupation, name and address of employer, Social Security number, telephone number of person responsible for payment, health insurance policy numbers, name, address and telephone number of the nearest relative or friend.

- After the registration form is filled out, make sure that it is complete. If you have problems communicating with the patient, ask an accompanying friend or relative to help. If no one is with the patient, you might have to call the patient's physician for the information you need.

NEW PATIENT
REGISTRATION FORM

Since this is the first time you have been to City Medical Center we would like to make sure that we enter the correct information into our computer. Please take a moment to complete the following questions.

Patient Name _____

Birth Date _____ Maiden/Other Name _____

Street Address _____

Home Phone _____ Marital Status _____

Social Security number _____ Religion _____

Employer _____ Occupation _____

Next of Kin _____ Home Phone _____

Work Phone _____

Relation to Pt. _____

Person to Notify _____ Home Phone _____

Work Phone _____

Relation to Pt. _____

Who is responsible for payment of bill? _____

_____ Patient? We can use information provided above.

_____ Other? Enter name and address below.

_____

_____

_____

_____

Relation to Pt. _____

Language spoken by patient _____

Is this related to an auto accident? _____ If so, please give date _____

Figure 20-3: A Patient Registration Form

Laboratory Test Requisitions

Along with a properly filled out registration form, you will also need a **laboratory requisition form** from the patient's physician. Often patients will come into a drawing area and request a test that they have done weekly. If there are no standing orders on file or if the physician has not given the patient a requisition, you must contact the physician before drawing blood. Many "regulars" have standing orders on file, which should be filed nearby for your easy access. Remember: if there is no requisition, there can be no blood draw.

laboratory requisition form: a form filled out by physicians or nurses to order clinical laboratory tests.

The Reception Room

The area where patients wait for service in a medical facility should be pleasant, well-lit, and comfortable. In a satellite blood drawing station, you may have a reception area that is cleaned on a nightly basis by a building maintenance crew. However, throughout the day you should be aware of the reception area to make sure that the space is uncluttered. People much prefer to wait in an area that is not littered with torn magazines, candy wrappers, soft drink cans, newspapers, and other debris.

The following are ideas that can help create a pleasant environment for waiting patients:

- Straighten the reception area several times a day, rearranging magazines, adjusting lighting, and so forth. Patients often rearrange chairs; so return furniture to its original location for maximum use of the room's space.

- Place a "Thank You For Not Smoking" sign in full view of the waiting patients. Even though the facility may be a nonsmoking facility, people may still be tempted to smoke.

- Make sure that the temperature is approximately 70° F at all times.

- Magazines should have vinyl covers to prevent soiling and tearing. Make sure that some up-to-date magazines are available for your patients.

- If your station has a significant number of children as patients, set aside a corner for children with a small table and chairs, children's books in good condition, and a few toys that can be washed easily and played with quietly. Make sure that safety caps are installed in all electrical outlets.

- Music at a low volume can soothe patients. Radio stations are generally not recommended.

- Office furniture should be cleaned frequently and replaced if needed.

- The walls should be clean and mar-free. Subtle wallpaper is often a nice addition to a reception room. Soft colors such as blues and warm browns are preferable to loud colors that can make patients uneasy.

- Wall decor can include pastoral scenes or other pictures that make the patients feel welcome and relaxed. Some waiting areas include a small television and a well-kept aquarium.

Communicating on the Telephone

Anyone who works in some aspect of the healthcare environment can tell you that the telephone is a critical part of the medical world. Developing good telephone communication skills is essential for most healthcare workers, including the clinical laboratory assistant.

Telephone Etiquette

When you communicate on the telephone at work, you may be speaking to a nurse who wants you to draw blood immediately. A patient might want information about your drawing station. A physician wants to give you a verbal order for a blood test, or a fellow employee needs your help immediately. Speak as you would in a face-to-face encounter. The person on the other end should get the impression that you are glad to accept the call and that any needs that are being expressed will be acted upon with efficiency and care. Avoid excess conversation. The following are hints to improve your delivery over the telephone:

- Speak in a regular voice, not too loud or too soft, keeping the mouthpiece about one inch from your lips.

- Speak distinctly and clearly. Patients may be on medication, hearing-impaired, or limited in their English proficiency.

- Concentrate specifically on the call. Do not try to do several other things while speaking to the caller.

- Avoid a monotone voice pattern. Be expressive in your speech, but avoid excessive drama.

- Be polite to the caller even if you are hurried, and the call is an inconvenience.

- Avoid being flippant and casual. You are a professional, and your language should be reflective of that role.

- Give feedback so that the caller is confident that you received the message.

- Answer the telephone promptly on the second ring.

- Answer the telephone by giving the name of the department and your name. An example: "Clinical laboratory, this is Jake Martin speaking." You may get slightly different instructions from your employer about how to answer the telephone.

Taking a Message

As a clinical laboratory assistant, you may take messages that are detailed and important. Do not rely on your memory to remember all the tests that a physician just ordered or the address of a location where a blood test should be sent. To avoid any omissions or inaccuracies, always have a pad and pencil nearby to take a message immediately. Also, a preprinted message pad can be invaluable to separate messages and make sure all information is taken (Figure 20-4).

```
                    WHILE YOU WERE OUT

  ☐ URGENT


  FOR: _____     DATE: _____
  FROM: _____    OF: _____
  PHONE: (      ) _____   (EXT.) _____   ☐ RETURN
                                                     CALL


  ☐ REQUESTS YOU CALL BEFORE/AFTER    _____  A.M., P.M.
  ☐ WILL CALL              CALLED AT  _____  A.M., P.M.
     AGAIN           CAME TO SEE YOU  _____  A.M., P.M.

  MESSAGE _____
  _____
  _____
  _____
  _____
  _____
  _____

  PERSON TAKING MESSAGE: _____
```

Figure 20-4: A Preprinted Telephone Message Pad

The Hold Button

Imagine that you are answering telephones to help out the laboratory clerical staff during a very busy lunchtime. You get three calls at once, putting two on hold. Try not to keep the callers on hold for more than 60 seconds without checking to see if they wish to remain on hold. Be sure to thank them for holding. If the callers do not want to wait, take their name and telephone number and tell them that you will get right back to them right away. If a call is from someone in your facility, ask the caller if he or she wants to do one of the following:

- Continue to hold.
- Call back.
- Leave a message.

Telephone Equipment

Telephones in the healthcare environment are becoming more and more sophisticated. The choice of telephone system depends on the type of facility, its size and complexity of the office, and the type of calls most frequently received and placed. If you are going to be answering the telephone or making calls in the laboratory, make sure that you are familiar with the system that the clinical laboratory or drawing station uses. Chapter Twenty-one goes into more detail about telephone systems in the healthcare facility.

Chapter Summary

Whether you are working in a satellite blood drawing station or in a healthcare facility taking blood from outpatients as a clinical laboratory assistant/phlebotomist, you will be involved with greeting the patients. In many cases, you may be the only person with whom patients interact in the clinical laboratory. So, even though you may be taking a telephone message or getting registration information, it is your responsibility to perform the best service for the patients. Greet them with a welcome when they arrive, and make them comfortable while they are waiting.

Name _____

Date _____

Student Enrichment Activities

Circle T for true, or F for false.

1. T   F   You should try not to keep a caller on hold for more than 90 seconds.

2. T   F   Loud colors in a reception area do not always make patients relax.

3. T   F   Smoking is not allowed in the reception area of a blood drawing station.

4. T   F   A temperature of 75° F is best for patients in a healthcare facility.

5. T   F   It is permissible to call patients by their first names as soon as you meet them.

6. T   F   Speaking slowly helps a limited English-speaking patient understand you better.

7. T   F   Speaking loudly helps a limited English-speaking patient understand you better.

8. T   F   Keep the telephone mouthpiece about 1 inch from your lips when talking on the telephone.

9. T   F   Using slang expressions while talking to patients on the telephone puts them at ease.

10. T   F   Your body language can give a completely different message to a patient than does your spoken word.

Complete the following statements.

11. An _____ practice deals with cancer patients.

12. Two times when an outpatient blood drawing facility could be very busy are during _____ and _____.

13. _____ is the ability to feel sympathetic to the pain of others.

14. _____ is one of the best ways to find out what a patient really feels.

15. A registration form and a _____ _____ _____ are the two documents that the laboratory assistant often needs before drawing blood on the outpatient.

Chapter Twenty-One
The Computer System and Other Office Machines

Objectives

After completing this chapter, you should be able to
do the following:

1. Define and correctly spell each of the key terms.

2. Describe some uses for the computer in the clinical laboratory.

3. Identify terms associated with the computer and its operation.

4. Explain the three types of computers.

5. Identify components of a computer system.

6. List several operations that a computer system can perform in the clinical laboratory.

7. Discuss the use of a fax, a photocopier, and a multibutton telephone system in the clinical laboratory.

Key Terms

- backup
- cathode ray tube
- central processing unit
- facsimile (fax) machine
- floppy disk
- hard copy

- hard disk
- hardware
- mainframe
- microcomputer
- minicomputer
- software

Introduction

One of the most important methods of communication in the healthcare facility today is the computer. Computers are connected throughout the hospital so that departments can communicate with each other. Physicians have computers that automatically receive results of tests from the clinical laboratory. The computer can print labels for specimens, automatically produce billing reports, assemble worksheets for lab employees to organize their work, produce appointment schedules, and perform many other tasks that help make the laboratory function in a timely manner.

It has never been more critical for ALL healthcare professionals to understand how to work with the computer while performing their jobs. Therefore, keyboard skills are mandatory. Anyone who does not know how to type should enroll in a course to learn or to improve upon his or her typing skills.

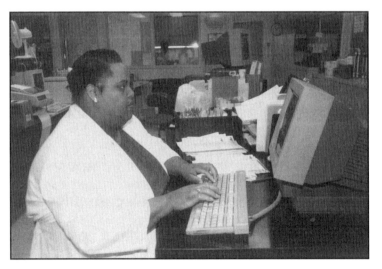

Figure 21-1: Clinical laboratory assistants have a great advantage if they have computer skills before becoming employed by a laboratory.

In addition to the computer, there are other machines in the front office of a clinical laboratory that you may have to operate on occasion. Satellite drawing stations may have equipment that you may be assigned to use, such as fax machines for sending and receiving information from physicians, copy machines to duplicate patient insurance information, and multibutton key telephones that receive several calls at once. Being familiar with office machines commonly used in healthcare facilities can make you a more flexible employee who can assist and even substitute for clerical workers when needed.

The Computer in the Healthcare Facility

Computers can be intimidating to anyone who has not had exposure to them. The healthcare industry today is fully computerized, and workers cannot afford to be overcome with computer fear. Computers DO make your job much easier and more efficient.

The uses of computers in healthcare are endless. Physicians use computers to keep track of patient information and charges, and to assist them in making diagnoses. Physicians can also send insurance information directly to insurance companies and have claims paid much faster without depending on the mail. Further, special programs allow the physician to enter symptoms of a puzzling illness in the computer and to receive a list of possibilities for diagnosis.

Usually, the clinical laboratory has computer terminals located in all departments (sometimes several in each department), in drawing stations, in the clerical area, and in managers' offices. Automated analyzers will often send results directly to computers after the lab employee has checked over the results for any errors. Most employees in the clinical laboratory will be assigned computer tasks daily.

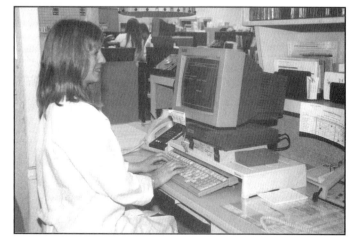

Figure 21-2: A computer can help keep track of patient information and can assist in a variety of other tasks as well.

When using computer systems, the clinical laboratory assistant/phlebotomist must always remember the importance of ethics and confidentiality. The computer, like medical records in the healthcare facility, contains **privileged information** that must be respected and protected.

Thinking It Through ...

Roseanne has always wanted to work in the medical field. She is delighted to take part in a training program to become a clinical laboratory assistant/phlebotomist. She really wants to work with patients, and she plans to become a nurse someday when her children are much older. Meanwhile, she just loves the patient contact of her new job as laboratory assistant.

However, Roseanne has one big problem: she hates computers. She has never felt that computers improved our society. She doesn't seem to be able to understand them at all, and her husband confirms this opinion. She hates it when her sons sit in front of her husband's computer and cut themselves off from the world. She has no keyboard skills ("I didn't want to be a secretary, so I didn't take typing"), and when she's at work she resents the time she must spend on the computer when she could be with patients. She feels that someone else who really enjoys computers and doesn't like the patients as well as she does should do the computer entry work, and she'll stick to the patients. What should Roseanne do?

1. Does Roseanne have any options here that could take her away from computer responsibilities?

2. Where might Roseanne have gotten her computer fears?

3. As a nurse, can Roseanne avoid computers?

Computer Terms

As in healthcare with its specific terminology, the computer world has its own unique language. In order to understand the computer and its multitude of functions, you should be familiar with many of the terms used frequently in conjunction with computers. Below is a brief glossary of the most common terms to which you may be exposed when using computers.

Commonly Used Computer Terms

backup: the duplication of files made to protect information; often done on a computer once or twice a day.

boot: to start up a computer.

CPU: central processing unit; the brains of the computer system.

CRT: cathode ray tube; a visual display unit with a screen that is connected to a computer.

cursor: a marker on the screen showing where the next letter, number, or symbol will be placed; can be a blinking underline, rectangle, or square.

disk: a magnetic storage device made of rigid material (**hard disk**) or flexible plastic (**floppy disk**).

disk drive: a device used to get information on and off a disk.

DOS: disk operating system; a program that tells the computer how to use the disk drive.

downtime: a period of lost work time when the computer is not operating or is malfunctioning.

electronic mail: e-mail; transmission of letters, messages, results, memos, and so on from one computer to another by the use of telephone lines.

font: an assortment of print characters of a given size or style.

hard copy: the readable paper copy or printout from a computer.

hardware: the electronic, magnetic, and mechanical equipment of a computer (keyboard, monitor, and so on).

input: data put into the computer via the keyboard or floppy disk.

interface: the hardware and software that allow computers to interact.

K: computer shorthand for 1,024 bytes; a term used to measure the memory capacity of the computer.

Commonly Used Computer Terms (Cont.)

keyboard: an input device like a typewriter keyboard that converts keystrokes into electrical signals displayed on the screen as letters and symbols.

memory: data that is held in storage.

menu: a list of available computer functions for selection by the operator; usually appears when the computer is turned on.

microcomputer: a self-contained computer system that uses a microprocessor as the CPU; often called a PC (personal computer).

modem: a peripheral device that allows the computer to communicate with other computers or terminals over the telephone lines.

monitor: a visual display unit with a screen called a cathode ray tube (CRT).

mouse: a handheld computer input device, usually separate from the keyboard, used to control cursor position.

output: what the computer produces after information is processed and printed out.

peripheral: anything plugged into the computer, including the printer, disk drive, monitor, and so on.

printer: a device that produces a hard copy; types include laser, dot matrix, and letter quality printers.

program: a set of instructions written in computer language, designed to tell the computer how to complete operations.

RAM: Random Access Memory; temporary or programmable memory that stops when the machine is turned off.

ROM: Read Only Memory; permanent memory in a computer determined by the computer manufacturer.

scrolling: moving the cursor up, down, left, or right through information on the computer display.

security code: a code you must enter before accessing a computer system; especially important in a healthcare facility where much information is privileged.

software: computer programs necessary to direct the hardware of a computer system.

terminal: a device used to communicate with a computer, usually a keyboard and a monitor; a medical office may have several terminals and one computer, which is located elsewhere in the office or building.

Types of Computers

Computers come in three different sizes: small (microcomputers), medium (minicomputers), and large (mainframes).

Mainframes

The largest computers are called **mainframe** computers. These computers are very expensive and are capable of performing many tasks at a very rapid rate of speed. Most large facilities own their own mainframe system and send information to other computers or terminals located off-site. For example, you may see only a keyboard and monitor at your workstation because the "brains" of the computer system are located in another building. Mainframe computers require environmentally controlled rooms and sophisticated electrical wiring.

mainframe: the largest of computers, capable of performing multiple tasks at rapid speeds; usually found in large facilities.

Minicomputers

Minicomputers are capable of processing data like a mainframe, but they do not need special environmental conditions or complicated wiring. Many clinical laboratories will have their own minicomputer system that can tie into the healthcare facility's mainframe system.

minicomputer: a computer system often used in a clinical laboratory setting; larger than a microcomputer and smaller than a mainframe computer.

Microcomputers

More commonly known as personal computers, the **microcomputer** is very popular with individuals who want their own computer system for personal needs. Small businesses and schools rely extensively on this computer. These computers are self-contained but can be linked to larger computers.

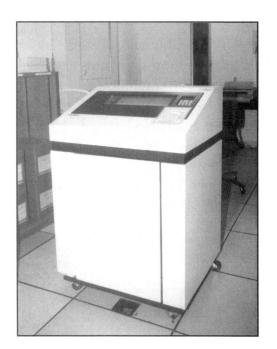

Figure 21-3: A minicomputer may be used in a clinical laboratory to communicate with the healthcare facility's mainframe system.

microcomputer: a self-contained computer system that uses a microprocessor as the CPU; often called a PC (personal computer).

All three computers have much in common and operate in much the same way. They can be linked together to communicate with each other in order to share information.

Computer Components

It is helpful to understand the basic role of each main component of the computer. All computers have a means to enter (input) information, a means to process information, and a means to output information.

Entering Information

The most common way to enter information into a computer is with a keyboard. This keyboard is similar to a typewriter keyboard, but there are special keys that differ from the typewriter. An important key on some computer keyboards is the ENTER key. After you have put information into the computer, you press the ENTER key. Scanners also may be used to enter information into a computer. In addition, **floppy disks**, **removable disks**, **compact disks**, and **magnetic tapes** may be used to transfer data from one computer to another.

Processing Information

After the information is entered into the computer, the information can be displayed on the computer screen, also called the **CRT (cathode ray tube)** or the monitor. The computer takes the information and processes it through a critical part of the computer, called the **CPU (central processing unit)**. The CPU consists of many electronic components and microchips. The computer performs in computer or machine language. So, you do not have to know its "machine language." However you must be extremely careful when inputting your own information because the information in the computer is only as accurate as the person who enters it.

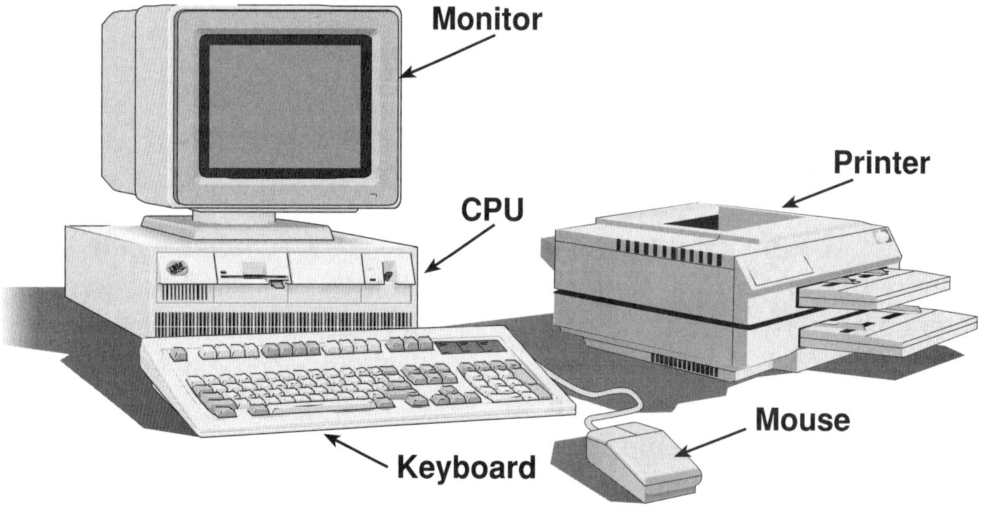

floppy disk:
a flexible magnetic storage device for computer programs and information; usually 3½ inches.

cathode ray tube:
CRT; a visual display unit with a screen that is connected to a computer.

central processing unit:
CPU; the central processing unit or the brains of the system; the CPU's memory is made up of bits.

Figure 21-4: A Computer System's Hardware Components

The **hard disk** is the fast storage device that is usually mounted inside the computer or in its own case outside a computer. There are a wide variety of sizes for the hard disk, depending on the storage needs of the facility. Hard disks can malfunction, causing a "crash" of the system, and information can be permanently lost. **Backup** programs should be run continually to save information in case of a crash in the system.

Outputting Information

There are several ways to get information (output) from the computer. You can see information on the CRT (computer screen), as you would view information on a television set. You can print this information to receive a **hard copy** of the material you need, printed on paper. Information can also be transferred to floppy disks, removable disks, compact disks, and magnetic tapes.

The computer machinery (the electronic, magnetic and mechanical equipment such as the keyboard, central processing unit, monitor, and so forth) is called **hardware**. **Software** includes the computer programs that instruct the computer about what to do and how to do it. Examples of software include **word processing** programs, **spreadsheets**, presentation graphics, and **database** programs.

Be aware that hardware and software are being produced at an astonishing rate of speed. You may get used to one computer system in your laboratory, and then a decision may be made to overhaul the system completely. Sometimes the laboratory computer stays the same, but the hospital mainframe computer is altered. The former commands that you had to learn in order to interface with the hospital's computer may be completely changed. Be flexible and learn new programs without complaining. You will find that all programs have a great deal in common.

hard disk:
a magnetic storage device for information, usually located inside of the computer.

backup:
the duplication of files to protect information; often done on a computer once or twice a day.

hard copy:
the readable paper copy or printout from a computer.

hardware:
the electronic, magnetic, and mechanical equipment of a computer (keyboard, monitor, and so on).

software:
computer programs necessary to direct the hardware of a computer system.

Specific Clinical Laboratory Tasks for the Computer

There is significant variation among healthcare facilities as to how each facility uses its computer system in the clinical laboratory. Some departments lend themselves more to being hooked into computer systems, such as the clinical chemistry department with their huge autoanalyzers. Other departments, such as microbiology, have taken longer to computerize. In spite of variation, the following list summarizes many of the functions that a clinical laboratory assistant can perform on the computer in the clinical laboratory:

- Enter patient data, such as name, address age, sex, physician, healthcare facility identification number, and so on.
- Input clinical laboratory tests ordered by the physician. This information can be processed in various ways, including producing labels for specimens, creating worksheets for the employees who run the various tests, and so on.
- Enter test results under the supervision of the clinical laboratory technologist.
- Operate machinery that files quality control information in the computer, and initiate the electronic filing of test results after they have been checked.
- Print patient results for physicians and nursing floors.
- Print interim and final reports that batch individual patient results.
- Perform inventories on supplies.
- Order supplies through the computer.
- Inquire about test results in the computer to relay to physicians and nursing stations.
- Delete errors.

Each task is performed in an exacting manner according to the type of system your laboratory possesses. You MUST follow the procedures exactly. Carelessness can result in lost results, incorrect reporting of results, and many other problems.

The Facsimile Machine

Facsimile (fax) machines frequently are used by the clinical laboratory and other departments of the healthcare facility. This machine makes it possible to send and receive letters, medical reports, laboratory reports, insurance claims, and so on. Fax machines can also be used to order office and medical supplies.

A fax machine is connected to a telephone line. It scans a document and converts the image to electronic impulses, which are transmitted over the telephone lines. The receiving fax machine converts the impulse into an identical copy of the original; then, a printed copy is created.

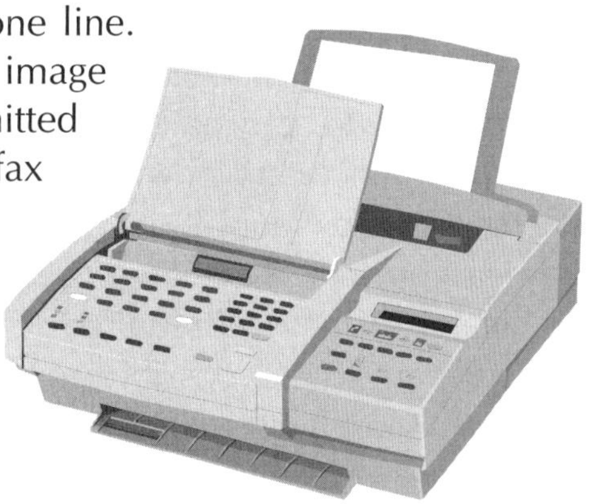

Fax machines may use a special thermally treated paper or just plain paper. Thermally treated paper fades eventually. Therefore, faxes on this type of paper must be copied on plain paper as soon as possible.

Figure 21-5: Fax machines send information over telephone lines, producing a printed copy.

facsimile (fax) machine: a machine that sends documents from one location to another by telephone lines.

Fax machines come with a variety of features, including a secret code that locks out unauthorized users to protect patient confidentiality. Some machines can store multiple documents. If paper runs out, some machines have a memory that stores messages until new paper is put in. You will have to learn the procedures for operating the fax machine that you will be assigned to use. General rules for using a fax machine follow:

- To avoid damaging the machine, remove all staples and paper clips before you place a paper into the fax machine.
- Do not use correction tape or fluid on faxed documents.
- If you are sending confidential material, the receiver should be notified so that he or she can watch for the material as it is transmitted.
- You will be required to state on the cover page of the fax how many pages you are faxing, your name and fax number, and the receiver's name and fax number.
- Be familiar with the error messages of your particular machine. You may have to resend documents if an error message states that the transmission did not go through.
- Make sure the transmission is complete before you leave the machine.

The Photocopy Machine

The copy machine is an extremely important machine in the clinical laboratory. A photocopier produces a photographic reproduction of printed or graphic material. When high quality copies are needed quickly and in limited quantities, using a copy machine is the best way to accomplish that task. Documents can be reproduced on ordinary paper stock or on specialty paper.

You may have a fax machine and a photocopier at your drawing station as well. You may have to copy patient information such as a Medicare card or another insurance card for your records. You may have to copy requisitions to retain a copy for your records. When using the machine, you may be required to put in more paper (and possibly toner) if necessary. Most facilities have a regular maintenance program for their copiers. However, paper jams often occur in copiers that are used continually. Get someone to help you when such a problem occurs.

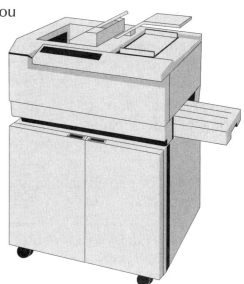

A photocopy is usually made by either feeding the original material into the copier or by placing it face down on the platen glass. After the numbers and size of the copies are selected, press the "print" button.

Figure 21-6: A photocopy machine can reproduce documents quickly and easily.

Please ask for training on the basics of the particular photocopier in your workplace. Minor troubleshooting tricks can avoid the embarrassment of delaying a patient or of not getting test results to a physician who needs a copy immediately.

The Multibutton Telephone

Telephones in such departments as the clinical laboratory are becoming more and more complicated and sophisticated. The choice of telephone systems used depends on the type of healthcare facility, its size and complexity, and the type of call most frequently received and placed. You may receive some training on your telephone system to make sure that you can use the system with ease.

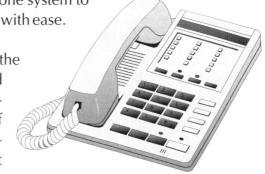

The multibutton telephone allows the user to handle several incoming and outgoing calls at the same time. Buttons may be placed on the bottom of the telephone, which flash intermittently. A steady light indicates that lines are in use. A flashing light means that the line is on hold.

Figure 21-7: A multibutton telephone makes it possible to handle several calls at once.

The hold button provides complete privacy by closing off all other extensions, so this button should always be used when the caller is asked to wait. If you put the receiver down for a moment without pressing a hold button, the caller may hear conversations in the background that can be confidential in nature.

Telephones can vary, but multibutton telephones are generally operated in a similar fashion.

To Place A Call

1. Choose a line that is not being used by someone else, as indicated by a lit or flashing button.

2. Push down the button for the line you want to use, pick up the receiver, and enter the number to be called by pressing the appropriate keys. You may have to enter one or more numbers to obtain an outside line if you are calling in a large facility.

3. If you accidentally press a line that is on hold, press the hold button immediately to re-establish the hold.

To Answer a Call

1. When the telephone rings, determine the line to be answered by the lighting of the button on the bottom of the telephone.

2. Before picking up the receiver, press the key for the line to be answered. Remove the receiver and speak.

To Put Someone on Hold

1. Ask the caller if he or she will "hold, please." Wait for a reply before you press the hold button. You may want to place someone on hold if two calls come in at once, or if you must be away from the telephone for a short length of time during the call.

2. Press the hold button for 2 to 3 seconds until you are sure the line is holding. The light will flash on the holding line if you have done it correctly. To release the hold, push the button on the hold line and speak to the caller.

Chapter Summary

A very important skill for the clinical laboratory assistant is the ability to use the computer. In order to operate a computer with ease, you should be familiar with the uses, terms, and components of the computer in the healthcare environment. The computer makes laboratory work more efficient and allows faster access of test results by physicians, nursing stations, and so on.

It is also wise to be familiar with the office machines that are used routinely in the clinical laboratory. These include the fax, the photocopier, and the multibutton telephone.

Name _____

Date _____

Student Enrichment Activities

Define the following terms.

1. ROM: _____

_____

_____

2. RAM: _____

_____

_____

3. CPU: _____

_____

_____

4. cursor: _____

_____

_____

5. hardware: _____

_____

_____

6. software: _____

_____

_____

7. input: _____

_____

_____

8. backup: _____

_____

_____

9. security code: _____

_____

_____

10. downtime: _____

_____

_____

Circle T for true, or F for false.

11. T F   Laboratory assistants rarely use the computer at work.

12. T F   Microcomputers are also known as personal computers.

13. T F   Hardware includes computer programs.

14. T F   A fax machine sends messages over the hospital intercom system.

15. T F   Photocopiers can often have operational problems.

16. T F   You do not need to know how to type to use a computer well.

17. T F   Floppy disks are hard disks.

18. T F   A hard copy refers to information printed from a computer to paper.

19. T F   There are several different types of printers that may be used in a
               a healthcare facility.

20. T F   You can print patients' blood specimen labels from a computer.

Name _____

Date _____

Complete the following statements.

21. The fax machine works by _____

_____.

22. Two ways to input information on a computer are by _____
     and by _____.

23. Processing information in the computer is done by the _____.

24. The information obtained from the computer is called the _____.

Complete the following exercise.

25. Name five tasks that a computer can perform in the clinical laboratory.

A. _____

_____

B. _____

_____

C. _____

_____

D. _____

_____

E. _____

_____

Chapter Twenty-Two
Health Insurance

Objectives

After completing this chapter, you should be able to do the following:

1. Define and correctly spell each of the key terms.

2. Describe the three general categories of healthcare insurance.

3. Discuss the federal health insurance programs: Medicare, Medicaid, TRICARE, CHAMPVA, and Workers' Compensation.

4. Describe how an HMO works.

5. Identify IPA, PPO, EPO, and POS group healthcare programs.

6. Describe what unemployment compensation disability insurance covers.

7. Discuss confidentiality and potential fraud in relation to patient healthcare insurance.

Key Terms

- CHAMPVA
- COBRA
- deductible
- diagnosis related groups
- health maintenance
  organization

- Medicaid
- Medicare
- TRICARE
- Workers' Compensation

Introduction

Approximately 85% of a physician's income comes from some form of health insurance payment. Fees for clinical laboratory tests are also paid by many insurance companies. The clinical laboratory assistant/phlebotomist does not prepare and submit insurance claims for patients. However, in an outpatient setting, the clinical laboratory assistant may be responsible for patient registration and for obtaining insurance information from the patient. Therefore, it is important to understand basic insurance coverage and related terms. Often, though, patients will have questions about coverage that you may have to refer to their physicians. However, the more knowledge that you obtain in this area, the more helpful you can be to the patient and the more flexible you can be when clerical cross-training opportunities arise.

Categories of Insurance Plans

There are basically three options for a patient seeking health insurance. Within these three options, there are many variations.

1. GOVERNMENT PROGRAMS: These programs are financed and controlled by either federal or state government for specific categories of patients. Common programs in this category are Medicare, Medicaid, TRICARE (formerly known as CHAMPUS), Civilian Health and Medical Program of the Veterans Administration (CHAMPVA), and Workers' Compensation.

2. GROUP-SPONSORED AND INDIVIDUAL POLICIES: These policies are purchased by a group (employers, unions, organizations) or an individual through commercial insurance companies.

3. FIXED, PREPAID FEE PLANS. These health insurance plans are arranged with contracted healthcare providers for both groups and individuals.

Government Health Insurance

Medicare

Medicare was created by the United States Congress in the mid-1960's. It is a federally funded healthcare program originally designed to help senior citizens pay for medical care. Although Medicare primarily pays for medical costs for those 65 and older, it now also covers medical costs for anyone with end-stage kidney disease, for organ donors, and for patients with a total disability lasting longer than 29 months.

Figure 22-1 is an example of a Medicare card that is carried by all Medicare subscribers. In an outpatient setting, you may be required to make copies of insurance cards submitted by patients.

Medicare: a federally-funded program enacted in 1965 that provides health-care to people over the age of 65 as well as to the disabled, regardless of financial status.

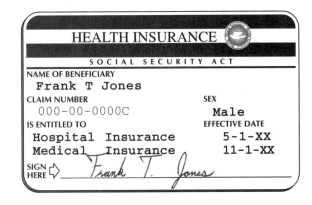

Figure 22-1: An Example of a Medicare Card

In 1991, in an effort to help curb the rising cost of healthcare, payment plans called **diagnosis-related groups (DRGs)** were added to Medicare that impose fixed payment amounts for different types of patient care. DRGs are based on the idea that similar medical diagnoses could generate similar hospitalization costs.

DRGs have significantly impacted the clinical laboratory. Before their imposition, physicians could order batteries of tests for a condition with the assurance that Medicare would pay for any tests ordered. Today, there are only certain laboratory tests allowed with each diagnosis that will be paid by Medicare. Physicians are much less likely to order tests that are not covered by Medicare, as patients must pay in full for tests not authorized. Other insurance companies have adopted the DRG concept.

diagnosis related groups: DRG; a system of disease classification used to determine reimbursement rates.

Medicare coverage is divided into two parts. *Part A* covers inpatient hospital services, some post-hospital care, and care at an extended care facility. *Part B* is purchased by the patient (who pays a monthly premium) and covers physician charges for inpatient and outpatient services, outpatient diagnostic services, drugs administered by a physician, kidney dialysis, home health care, and prescription medical supplies. Routine physical examinations and hearing aids are excluded.

Clinical laboratories that are not Medicare-certified laboratories are laboratories that have not accepted Medicare assignments. If you work at a clinical laboratory that does not accept Medicare patients, they should be informed immediately of that policy.

Medicaid

Medicaid: a program funded by the state and federal government for providing medical care to the poor and disabled.

In 1965, the United States Congress mandated that each state must establish a program to assist a certain population with medical expenses. The federal government gives each state compensation for this purpose. People eligible to receive **Medicaid** benefits include welfare recipients, low-income people who are medically needy but not disabled, people receiving aid to dependent children, and people who are disabled and blind. Eligibility and benefits vary greatly from state to state. Physicians who accept Medicaid patients (they are not required to accept Medicare or Medicaid patients) agree to accept state reimbursement as payment in full. Some states require the patient to make a **co-payment.** (With Medicare, there is a 20% co-payment of the charges made by the physician that is paid by the patient.)

TRICARE and CHAMPVA

TRICARE: formerly known as CHAMPUS; a government healthcare insurance program that covers dependents of active-duty and retired military personnel.

CHAMPVA: the Civilian Health and Medical Program of the Veterans Administration; a governmental healthcare insurance program for surviving spouses and dependent children of persons who died or are permanently disabled as a result of military service.

TRICARE is a federal government medical program covering the dependents of active-duty and retired military personnel. **CHAMPVA** is a federal program covering the surviving spouses and dependent children of persons who died as a result of military service and veterans who are totally or permanently disabled as a result of military service.

Workers' Compensation Insurance

The United States Congress has set up minimum requirements for employees to cover the cost of on-the-job injuries or illnesses. Congress added this program because regular health insurance does not cover job-related illness or injury. The employer purchases this compensation insurance (**workers' compensation**) from an insurance carrier. Patients are required to report job-related illness or injury to the employer before getting medical help.

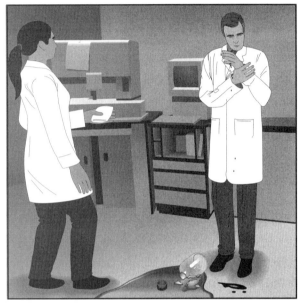

Figure 22-2: Workers injured on the job are eligible for Workers' Compensation.

workers' compensation: a program established by law in each state providing income and healthcare insurance to persons who become ill or injured in the course of their employment.

Group Health Insurance Programs

Most often, group medical plans can be obtained through a person's employer, union, or professional organization. There are several different types of plans. Group health insurance can be considered managed care, or it can be commercial insurance. Examples of such plans are listed below.

Health Maintenance Organizations (HMOs)

Health Maintenance Organizations, better known as **HMOs**, are prepaid healthcare provider group practices serving a specific geographical area. HMOs are generally concerned with promoting "wellness" with the idea of cutting down costs of medical care. Yearly physicals are often encouraged and are fully covered. The subscriber is assigned to a primary care physician who is responsible for authorizing all referrals to other providers. Total health maintenance is available for a predetermined premium, although some HMOs require the patient to pay a small charge for each visit, normally between $5 and $15. Insurance forms are not used. Outside specialists who care for HMO patients bill services to the HMO itself. Examples of HMOs include Kaiser Permanente, FHP, Secure Horizons, and Health Net.

Health Maintenance Organization: HMO; a type of prepaid group healthcare program that provides health maintenance and treatment services to its members.

HMOs are often criticized for requiring long waits for patients to obtain appointments and lack of flexibility in choosing a physician. Some members of HMOs also feel that critical diagnostic tests are sometimes not ordered in the interest of saving money. Other HMO subscribers praise the lack of insurance forms and large co-payments often demanded by other types of healthcare insurance. HMOs are among the least expensive of health insurance offerings. Many have their own hospitals.

Individual Practice Associations (IPAs)

Individual Practice Associations (IPAs) are composed of individual practitioners who have joined together to provide prepaid healthcare to individuals and groups who purchase coverage. Healthcare providers in IPAs hire their own staffs and maintain separate, private offices.

Major Medical Plans

deductible:
the amount
of medical
expenses that
must be met
before an
insurance
policy begins
to pay.

Group major medical plans have both basic medical insurance coverage and catastrophic coverage. The costs of illness and injuries beyond those covered in the basic medical plan are provided for under catastrophic coverage. An employer and employee may share the cost of the insurance premium, or the employee may pay all of it. These plans usually have an annual individual and family **deductible** fee. Payment for services might include the employee paying 20% of expenses and the insurance company paying 80% of the expenses. The patient is free to choose a healthcare provider who accepts his or her particular insurance plan. Major medical plans include Blue Cross/Blue Shield, Aetna, and Prudential.

Other Managed Care Networks

In addition to the types of plans already described, other managed care networks operate today that are variations of those plans:

- The PPO (Preferred Provider Organization) is a variation on the HMO theme. A formal agreement is drawn up among healthcare providers to treat a certain patient population, such as employees of a large corporation. The patients are offered discounts if they seek services from a PPO provider. A PPO can allow the subscriber more freedom of choice than an HMO. Fees are usually higher than an HMO.

- The EPO (Exclusive Provider Organization) differs somewhat from an PPO. PPO subscribers can get limited benefits if they receive care from a non-PPO provider; however, in an EPO, subscribers may not receive any benefits if they go to a non-EPO provider.

- The POS (Point-of-Service) has many variations. Patients do not have to decide how they receive services at the time they enroll in this plan. Enrollees can use another provider for reduced payments.

Individual Health Insurance Plans

If a person is not eligible for health insurance through the government, an employer, or some type of organization, he or she has to apply to a commercial insurance company that provides individual medical insurance policies if coverage is desired. This insurance is generally the most expensive type of coverage.

When a person's employment is terminated or when employees' spouses are left without insurance due to divorce, group plans are required to provide healthcare continuation coverage temporarily. This extension is made possible by **COBRA**, the **Continuation of Benefits Reconciliation Act**. The person must pay both the employer's and the employee's contribution to the plan. This coverage can extend from 18 to 36 months, depending on how the person qualifies for COBRA benefits.

COBRA: Continuation of Benefits Reconciliation Act; provides healthcare continuation coverage to employees when employment ends, or to employee spouses who become divorced or separated.

Unemployment Compensation for Disability

Several states have a state disability insurance program. Examples of these programs are UCD, TDI, and SDI. Most state programs do not allow for hospital benefits. Payments often begin after 70 consecutive days of a disability. Filing deadlines vary, but most states require filing within 20 days of receiving a disability. There is a restriction on how much compensation one disability can bring, usually up to six months of compensation for the same disability.

Ethical and Legal Considerations Regarding Health Insurance

Although a clinical laboratory assistant/phlebotomist does not process or file insurance claims, you may be required to obtain insurance information from outpatients. All insurance information must remain confidential and cannot be released to a third party (anyone other than the patient, physician, or staff member) without written authorization by the patient.

Insurance fraud is a very real concern in today's healthcare environment. Many cases exist in which a patient asked a healthcare worker to misrepresent facts about patient treatment, such as changing diagnoses to receive more compensation, or changing the date of a visit to ensure that coverage will be provided. Although the clinical laboratory assistant may not be asked to alter insurance information, you should know that there are patients who may try to abuse the insurance system. Fraud on a large scale (such as unwarranted Workers' Compensation claims) can cause healthcare costs to rise. This affects everyone.

Thinking It Through ...

Dennis is a laboratory assistant who is about to draw a patient's blood for several tests. He calls her name and is surprised to see a high school classmate whom he hasn't seen for several years.

"Hi, remember me?" Dennis asks the young woman called Claire. "Except, I don't remember your name being Claire. Weren't you known as Julie in high school?"

Dennis notices that the young woman becomes very uncomfortable and blushes. She mutters something about changing her name and looks down. She looks like she is going to cry. Dennis then remembers that this woman had a sister who was a year behind them in school. He remembers that the sister's name is Claire.

1. What could be happening in this case?

2. If fraud is suspected, what should Dennis do now?

The clinical laboratory assistant/phlebotomist may be asked by a patient (often a friend) to draw a test but not to enter it into the computer system so that it is not charged to the patient, especially if the patient's insurance will not cover an expensive test. This is not a practice that is welcomed by the facility as every test requires valuable employee time as well as the instrumentation and reagents used to run each test.

Chapter Summary

Although the clinical laboratory assistant/phlebotomist does not handle insurance claims directly, knowledge of different insurance coverage is helpful when interacting with patients. Some patients may be nervous about what laboratory tests are covered by their insurance companies and which ones the patients will have to pay for themselves. In these cases, you should refer questions to the patient's physician or insurance company. If you work in an HMO environment, the patient is probably not paying anything for the tests and will not be asking this type of insurance question.

Some patients may try to outsmart the system by using fraudulent means to receive insurance benefits to which they are not entitled. You must never participate in insurance fraud of any kind.

Name _____

Date _____

Student Enrichment Activities

Complete the following exercises.

1. HMO stands for _____ _____ _____.

2. DRG stands for _____ _____ _____.

3. Medicare was created in the 1960's by the _____.

4. Medicare is divided into two parts: Part _____ and Part _____.

5. What is the difference between CHAMPVA and TRICARE?

   _____

   _____

   _____

   _____

   _____

   _____

   _____

6. Workers' Compensation covers _____

   _____.

7. Two examples of major medical plans include _____

   and _____.

8. Generally the most expensive type of insurance coverage is _____

   _____.

9. COBRA insurance coverage is _____

   _____

   _____.

10. Insurance information is _____ and must not be revealed to a third party.

Circle T for true, or F for false.

11. T F   The states administer Medicaid programs with federal funds.

12. T F   Workers' Compensation insurance is purchased by employers.

13. T F   The deductible fee is the amount an insured person must pay before the insurance company begins paying benefits.

14. T F   HMOs emphasize "wellness" by encouraging yearly physical examinations.

15. T F   Major medical plans never have a deductible payment.

Circle the correct answer.

16. DRGs:
   A. are Workers' Compensation funds.
   B. refer to veterans' insurance.
   C. were designed to help curb the rising cost of healthcare.
   D. is another name for health maintenance organizations.

17. An IPA health insurance plan:
   A. is made up of individual practitioners.
   B. allows individual doctors to hire their own staff.
   C. includes doctors who have their own separate offices.
   D. includes all of the above.

Name _____

Date _____

18. Defined as a managed care network:

    A. PPO.

    B. CHAMPVA.

    C. DRG.

    D. Medicare.

19. UCD, TDI, and SDI are all examples of:

    A. Workers' Compensation.

    B. individual insurance company policies.

    C. HMOs.

    D. unemployment compensation disability insurance.

20. All the following statements are true about Medicare except that:

    A. Medicare was created in the 1960's.

    B. Part A and Part B are the two parts of Medicare.

    C. Medicaid is another term for Medicare coverage.

    D. Medicare will pay for kidney dialysis for those with end-stage kidney disease.

22-14

Chapter Twenty-Three
Customer Service Skills

Objectives

After completing this chapter, you should be able to
do the following:

1. Define and correctly spell each of the key terms.

2. Explain why customer service is one of the most important tasks of the clinical laboratory assistant/phlebotomist.

3. Explain components of verbal and nonverbal communication.

4. Identify key aspects of active listening.

5. Discuss questions that clinical laboratory assistants/ phlebotomists should ask themselves often in order to provide the best customer service possible.

Key Terms

- active listening
- articulation
- customer service
- feedback

- nonverbal communication
- proxemics
- verbal communication

Introduction

Think about the people around you whom you admire for their excellence. Perhaps you have the world's best mother-in-law; your best friend has been faithful for many years; your spouse makes you very happy; your former boss was the best you ever worked for; or your minister really inspires you. Ask yourself what the special people in your life have in common. Chances are that these admired people all give time to listen well, have clear, tactful communication skills, and make listeners feel they care.

customer service: efforts made to provide the customer (patient) with the best service available in the facility.

As a clinical laboratory assistant/phlebotomist, you are the clinical laboratory's ambassador to the patient. The patient's satisfaction with the laboratory can be related directly to the quality of **customer service** you provide the patient. Will you be remembered by the patient as a professional who made the patient feel welcomed in, listened to, and cared for? Or will you be someone whom the patient remembers as dismissive, distracted, careless, and uncaring?

verbal communication: communication by the spoken word.

As discussed in Chapter Sixteen, quality assurance programs in the healthcare facility are designed to serve the customer, assuring that every procedure in that facility has the patient's best interest at the core of the procedure. The clinical laboratory assistant/phlebotomist must keep customer service in mind constantly, and must understand thoroughly what it takes to be a professional — one who is dedicated to putting the patient first.

nonverbal communication: a form of communication that involves body language, tactile stimulation (touch), and facial expressions.

The Excellent Communicator

Communication is the verbal and/or nonverbal exchange of messages, ideas, thoughts, feelings, and information. Good communication is both an art and a well-practiced skill. Learning such skills promotes a positive, healthy relationship among people. Becoming an excellent communicator requires knowledge of three aspects of communication: **verbal communication**, **nonverbal communication**, and active listening.

Verbal Communication

Verbal communication involves the use of the spoken word. Expressing oneself through words is the most obvious form of communication. It involves a sender (speaker), a receiver (listener), and when completed, a process called **feedback**. Feedback gives the receiver a chance to correct any miscommunication during the interaction between the speaker and listener.

feedback: receiver's way of assuring that the message that was understood is the same as the message that was sent.

articulation: speaking in a clear, precise manner.

One of the most important things to remember as a speaker is to be **articulate**. Many of us are lazy in our everyday speech by slurring, mumbling, dropping syllables, or leaving off endings of words. This type of speech may be effective among your peers and people who have known you for several years. However, it will not help you deal with patients who for many reasons may not be able to understand you.

Enunciate your words. Choose your words carefully, and focus on clarity of delivery. Practice in front of a mirror. Record your own voice and listen to your words. Are some words sloppy? Do you speak so quickly that words run together? Are you so soft-spoken that your words come out indistinctly? Pay special attention to your articulation when you speak to friends. Does your speech vary with different groups?

Normal human behavior may set up many barriers during verbal communication. Several potential barriers can occur during a conversation:

- language limitations (inability to fully understand the speaker's language)

- cultural diversity (misunderstandings due to words having a different meaning in the speaker's or listener's culture)

- emotion (emotions can cause a listener to hear something completely different than what was spoken)

- age (individual generations may use the same words very differently)

- physical problems (hearing impairments can be a serious block to communication)

As a clinical laboratory assistant, you should be aware of all of these barriers to verbal communication when you are interacting with a patient. Ask yourself the following questions when you are giving important directions to patients.

Are you speaking clearly and slowly to someone who has limited knowledge of English? Are you refraining from speaking loudly, a reaction that does not help the process?

Are you watching the listener carefully to make sure he or she is not misunderstanding what you are saying? If the listener is from another culture, could he or she misunderstand anything you have said?

Are you giving complicated verbal directions to a patient who is very upset? The emotions that the patient is feeling may block most of the words you are saying. In this case, written directions might be a better choice.

Are you in the habit of using lots of slang in your speech? Can an 80 year-old woman understand your slang? Remember to articulate well. Are you being too scientific when you explain a procedure to a child? In other words, are you choosing the proper words for the situation?

Are you raising your voice to a hearing-impaired person? Chances are that a louder voice will not help, especially with someone who has a hearing aid. Are you speaking slowly and clearly, and not covering your mouth with your hand while you talk?

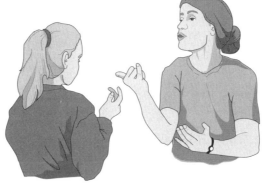

Figure 23-1: Some hearing-impaired people use sign language as one of their communication systems.

Nonverbal Communication

Nonverbal communication involves body language, tactile (touch) stimulation, facial expressions, and the written word. Both the sender and the receiver will often use both verbal and nonverbal methods when transmitting and receiving a message.

Some researchers state that 80% of language is unspoken. Unlike verbal communication that uses words only, nonverbal communication is multi-dimensional and involves several elements, including facial expressions, gestures, and eye contact.

The patient's face often tells the health professional what the patient will not reveal verbally. For example, when you approach a person to draw blood, observe the face for signs of pain, such as a frown, eyes that are full of pain, or a downcast mouth. Many patients automatically say "Fine" when you ask them how they are feeling. However, their expressions and the way they hold their body may tell you differently.

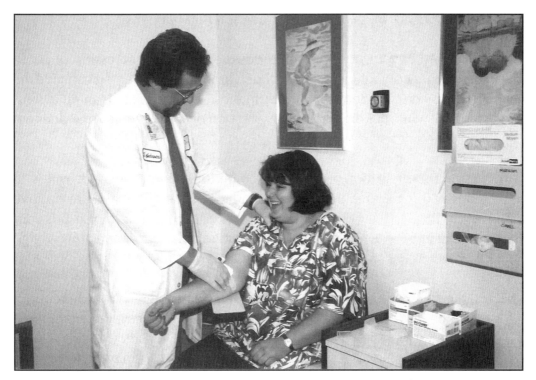

Figure 23-2: Some patients will provide nonverbal clues about their attitude toward a venipuncture. In this instance, the patient is comfortable and relaxed about the procedure.

As discussed in Chapter Twenty, your body language can convey a great deal to the patient. You may be busy trying to read the body language of a patient while you are communicating negative messages to the patient unintentionally. There are several ways you can improve your body language to make the patient feel welcomed and supported.

1. Your personal appearance is a part of communicating to the patient about your professionalism and pride in your job. You should be clean, well-groomed, and neatly dressed. Careless dress can be interpreted by the patient as reflective of your work habits.

2. Establish immediate eye contact if possible. If you look at a patient squarely in the eyes, you are showing sincerity and interest. Eye contact with the patient can create a bond, and it enables you to get feedback immediately from the patient about what is going on with him or her. Eyes say a great deal about confusion, anger, pleasure, boredom, pain, and so on. Also, you should know that in some cultures, immediate eye contact can be a sign of aggression and may cause the patient to look away and be frightened. Be gentle with a patient if that happens.

3. Be aware of your posture. Good posture gives the impression of confidence and competence. If you slouch around the patient, it can give the impression of inadequacy and disinterest. For instance, leaning against the wall while talking gives the impression of lack of energy and does not inspire confidence.

4. A smile is a great form of nonverbal communication. A pleasant smile will convey the message that you are glad to see the client and are positive about the service you are about to give. A smile should also put your patient at ease. It also is a good indication that your interaction will go well when the patient responds with a warm smile.

5. Make sure your gestures match your verbal message. When there is not a match, the patient can become confused and uneasy. For example, if you sound pleasant in greeting your patient, but you are glancing at your watch, frowning, and not making eye contact, you may be telling the patient, "I sound friendly, but really I am eager to get to lunch. I don't want to be here right now." Crossing your arms, rolling your eyes, and drumming your fingers on a table while a patient is trying to tell you about a past unpleasant blood draw conveys an uncaring attitude that will not put the patient at ease.

6. **Proxemics** is the study of an individual's concept and use of space. Have you ever had an uneasy feeling when someone moved too close to you while talking? Did you feel that your space was violated? Every individual maintains an invisible zone defined as personal territory. The size of this zone varies with the individual's needs at the time. For instance, if you are intimate with someone, your zone could be from 1 to 18 inches. If you are socializing with a group of people, the zone radius can be from 4 to 12 feet. Since you often come very close to people when drawing blood, leaning over their bed to check their veins, and so on, you should be aware that the patient may feel threatened and insecure if you get too close. Some cultures have large zones, and any penetration into that zone can be considered an act of aggression. However, most people will step back if you get too close.

proxemics: the study of an individual's concept and use of space.

Active Listening

You will find that many of your patients want to talk. Some are lonely, some want to put off the blood draw as long as possible, and some feel the need to let you know their entire health history. There will be days when you are in a hurry, or when you have heard a patient tell the same story many times. Regardless of this, you must try to have a sincere interest and concern regarding the message the patient is giving to you. Sometimes loneliness is really the only message. The patient wants someone to just make eye contact and show concern.

Active listening is a technique in which the listener gives the communicator his or her full attention, responding to the words spoken and asking pertinent questions. Your questions, however, should not interrupt the speaker's train of thought or lead the conversation. An active listener lets the speaker lead the conversation and gives responses that encourage further conversation and relay acceptance.

active listening: making a conscious effort to hear what the sender is communicating; an essential element of effective and meaningful communication.

Thinking It Through ...

"And then I told my neighbor, Sadie, that my hysterectomy was far more painful than hers, and she should stop belly-achin' and get on with it....." says Mrs. Milton to Daniel, the laboratory assistant.

Mrs. Milton has her blood drawn twice a week by Daniel. Mrs. Milton has poor veins, but Daniel can always get her blood sample on the first venipuncture. Mrs. Milton has been widowed for a year and is very lonely. She really wants Daniel to listen to her latest problems. When she leaves, she seems to be much more cheerful if Daniel gives her some time to talk.

1. How does Daniel listen actively to what Mrs. Milton is saying when Daniel is a 25 year-old man with no interests in common with Mrs. Milton, who loves to talk in depth about her neighbor and her own favorite soap opera?

2. What if Daniel has blood draws piling up and Mrs. Milton has just started a long story? How does he make Mrs. Milton think he is listening and still end their conversation quickly?

Here are some hints to help you become a better active listener:

1. Keep constant eye contact with the speaker. If you let your eyes roam, a distraction will surely come into your vision and your ability to focus on what is being said will lessen.

2. While the patient is making a point, keep an open mind, free from judgment.

3. Pay attention to all aspects of communication, not only to the speaker's voice and voice tone, but also to the nonverbal signs as well. You may pick up hidden messages in this manner.

4. When a patient is talking, make sure there no loud noises, ringing telephones, uncomfortable room temperatures, or other distractions for both you and the patient.

5. Make reflective statements that show the communicator that you are hearing and receiving the message given. For example, a patient may say, "I had the worst blood drawing experience the last time I was here." If you respond with a "too bad," you may sound like you are being dismissive. A better reflective response would be ,"I would like to hear about it so that we can make sure it doesn't happen to you again."

6. If the patient says something confusing, ask for clarification. You want to make sure that you are hearing the message clearly. After the clarification has been given, you might want to repeat the answer back to the sender. For instance, you might say, "Mrs. Brown, what you are saying is that the directions for the urine collection are unclear, and you were not able to collect the specimen according to the directions."

7. Show compassion for a speaker whose message is clearly reaching out for sympathy. The patient may need a dose of warmth before facing a serious surgery or before hearing the results of a biopsy. By being a good listener, you might have the opportunity to respond with an encouraging word that will get the patient over the next difficult task facing him or her in the healthcare facility.

Customer Satisfaction

Since EVERYONE in a healthcare facility is working to provide the best customer service possible, it is helpful for everyone in the health field to get in the habit of asking his or her self the following questions frequently.

1. Am I a positive reflection of my employer's goals?

2. Do I listen and respond to patients who have problems, questions, or special requests? Or am I quick to say, "It's not my responsibility."

3. Do I take action to help solve problems, answer questions, and handle special requests? Or do I pass the buck to someone else with more experience and more responsibility and immediately forget about the problem?

4. Do I accept blame when my carelessness or disorganization causes inconvenience to others?

5. Do I dedicate myself to doing everything within my power to serve the needs of the patient?

6. Do I look for ways to improve customer service for the patient? Do I share such ideas with supervisors?

Chapter Summary

The clinical laboratory assistant/phlebotomist often interacts with a large number of patients on a daily basis, as well as with friends and family members of patients, coworkers, physicians, and potential clients. Therefore, being a good communicator is mandatory for this position. Being aware of the differences in verbal and nonverbal communication can help the employee understand what patients are communicating and what the laboratory assistant is saying to the patient. The ultimate goal of the laboratory assistant/phlebotomist is to be a good listener who is dedicated to providing the best customer service possible.

Name _____

Date _____

Student Enrichment Activities

Complete the following exercises.

1. What are the differences between verbal and nonverbal communication?

    _____

    _____

    _____

    _____

2. Give five examples of nonverbal communication that can make a patient feel welcome.
    A. _____
    B. _____
    C. _____
    D. _____
    E. _____

3. What is the significance of proxemics when interacting with patients?

    _____

    _____

    _____

4. Name four ways to listen actively to a patient.
    A. _____
    B. _____
    C. _____
    D. _____

5. Why is good articulation so important in verbal communication?

    _____

    _____

    _____

Circle the correct answer.

6. If a patient begins to cry, the best thing you can do is to:
   A. Tell the patient to stop crying because you need to draw his or her blood.
   B. Ask the patient to come back when he or she can get his or herself together.
   C. Give the patient a hug and tell him or her everything will be fine.
   D. Listen carefully to the patient about what is wrong, showing sympathy.

7. A laboratory assistant is listening to the patient while drumming his fingers, yawning, and looking at his watch at 30 second intervals. The patient is getting the impression that the laboratory assistant is:
   A. tired or bored.
   B. in a hurry.
   C. impatient.
   D. all of the above.

8. All are important in communication except:
   A. being a good listener.
   B. being a compassionate individual.
   C. being stone-faced at all times.
   D. being aware of proxemics.

9. All are examples of nonverbal communication except for:
   A. the written word.
   B. facial expressions.
   C. a good vocabulary.
   D. gestures.

10. A good listener does all the following except:
    A. keep constant eye contact with the speaker.
    B. laugh lots when listening to the speaker.
    C. watch for nonverbal communication clues.
    D. make reflective statements.

Chapter Twenty-Four
Conflict Management in the Clinical Laboratory

Objectives

After completing this chapter, you should be able to do the following:

1. Define and correctly spell each of the key terms.

2. Discuss various styles of dealing with conflict, including accommodation, avoidance, collaboration, compromise, and control.

3. Identify sources of conflict for the clinical laboratory assistant/phlebotomist.

4. Discuss ways to deal with conflict that can lead to a satisfactory resolution for all parties involved.

Key Terms

- accommodator
- avoider
- collaborator

- compromiser
- controller

Introduction

Few things can interfere more with good customer service more than an angry employee. Patients expect to be treated with respect and consideration. Their anxiety level may be high as they face procedures, surgeries, or painful treatments. A tense, angry employee can heighten the patient's anxiety level.

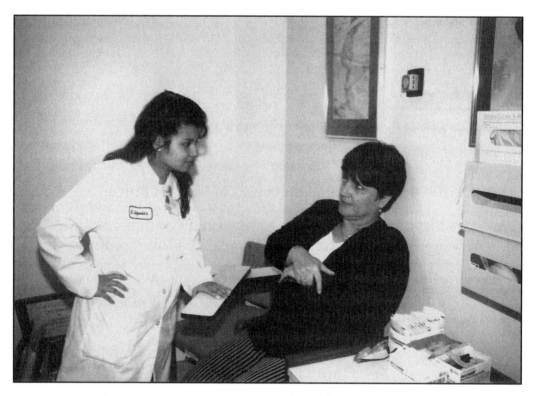

Figure 24-1: An angry employee may not be able to give a patient the customer service the patient deserves.

Working in a healthcare environment is often stressful. In the clinical laboratory environment, some physicians order tests and want the results before the blood is even drawn. Staffing can be reduced due to budgetary considerations, often putting you in the position to work very hard during your entire shift. Staffing can also be reduced due to illness, and you can feel resentment toward a fellow laboratory assistant who calls in sick on a weekend shift when the staff is already reduced.

Conflict is inevitable in an environment that requires a person to interact with patients, their families, and fellow employees, any or all of whom may be under stress. Continual conflict can result in unhappiness with your job, and can lead to poor customer service. Learning to manage conflict skillfully is very important for the clinical laboratory assistant/phlebotomist.

Styles for Handling Conflict

As a clinical laboratory assistant/phlebotomist, you may experience conflict with people in a variety of situations. For example, patients who do not want their blood drawn may be verbally abusive, or a nurse may be angry at you because you did not arrive for a blood tests exactly when requested. A physician may get angry with you on the telephone about a blood test you did not draw, even if he or she failed to order it; or a fellow laboratory assistant may not carry his or her share of the workload, leaving you with more work to do. Everyone has his or her own methods for handling such conflicts. The following are styles that are used by people to deal with conflict.

Accommodation

A person who is an **accommodator** will try to avoid the source of conflict and try to maintain all relationships on an even keel. The accommodator gives in, appeases, and keeps smiling. Being a peacemaker is foremost in the accommodator's mind. Unfortunately in this situation, resolving the conflict is often not accomplished.

accommodator: one who assists, aids.

Avoidance

avoider:
one who
evades, shuns,
or bypasses.

The **avoider** finds any conflict distasteful, something to be avoided. Displays of anger are seen as unhealthy. This person feels that it is hopeless to work for a resolution. Personal goals cannot be met in conflict situations, and everything should be done to postpone, divert, or withdraw from the problem. This is a dangerous reaction to conflict, because eventually the avoider can become unhappy and spread that attitude to others.

Collaboration

collaborator:
one who
assists,
acting as a
partner.

The **collaborator** wants to solve a conflict situation. The collaborator tries to identify what each party wants in the conflict, and tries to achieve a "win-win" resolution. The collaborator uses appropriate problem solving techniques (see next section) to promote a positive outcome for everyone involved. This style is invaluable in solving conflict.

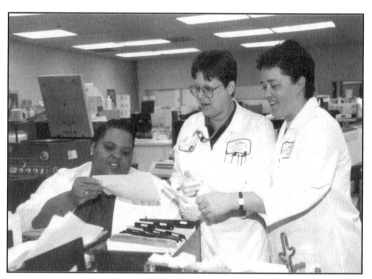

Figure 24-2: Collaboration can result in a resolution that pleases all parties.

Compromise

compromiser:
one who
adapts, adjusts,
and negotiates.

The **compromiser** is dedicated to having all parties bargain to reach a resolution of the conflict. The compromiser may use persuasion and manipulation to get each party to give up something in order to resolve the problem. The goal is to partially satisfy all parties in the conflict. The problem with this approach is that partial satisfaction often is not enough for some parties, which may cause the conflict to flare up again.

Control

The **controller** is a very common type of problem solver, and control is often a laboratory manager's conflict management style. This is a power-oriented style, based on the opinion of the controller that his or her analysis of the conflict is not to be questioned. Often blame is placed, and the

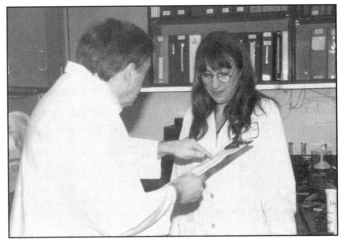

controller:
one who rules
and manages.

Figure 24-3: Authoritarian resolution of conflict can lead to more conflict.

perpetrator is punished. Unfortunately, when the controller exerts this type of judgment, there is little or no discussion of problem solving techniques. In other words, in the control method of conflict management, instead of focusing upon resolving the conflict, the manager focuses upon winning the conflict.

Thinking It Through ...

Holly has found the job of her dreams. She is working for a doctor's complex laboratory where she doesn't have to work weekends. Her salary is significantly higher than it was at her last job, and she can walk to work. She really likes working with the other laboratory assistants at the laboratory, and she is given quite a bit of responsibility that she didn't have at her last job. She feels challenged every day.

However, Holly's boss is a "control freak." He insists on making all decisions at the laboratory, and he involves himself in all conflict situations without allowing anyone else to participate in any resolutions. He gets angry at situations and yells at the employees before finding out exactly what is happening. He is always searching for someone to blame.

1. What should Holly do about her boss?

2. With all of the positives of Holly's job, would it be worth it to quit?

Most of us at one time or another have used most or all of these styles when confronted with a conflict situation. No one can be a pure collaborator in every case. If you are already stressed from personal or health problems, you may not see the conflict at work as clearly as you would if you were unburdened by other stresses. The importance of identifying styles is to see where you fit and how you can cooperate more fully in reaching a resolution that truly is comfortable with all parties, although sometimes this is not possible.

Problem Solving

Clinical laboratory assistants/phlebotomists may have complaints regarding problems associated with their job as follows:

- "We feel like we don't get enough respect from other healthcare professionals. Technologists bark orders at us, nurses ignore us, physicians yell at us. Sometimes we feel we are not treated like intelligent human beings."

- "Sometimes we feel like we are doing our jobs without support from others. When we are overwhelmed with blood draws, the other laboratory professionals turn away and refuse to help us."

- "I get tired of carrying more than my share. My fellow laboratory assistant is always disappearing, refusing to perform difficult blood draws and making my job much harder."

- "I'm tired of my fellow workers always calling in sick on weekends. Don't they know how hard it is when we are short on staff anyway?"

- "I get tired of being blamed for everything that goes wrong in the laboratory. Sometimes I feel like a scapegoat."

How do such problems get resolved? How does a clinical laboratory assistant/ phlebotomist approach these problems without endangering his or her position? The following problem-solving ideas might help in reaching a resolution.

1. Blaming others should not be the first approach in attempting to solve a conflict. The parties in the situation should be considered part of a team instead of individuals who must assess blame and assign punishment. It is helpful to think of the parties as "we" instead of defending "me." This way, the parties should not feel threatened.

2. All parties involved must be given a chance to describe the problems in terms of how to improve teamwork. Identify all possible options that are satisfactory to all parties.

3. Goals and benefits agreed upon should reflect the thoughts and ideas of all parties involved. A resolution should not come automatically from those in management, without feedback from others involved as well.

4. Facts and issues should be discussed. Name calling cannot be tolerated. Stay away from personal attacks. Concentrate on the specific issues.

5. Try to work for the long-term conflict resolution rather than solving a problem only temporarily. Try to look forward and see if the resolution will hold up in the future. Otherwise, the conflict may arise again in a short time.

6. Make sure everyone understands how the implementation of the resolution is going to be accomplished. Have each party explain what he or she perceives is the resolution. Some people may agree to anything to avoid more problems, when the fact is that they really do not understand what happened in the conflict resolution.

People need to be appreciated and validated, especially in their professional lives. Always try to keep a positive attitude and try to keep working for resolutions. Becoming convinced that a situation is hopeless is what makes unhappy, difficult employees. So, work for satisfactory resolution to problems whenever possible.

Thinking It Through ...

Debbie has been working for Sunnyside Reference Laboratory for several months. She is a very hardworking employee, always on time and eager to learn new skills. Debbie especially enjoys dealing with the patients, and she seems to have great success with them. In fact, several patients now ask for her when they come into the laboratory to have their blood drawn.

Diana is the laboratory manager. From the beginning of Debbie's employment, Diana has not been very friendly to her. Diana has never complimented Debbie and has often been impatient with her when Debbie has asked questions. As a result, Debbie does not know where she stands with her boss and really would like to find out if Diana thinks she is doing a good job. How should Debbie proceed?

1. Should Debbie march up to Diana and demand a hearing?

2. Should Debbie get a third party involved to find out indirectly what is going on?

3. Should Debbie ask for an evaluation from Diana?

Chapter Summary

Working in a fast-paced healthcare environment will inevitably lead to conflict in the workplace. The clinical laboratory assistant must always make sure that conflict does not interfere with the main concern of the healthcare worker: providing the best customer service possible. Conflicts should not be ignored as the pressure of conflicts can build until the employee is no longer an effective professional. So, understand your style of dealing with conflict, and work to be a collaborator in solving problems.

Name _____

Date _____

Student Enrichment Activities

Complete the following exercises.

1. Describe five methods of dealing with conflict. Which method most accurately describes your style of dealing with conflict most accurately?

   A. _____

   _____

   B. _____

   _____

   C. _____

   _____

   D. _____

   _____

   E. _____

   _____

   F. My method of dealing with conflict is: _____

   _____

2. Identify three potential sources of conflict in a clinical laboratory assistant's work day.

   A. _____

   B. _____

   C. _____

Circle T for true, or F for false.

3. T   F   Often the best way to resolve conflict is for the big boss to decide what is best for all parties.

4. T   F   Name calling has no place in conflict resolution.

5. T   F   Sometimes it is necessary to establish blame immediately when discussing a problem.

6. T   F   Avoiding the conflict can make it go away.

7. T   F   Feeling hopeless about conflict resolution can lead to being a very unhappy employee.

8. T   F   Considering a person with whom you are in conflict as a part of "we" instead of "he or she" and "me" is helpful in conflict resolution.

9. T   F   Compromise is the only answer in conflict resolution.

10. T   F   A collaborative approach can insure that both parties achieve their own goals in conflict resolution.

Chapter Twenty-Five
Obtaining the Right Job for You

Objectives

After completing this chapter, you should be able to do the following:

1. Define and correctly spell each of the key terms.

2. Identify employment conditions that most match your personal needs.

3. List as many potential employers as you can identify in your area.

4. Prepare a resumé of your qualifications.

5. Prepare a cover letter.

6. Discuss the importance of filling out an application properly.

7. Identify ways to prepare for a successful interview.

8. Answer questions frequently asked by interviewers.

9. Prepare a follow-up thank you letter for an interview.

Key Terms

- cover letter
- employment agency

- pocket resumé
- resumé

Introduction

You have completed a great deal of hard work and may have become certified as a clinical laboratory assistant/phlebotomist. You now begin a new adventure. If you were trained outside of a healthcare facility, you must find a position as a clinical laboratory assistant/phlebotomist. Or, if you were trained in a facility that has hired you, you must keep the position you have just obtained. Finding and keeping a position is indeed a challenge and requires more hard work and persistence, as well as a great deal of professionalism and preparation.

Introduction to Clinical Allied Healthcare, the core text of this series, has an extensive discussion of career planning in Chapter Twenty. That chapter will focus on how to get and keep a job.

Your Ideal Job Situation

Before you obtain your first job as a clinical laboratory assistant/phlebotomist, you need to do some serious thinking about your unique needs and expectations. There are several questions you might consider before beginning a job search:

- What hours do I want to work? Days? Evenings? Graveyard shifts? Weekends? Hospitals usually have all these shifts available as they are open 24 hours a day. A smaller private laboratory may function only on weekdays, with no weekend or evening work. Keep in mind that as a new employee, you may not be offered the shift you want but might have to start by working the less popular shifts, like graveyard or weekend shifts.

- How many hours do you want to work? If you are the sole financial support of yourself (and perhaps your family), you may need to work full-time. Also, you might want the opportunity to work overtime. If you are going to school, you might want to work only on weekends or nights. If you have a family, part-time days might be ideal. If your children are very young, the evening shift might be right for you.

- Are you willing to commute? How far away will you travel to a job? Is your car in good working order to travel on a freeway? Would you rather be close to work so that you can take public transportation? Have you considered the cost of the commute?

- Is this employment opportunity going to be a job or a career? Is working secondary to other considerations right now, such as your family? Or do you want as much responsibility and challenge as possible right away? Some clinical laboratory assistant positions are much more demanding than others. Some offer a much greater potential for career advancement and cross-training.

- What are your salary needs? Will childcare costs take up most of your salary if you accept a position with a low salary? Hospitals often pay more than private laboratories. Plus, premiums are attached to the less popular shifts such as graveyard. Do not bother to interview for a position that does not come with a salary you can accept. Also review your benefit needs. If you have a spouse who already provides your benefits, you might consider taking a short hour position that offers no benefits but that might work into a better position in the future.

Where the Jobs Are

Many first-time clinical laboratory job seekers are not aware of the variety of employers who should be considered in an employment search. Being aware of all the possibilities will improve your chances of finding a job suited to your needs.

- INSTRUCTORS AND COUNSELORS: Your instructor has observed you during your training and may offer some valuable advice as you search for a job. Instructors often have contacts on a professional level who may be interested in you. Often, employers may call your instructor if past students of the instructor have been good employees. Your training site may also have a counselor on staff who keeps track of job opportunities and can give you help.

- NEWSPAPER ADVERTISEMENTS AND POSTINGS: Many employers advertise for clinical laboratory assistant/phlebotomists. Look through the entire medical/healthcare listing in the classified section in case there are different titles for the position: phlebotomist, medical laboratory assistant, clinical laboratory assistant, lab assistant, and so on. Some training sites and healthcare facilities also have bulletin board postings. Professional laboratory magazines may have listings too.

- FAMILY AND FRIENDS: You do not have to look very far to find a person who got a job through family or friend connections. Many good job leads come from such places. Often an employer would prefer to hire someone who has been recommended by a trusted employee rather than hire someone based on references from people who are unknown to the employer. Therefore, tell everyone you know that you are looking for a job.

employment agency: a business that connects job seekers with potential employers.

- EMPLOYMENT AGENCIES: Every state has an **employment agency** that is responsible for helping people find jobs in their field. They interview applicants, test abilities, and attempt to match interests with an appropriate job. Because these are state programs, there is no fee for the applicant. There are also many private employment agencies that provide the same type of services, but these agencies often ask the applicant to sign a contract and pay a fee for the employment help. MAKE SURE YOU UNDERSTAND ALL CONTRACTS BEFORE YOU SIGN THEM! Some private employment agencies have much better rates than others, so shop around if you use these types of agencies.

- HEALTHCARE FACILITY HUMAN RESOURCES DEPARTMENTS: Most healthcare facilities have a human resources department that has the difficult task of filling jobs in every department of the facility. Human resource officers are constantly looking for responsible employees. If you are targeting a facility, contact the person in charge of Human Resources. Send that person a letter, indicating that you are interested in being interviewed for a clinical laboratory assistant/ phlebotomist position. You might ask for an interview even if there are no open positions available in your field at the time. This way, you will be introduced to the interviewer and will have your application on file for future reference.

The Resumé

resumé: a brief, written account of personal and professional qualifications and experience that is prepared by an applicant for a position.

The **resumé** is a summary and a biographical sketch of your work experience and personal talents which you present to a potential employer. Producing a resumé that truly represents your talents and valuable experiences takes time and skill. Most beginning resumé writers want to put down every detail of their lives in the resumé, but the resumé must be concise. In most instances, it should not be more than one page.

Employers want to know about your education, work experience (especially relating to the clinical laboratory), personal qualities and attributes, career objectives, references, and recommendations. You will need to put down much of this information in a small space, and you must sell yourself in the most positive, intelligent manner. This indeed is a challenge!

Organizing the Resumé

There are several different formats that you can use for the resumé. Check out books from the library that illustrate the different resumé formats that can be used. If your job history is limited, this section of your resumé will not be your main focus. Instead, you might focus on your education and training, with emphasis on the skills that you have mastered in order to be a clinical laboratory assistant/phlebotomist.

You must include in a resumé:

1. YOUR FIRST AND LAST NAME along with your middle initial. You also must have a COMPLETE ADDRESS listed. Do not forget your zip code. If you list a post office box, some employers may see it as a red flag indicating instability of residence on the part of the potential employee.

2. You need to provide a COMPLETE TELEPHONE NUMBER, including the area code, of a place where you can be easily reached. Your name, address, and telephone number can be centered at the top of the resumé. Some people also like to add their fax number as well as an e-mail address.

3. A CAREER GOAL/OBJECTIVE can be listed below your personal information. This is to aid the employer in knowing immediately the position you wish to obtain. Some employers read applicants' resumés for many different positions. For example, the prospective employer might be hiring for both part-time and full-time clinical laboratory assistants/phlebotomists. So, be sure you know the exact title of the position for which you are applying. And remember, laboratory positions often have a variety of titles.

4. A SUMMARY OF QUALIFICATIONS highlights strongest attributes such as integrity, initiative, communication skills, leadership ability, and so on. If you have held a previous job, employment history appears here as well. Jobs are listed in reverse chronological order, with the most recent job listed first. All applicable experience should be listed, along with responsibilities and duties. Unless your employment was short, list the dates you started and ended your employment.

5. EDUCATIONAL BACKGROUND should start with your most recent educational experience (including seminars and additional training). If you have been out of high school for more than five years, it is not necessary to list high school information. Vocational training, college education, and any degrees all are important to potential employers.

6. ADDITIONAL INFORMATION might include community activity involvement, volunteer leadership positions held (indicating leadership potential), and any languages spoken besides English. It is not necessary to state "references available upon request" as that is obvious for any job applicant and is considered out-of-date. Never put down a specific salary unless the potential employer requests that you do.

An example of a potential resumé format follows (Figure 25-1). Make sure that all margins are the same size (1-inch right and left margins, 1-inch top and bottom margins). Make the document look balanced, filling the entire page. Proofread the document at least twice, and have someone else proofread it as well. Neatness is mandatory.

Brenda Blood Drawer
3254 Nottingham Court
Laguna City, CA 92666-7507
714 555-3716

CAREER OBJECTIVE: A responsible position as a full-time clinical laboratory assistant/phlebotomist.

SUMMARY OF QUALIFICATIONS: I have obtained and developed the following professional and interpersonal skills through my training, education, intern work experience, and participation in various community activities.
• 3 month internship as a clinical laboratory assistant/phlebotomist
• 120 hour training program resulting in certification as a clinical laboratory assistant/phlebotomist
• Phlebotomy certification
• Cardiopulmonary Resuscitation (CPR) certification
• Excellent computer skills
• Self-motivated
• Well organized
• Excellent communication skills

WORK EXPERIENCE:
Good Samaritan Hospital
3451 Goodwill Avenue
San Clemente, CA 93330
Internship/Clinical Laboratory Assistant: Duties and responsibilities included performing venipunctures and capillary sticks; transporting specimens to the clinical laboratory; assisting clinical laboratory clerical staff with answering telephones and computer entry; preparing specimens for laboratory testing; setting up microbiology department specimens; preparing specimens for transport to other testing sites.

EDUCATIONAL BACKGROUND:
19__: Graduate of Beach Cities Clinical Laboratory Assistant Program.
Graduated 2nd in class standing.
19__: Graduate of Laguna City High School

COMMUNITY ACTIVITIES:
19__: Student volunteer for Coastal Medical Center; Volunteer of the Month in May, 19__
19__: Secretary, Student Volunteers of America

Figure 25-1: A Sample Resumé

Electronic Resumé Transmission

In this day of electronic transmissions, some employers may request that you send your resumé by e-mail or by fax. If you do not have access in your home to either method of transmission, copy centers in your area may have both capabilities.

The Cover Letter

cover letter: a letter that accompanies a resumé to explain or introduce its contents.

A **cover letter** should be included with every resumé that is sent to an employer. It should be on top of the resumé in the envelope. A cover letter introduces you to the employer. It must be short and simple. Most information about you will be in the resumé. The letter should be formatted in business style, as in the example shown in Figure 25-2.

Brenda Blood Drawer
3254 Nottingham Court
Laguna City, CA 92666-7507
714 555-3716

January 2, _____

Ms. Jane Hathaway
Director of Human Resources
Good Samaritan Hospital
3451 Goodwill Avenue
San Clemente, CA 93330

Dear Ms. Hathaway:

I am responding to your advertisement in the Los Angeles Times on (date of advertisement) for the position of clinical laboratory assistant. I am a recent graduate of Beach Cities Clinical Laboratory Assistant Program, placing second in my class.

Enclosed is my resumé. Please consider me for an interview for the above position. I have experience as a clinical laboratory assistant intern at your hospital. I am eager to begin a full-time career.

If you desire additional information or would like to schedule an interview, please contact me at the telephone number in the letterhead.

Thank you for considering me as a potential employee.

Sincerely,

Brenda Blood Drawer
Brenda Blood Drawer

Enclosure

Figure 25-2: A Sample Cover Letter

The Application

Most healthcare facilities require that you fill out an application form, a standard document that is completed by all potential employees. These forms require much more detail than is placed on the resumé. Applications are often used to screen applicants, so it is very important that your application be as neat as possible. Read the application CAREFULLY before filling it out to avoid errors. If you do not follow directions well in preparing the application, employers may reject the application immediately. As a clinical laboratory employee, following directions carefully is extremely important.

Sometimes an employer will send you an application in the mail, allowing you to complete the document at home. Other times, you will be asked to fill out an application at a facility. The application will ask for information that you may not have with you, such as specific dates of employment, former employers' addresses and telephone numbers, and so on. It is best to put together a **pocket resumé**, which you carry with you at all times during the job search. A pocket resumé might contain:

pocket resumé: a list to carry with you of important details that are usually requested on job applications, such as a Social Security number, names and addresses of schools attended, and so on.

- your Social Security number if you do not know it

- names and addresses of all schools attended, with dates of attendance

- names, addresses, and telephone numbers of all employers as well as dates of attendance

- names, addresses, and telephone numbers of references

On an application, you may be asked to name a salary that you require. Many people recommend putting "Open" in response to this query. You may disqualify yourself by asking for too much salary or undersell yourself by requiring too little.

You must tell the truth when filling out an application. When you are asked why you left each of your jobs, word your answers carefully. It is best to be as positive as possible on an application.

When a question is not applicable to you, such as term of military service, put "N/A" (not applicable) in such a space. This shows the potential employer that you did not forget to fill out the space.

References

You should always have a prepared list of references with you during the job search. References include people who have given you permission to use their names, addresses, and telephone numbers in case a potential employer wants to contact them about you as an employee. Do not ever list a reference who has not been confirmed by you beforehand. People who are excellent references include the following:

- a former employer who thinks highly of you

- a co-worker with whom you had an excellent working relationship

- someone who has known you for several years and can attest to your character (in this case, it would be wise to choose someone in the healthcare field)

- a clergyperson who can attest to your character

Never list relatives, best buddies, or people you feel might not speak well of you. Some applicants do not list current employers if they feel that the employer might resent their actions and place their current job in jeopardy.

The Job Interview

The job interview is possibly the most critical phase of your job search. You could produce the most impressive resumé, turn in the neatest and most complete application, and submit glowing references. However, if the interview goes poorly, it is likely that you will be eliminated from consideration for the position. You must give your prospective employer a good first impression by presenting yourself as a positive, competent person who is right for the job.

To prepare for the interview:

1. Review your most positive characteristics, the ones that will be selling points in the interview. For example, your ability to get along with different types of people, your work ethic, your punctuality, your natural enthusiasm for patient interaction, and so on, are positive characteristics.

2. Research the healthcare facility's accomplishments and community contributions. You can then use that knowledge in the interview. For example, the facility has just gotten a high rating as a result of its success with heart surgeries. You might express interest in working for a facility that is obviously dedicated to such excellence.

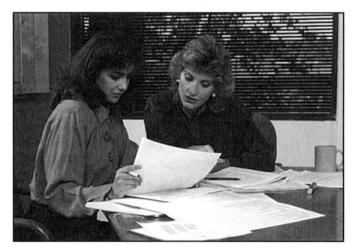

3. Select clean, well-fitting clothes that are businesslike in appearance. A conservative suit with a knee-length skirt (not too short!)

Figure 25-3: Being prepared for the interview will give the employer a favorable image of you.

might be appropriate for a woman. A man might wear a sports coat, tie, and slacks for the interview. Make sure clothes are well pressed with no missing buttons or tears.

4. Be prepared to answer questions that will be given to you by the interviewer. Figure 25-4 lists some frequently asked questions at an interview.

Frequently Asked Interview Questions

- Why are you qualified for this position?
- What are your strengths?
- What are your weaknesses?
- What do you know about this facility?
- What made you want to work in a clinical laboratory?
- Why do you want to work here?
- Why did you leave your last job?
- What are your long-range career goals?
- What were your favorite subjects in school?
- What is the most difficult problem you ever had as an employee? How was it solved?
- What makes a good supervisor?
- Do you work well under pressure?
- What two things are most important to you in a job?
- How would you define success for you?
- What does the term "patients' rights" mean to you?

Figure 25-4: Frequently Asked Interview Questions

5. Arrive at least 15 minutes early to an interview. Give yourself plenty of time to find the facility, to locate the interviewer's office, and to gather your thoughts before the interview starts. If possible, make a trial run to the location before the date of the interview to make certain you do not get lost.

6. Be prepared to complete an application if possible. Remember to bring your pocket resumé with all the dates, addresses, and telephone numbers necessary. Be sure to write neatly!

7. When you enter the interviewer's office, put out your hand for a handshake. Make sure your hand is dry and that your handshake is firm. A weak, damp handshake will make a poor impression. Practice your handshake with several people before you interview. Do not sit down until you are asked to do so. Also look the interviewer directly in the eyes. Do not look down as you are talking.

8. Answer all questions directly and honestly, maintaining eye contact. Always tell the truth. Be positive. Do not answer questions with long, rambling answers. Your interviewer will appreciate concise, well thought out answers.

9. The interviewer will probably ask you if you have questions for him or her. Figure 25-5 summarizes some questions that are proper to ask the interviewer.

Questions for the Applicant to Ask

- May I see a job description? (If you haven't seen one already.)
- What hours would I be working?
- What would my work schedule be?
- What are my chances for promotion?
- What about continuing education?
- What benefits are offered for this position?
- How often would job performance evaluations be performed?
- What would the salary be? (Usually asked late in the interview.)

Figure 25-5: Questions for the Applicant to Ask

10. Be alert to when the interview is over. It is likely in a healthcare facility setting that the interviewer will have a limited amount of time for the interview. When you see that the interviewer is wrapping up the discussion ("Well, I think we have covered all the necessary subjects I wanted to touch upon,") do not engage in further lengthy discussion. Get up from your chair, extend your hand with a polite "thank you so much for your time." Then say, "I'm looking forward to hearing from you," and leave the office.

Thinking Jt Through ...

> Monica is interviewing with the laboratory manager of a large healthcare facility. Monica really wants to be hired as a clinical laboratory assistant/phlebotomist.
>
> Monica is aware that by law she is not required to answer certain questions such as her age, marital status, family planning goals, child care provisions, religious preference, height, weight, and dependent situation.
>
> The laboratory manager immediately asks Monica, "Are you going to get pregnant in the near future, Monica?"
>
> How should Monica respond to this clearly illegal question?

The Thank You Letter

A most important part of the interview process is the follow-up thank you letter. It is conceivable that your interviewer could have seen five to ten other people for the same position that day. You want to keep the memory of your interview fresh in the prospective employer's memory. The letter should express your appreciation for the interview and the interviewer's time. Repeat your interest in the position and express the desire to get back in touch. Figure 25-6 illustrates a thank you letter after an interview.

Brenda Blood Drawer
3254 Nottingham Court
Laguna City, CA 92666-7507
714 555-3716

January 4, _____

Ms. Penny Beitler
Clinical Laboratory Manager
Good Samaritan Hospital
3451 Goodwill Avenue
San Clemente, CA 93330

Dear Ms. Beitler:

Thank you so much for taking time out of your busy schedule last Monday to meet with me. I found your description of the clinical laboratory assistant position to be comprehensive and informative.

I am very enthusiastic about working in the environment you described in our interview. Particularly, I am pleased to know that I will be working extensively with computers. I have just completed an intermediate computer course at Sam Hill Community College.

I am confident that I have the skills and enthusiasm to make a significant contribution to your department. I would appreciate the opportunity to work for you.

Sincerely,

Brenda Blood Drawer
Brenda Blood Drawer

Figure 25-6: A Sample Thank You Letter

Chapter Summary

Finding the right job is not an easy task. First, you must decide what you need in a job. Do you want to be full-time? Are you willing to commute? What shifts will you work? Is this a job or a career? Then you must use all the resources available to identify a good employer, create your resumé, fill out an application properly, assemble recommendations, and prepare for the interview. Courtesy, self-confidence, a positive attitude, and common sense will get you far in an interview situation. Good luck!

25-18

Name _____

Date _____

Student Enrichment Activities

Complete the following exercises.

1. List five things you desire most in an employment situation.

    A. _____

    B. _____

    C. _____

    D. _____

    E. _____

2. Name five places in your community where you can obtain job listings.

    A. _____

    B. _____

    C. _____

    D. _____

    E. _____

3. Prepare a resumé using the format listed in Figure 25-2.

4. Prepare a cover letter to go with your resumé, following the example in Figure 25-3.

5. Prepare a pocket resumé in a notebook or on separate sheets of paper.

6. Assemble a reference list (using at least 5 names).

7. On a separate sheet of paper, answer the Frequently Asked Interview Questions in Figure 25-4.

8. Prepare a thank you letter for an interview.

Chapter Twenty-Six
The Excellent Clinical Laboratory Employee

Objectives

After completing this chapter, you should be able to
do the following:

1. Define and correctly spell each of the key terms.

2. List several desirable qualities that employers seek
   in an employee.

3. Discuss several ways to get a good start at a new job.

4. Identify the Ten Commandments of Human Relations.

5. Explain how to terminate employment.

Key Terms

- employee evaluation

Introduction

Everyone has known somebody who is good at getting hired but not so good at keeping the job. The same talents that are needed to be a good student are not necessarily the same as those required to sustain good work habits on the job. What is needed is a dedication to teamwork, a strong work ethic, and a desire to do the very best job for each and every patient.

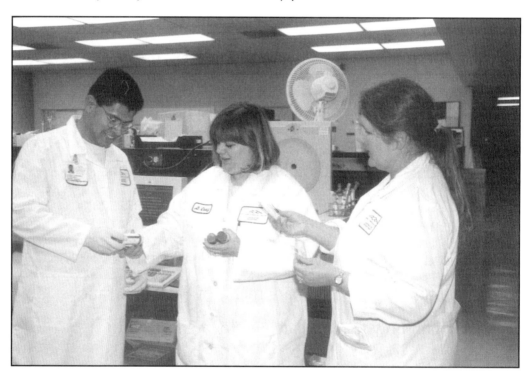

Figure 26-1: Cooperation and enthusiasm are among the qualities that are necessary to be a valuable employee.

What Employers Want from an Employee

You have invested much in your education and skills training. You have worked hard to assemble a resume and prepare for interviews. Now you have secured a position. An employer will expect you to perform with increasing expertise as a clinical laboratory assistant.

Desirable qualities that most employers would rank as most important in an employee include the following:

- excellent oral and written communication skills

- ability to cooperate with fellow employees (ie, teamwork)

- dependability (Arriving to work on time is especially important!)

- enthusiasm

- initiative (Employers love the employee who asks for tasks to perform when it is quiet.)

- time management skills (This is very important in the clinical laboratory where many tasks must be done quickly.)

- professionalism (You must be able to honor patient confidentiality, always acting as a professional.)

- detail-oriented (There is no room for careless performance in the clinical laboratory, as forgotten details could endanger a patient.)

- computer skills (Most clinical laboratories are computerized.)

Getting Off to a Good Start

It's likely that your first weeks on the job will be very stressful. Your new position may require some knowledge that you have not learned in an internship or in training. Also, each healthcare facility has its own ways of functioning. Computer systems vary from facility to facility. Further, many facilities may have a probationary period (usually up to six months). If the new employee does not perform well within this period, he or she may be dismissed. The pressure of being on probation may increase your stress levels.

To get off to a good start, the following suggestions may be helpful.

- While you are in training, try to get sufficient sleep each night.

- Read the employee handbook immediately. Get to know the unique characteristics of the clinical laboratory as soon as possible.

- Respond to training with a positive attitude. Do not moan and groan if asked to repeat a task several times during training.

- Accept criticism with a smile. No one likes criticism, but you will make mistakes during your training. Do not offer excuses for a mistake. Recognize the mistake and work hard to try not to make it again.

- Ask questions! If you are unsure about any directions, ask for clarification. You may think the question is stupid, but clarification may keep you from making a serious mistake that could affect a patient.

- Follow instructions completely. Do not take shortcuts.

- Save any suggestions for change until you are more experienced. In general, an employer does not want to hear immediately how your internship laboratory did things much better than this laboratory.

- Decide to get along with even the most difficult of your fellow employees. Make a pact with yourself to work well with all employees. If you remain positive with a difficult person, it will be harder for that person to continue to be difficult.

- Be a good communicator immediately. Speak slowly and clearly. Write down all communications legibly. Resist the urge to be bossy and argumentative. Be tactful.

- Create a businesslike image. Pay attention to proper hygiene from the beginning of your employment, reflecting pride in your new position. Proper clothing shows you are proud of yourself as well as your job.

- Accept all challenges. Be eager to learn new skills.

In addition to the above suggestions, these Ten Commandments of Human Relations can be extremely helpful when working with people.

The Ten Commandments of Human Relations

1. SPEAK TO PEOPLE. There is nothing as nice as a cheerful greeting.

2. SMILE AT PEOPLE. It takes 72 muscles to frown, only 14 to smile.

3. CALL PEOPLE BY NAME. The sweetest music to anyone's ears is the sound of his or her own name.

4. BE FRIENDLY AND HELPFUL. If you want to have friends, be a friend.

5. BE CORDIAL. Speak and act as if everything you do is a genuine pleasure.

6. BE GENUINELY INTERESTED IN PEOPLE. You can like almost everyone if you try.

7. BE GENEROUS WITH PRAISE; be cautious with criticism.

8. BE CONSIDERATE with the feelings of others. There are usually three sides to a controversy: yours, theirs, and the right side.

9. BE ALERT TO PROVIDE SERVICE. What counts most in life is what we do for others.

10. ADD TO THIS a good sense of humor, a big dose of patience, and a dash of humility, and you will be rewarded many times over.

Courtesy, Debra Garber, Zephyr Cove, NV

Figure 26-2: Practicing the Ten Commandments of Human Relations can help you become a valuable employee.

Thinking It Through ...

> You have been hired by a hospital with a large clinical laboratory. You realize right away that one of your co-workers (Tom) is not happy that you were hired. He had recommended a buddy of his for the position and is clearly disappointed that his friend was not hired. Tom barely speaks to you and refuses to answer questions you have about the job.
>
> **1.** How do you handle this employee?
>
> **2.** Do you confront Tom immediately?
>
> **3.** Do you tell your supervisor about Tom's attitude?
>
> **4.** How have you handled difficult employee to employee relationships in other jobs you have held?

Employee Evaluations

employee evaluation: an assessment of an employee's job performance by an employer.

Employee evaluations are performed periodically to assess how well you have performed your job. The first evaluation may occur as early as 3 months after you are hired. The time schedule for evaluations will vary from facility to facility, but you will probably have one near the end of your probationary period.

Usually, evaluations are performed by your direct supervisor. Or, in smaller facilities such as a physician's office, evaluations will be performed by the physician/employer or the office manager. Evaluations are set up to offer observations on both positive and negative areas of employee performance. Discussion topics during an evaluation might include the following:

- how well you are performing your tasks
- your general attitude
- suggestions for job performance improvement
- personal goals
- promotion opportunities
- possible increases in pay
- educational pursuits

CRITERIA-BASED PERFORMANCE EVALUATION

Phlebotomist
_____
(JOB TITLE)

EMPLOYEE: _____   DEPT: Laboratory   DATE: _____

MISSION *Translates the mission into specific behaviors.*	Does not Meet Standard*	Meets Standard	Exceeds Standard*
Demonstrates the Medical Center's Mission in everyday language and daily conduct.			
Answers the phone promptly with department and name, greets all callers in a friendly and professional manner.			
Consistently demonstrates positive attitude while performing job tasks.			
Consistently treats staff, patients, medical staff, peers, administrators and other customers in a nondiscriminatory and courteous manner regarding age, race, sex, religion, national origin, or disability.			
Displays appropriate professional behavior at all times, in all public places, throughout the Medical Center and while representing the Medical Center.			
Exhibits compassion and sensitive care to patients.			
Acknowledges patients who are waiting and provides service as quickly as possible.			
Demonstrates awareness of and/or participation in the Medical Center's CQI efforts.			

* Must be explained in space provided for Supportive Documentation & Comments

Figure 26-3: A Performance Evaluation Sheet can provide written documentation of your performance.

The most important thing to remember when going into your first employee evaluation is to have a positive attitude and an open mind. Defensiveness is immediately a turn-off for your employer. It is likely that the employer will offer suggestions on how to improve your performance because you are new at the position. Accept suggestions with grace, and let your employer know that you are eager to improve your performance.

Terminating Employment

There are many reasons that you may have to terminate employment, sometimes sooner than you had planned. Those reasons might include relocation of a spouse, a better job offer, illness, educational pursuits, pregnancy, a change in life-style, and so on. Regardless of the reason, you should give your employer at least two-weeks notice. This should be done to give the employer some time to fill your position. Notice should be sent to your direct supervisor. The letter of resignation should include the following data:

- date of your last working day
- positive comments about your position at the facility
- you may choose to include a sentence of two elaborating on the specific reason for leaving ("My husband has been transferred out of state.")

Keep the resignation letter on a positive note. You may want to ask for references from this facility. Also, consideration for your employer allows for a smoother transition and good feeling in case you ever want to come back to work.

When Employment is Terminated by the Employer

It is also possible that you may be released from your position by the employer. This is almost always an unpleasant experience for the employer and employee. Common reasons for termination include: tardiness, high absenteeism, continual errors, failure to get along with coworkers and patients, poor work habits, lack of knowledge about performing the job, dishonesty, poor attitude, and so on. Unfortunately, having a poor work record can follow you to the next job search.

Chapter Summary

As a clinical laboratory assistant, you are in the people business. You must get along with fellow employees, supervisors, and especially your patients. Just because you get hired, does not assure that you will keep the position without hard work, enthusiasm, and continual improvement of your skills.

Name _____

Date _____

Student Enrichment Activities

Complete the following exercises.

1. Describe what is meant by a good work ethic.

   _____

   _____

   _____

2. Name six desirable qualities of a good employee.

   A. _____

   B. _____

   C. _____

   D. _____

   E. _____

   F. _____

3. What steps would you take to be a good communicator at work?

   _____

   _____

   _____

   _____

4. Name five of the Ten Commandments of Human Relations.

   A. _____

   B. _____

   C. _____

   D. _____

   E. _____

5. What is an employee evaluation?

_____

_____

_____

_____

Chapter Twenty-Seven
Certification, Regulations, and Continuing Education Requirements

Objectives

After completing this chapter, you should be able to do the following:

1. Define and correctly spell each of the key terms.

2. Explain the purpose of certification for the clinical laboratory assistant.

3. Discuss various regulations and regulatory agencies that set standards for the clinical laboratory.

4. Explain why continuing education is important for the clinical laboratory assistant.

Key Terms

- certification
- continuing education

- National Accrediting Agency for Clinical Laboratory Sciences

Introduction

In today's healthcare environment, much is required of the clinical laboratory assistant. In some facilities, the assistant-level employee now performs tasks that were formerly in the job descriptions of the technician and even the technologist. Therefore, more knowledge is required as more tests are performed in the clinical laboratory. The clinical laboratory assistant/phlebotomist must be a highly skilled employee who can learn new skills to keep up with the rapid rate of change that occurs in the healthcare environment.

Certification

certification: a process resulting in completion of defined academic and training requirements and attainment of a satisfactory score on a national examination.

Today many healthcare facilities require national **certification** of their clinical laboratory assistant/phlebotomists to satisfy changing requirements at the state and federal levels. Certification requires a passing score on a national examination after completion of defined academic and training requirements. After certification, the phlebotomist is awarded initials that can be displayed after his or her name. The purpose of certification is to protect the patient by allowing only qualified personnel to work at specified levels of responsibility.

Certification in phlebotomy may be a real advantage in gaining satisfactory employment. Agencies that can certify clinical laboratory assistants/phlebotomists are listed below:

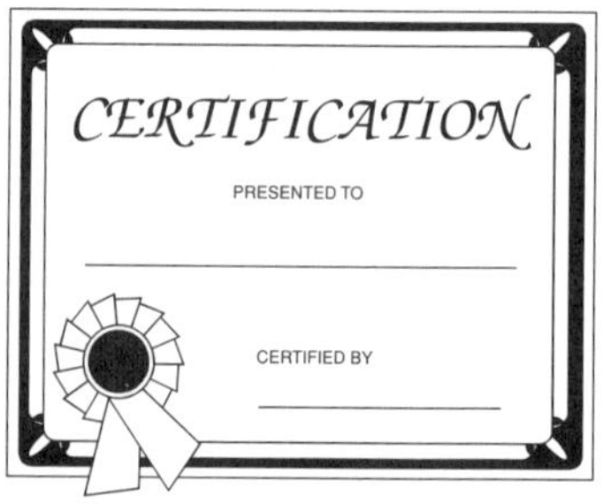

- The American Society of Clinical Pathologists (ASCP). The title given is Phlebotomy Technician or PBT (ASCP).

- The National Phlebotomy Association (NPA). The title given is Certified Phlebotomy Technician or CPT (NPA).

- The National Certification Agency for Medical Laboratory Personnel (NCA). This title is Clinical Laboratory Phlebotomist or CLP (NCA).

- The American Society for Phlebotomy Technology (ASPT). The title given is Certified Phlebotomy Technician or CPT (ASPT).

Figure 27-1: Certification protects the patients.

National Standards

In addition to certification, many regulatory considerations have an impact on procedures that the clinical laboratory assistant/phlebotomist performs. Regulations set standards of performance for all healthcare professionals. So in addition to certification, various regulations further define your position in the clinical laboratory.

The Clinical Laboratory Improvement Act of 1988 (CLIA '88)

As discussed in Chapter Seventeen, the Clinical Laboratory Improvements Act of 1988 is legislation that regulates all laboratory procedures, quality control procedures, and the laboratory personnel that perform such procedures. CLIA sets requirements and standards for every procedure used in specimen testing. A laboratory can be fined and even ordered to stop doing procedures if they are not performed according to regulations.

National Committee for Clinical Laboratory Standards (NCCLS)

The National Committee for Clinical Laboratory Standards (NCCLS) is an agency that develops national and international procedures for all areas of practice in the clinical laboratory including phlebotomy. Responsible clinical laboratories set up procedures based on such recommendations. Venipuncture procedures are often set up according to NCCLS standards.

National Accrediting Agency for Clinical Laboratory Sciences (NAACLS)

The **National Accrediting Agency for Clinical Laboratory Sciences (NAACLS)** is an organization that evaluates the quality of laboratory educational programs, including phlebotomy training. The process for accreditation involves external peer review to determine if certain standards of educational quality and student competency have been met.

National Accrediting Agency for Clinical Laboratory Sciences: NAACLS; an organization responsible for evaluating the quality of laboratory educational programs.

Continuing Education

continuing education: courses, workshops, and seminars offered to continually upgrade professional skills and knowledge.

New skills are needed on a regular basis in the clinical laboratory. New procedures are developed that must be learned rapidly. One of the best ways for the clinical laboratory assistant/phlebotomist to keep up with advances in the field is through **continuing education**. Continuing education for your field can be attained by attending a demonstration by a sales representative about a new technique involving a new product. It can also be gained through attending a workshop in your area, or by participating in an educational program at your place of work. Video conferences are also available, as well as self-instruction units.

Some professions require that members complete a certain number of continuing education units (CEUs) per year. If you are certified, organizations such as the American Society of Phlebotomy Technicians require the completion of a certain number of CEUs to maintain certification.

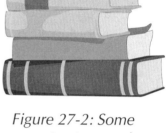

Figure 27-2: Some organizations and professions require a certain amount of continuing education each year.

Many opportunities are available for the clinical laboratory assistant/phlebotomist to acquire continuing education. Cross-training is often accomplished by attending seminars and workshops to learn new skills.

Chapter Summary

Adhering to the high standards of any profession gives employees pride in what they are doing. Being a professional with such standards makes employees more likely to receive offers of advancement. Furthermore, cross-training makes employees much more valuable to the employer. There are several types of certification processes for the clinical laboratory assistant/phlebotomist. Always take advantage of any continuing education offerings to make yourself a more informed and skillful clinical laboratory assistant.

Name _____

Date _____

Student Enrichment Activities

Complete the following exercises.

1. What does certification mean to the clinical laboratory assistant/phlebotomist?

   _____

   _____

   _____

   _____

   _____

2. Name three agencies that certify phlebotomists.
   A. _____
   B. _____
   C. _____

3. What are NCCLS standards?

   _____

   _____

   _____

4. What is the significance of NAACLS?

   _____

   _____

   _____

   _____

5. Why should the clinical laboratory assistant/phlebotomist participate in continuing education?

   _____

   _____

   _____

   _____

   _____

Complete the following statements.

6. _____ _____ _____ are earned when you attend a continuing education event.

7. _____ is the process that results in the completion of defined academic and training requirements.

8. _____ are initials that can follow your name after certification.

9. _____ is the abbreviation for the Clinical Laboratory Improvements Act of 1988.

10. _____ _____ is the process by which you learn new skills that can make you a more valuable employee.

Glossary

a-, an-: without or not.

ab-: away from, absent.

abandonment: the termination of supervision of a patient by a physician without adequate written notice or the patient's consent.

***accommodator:** one who assists, aids.

***accuracy:** the closeness of a result compared with the true or actual value.

acquired immune deficiency syndrome: AIDS; a viral disease caused by the human immunodeficiency virus (HIV), which damages the immune system leaving the patient susceptible to other infections. It is contracted through infected blood and other body fluids and sexual contact.

***activated partial thromboplastin time:** a frequently ordered coagulation test that assesses part of the coagulation mechanism in the body.

***active listening:** making a conscious effort to hear what the sender is communicating; an essential element of effective and meaningful communication.

ad-: near; toward.

adapter: also called the vacuum tube holder; a clear plastic cylinder with a small opening at one end to receive the threaded vacuum system needle.

aden-, adeno-, aden/o: gland.

***advance directive:** a legal document prepared when an individual is alive, competent, and able to make decisions. It provides guidance to the healthcare team if the person is no longer able to make decisions.

aer/o: air.

***aerobic:** requiring oxygen to maintain life.

***aerosol:** a substance released in the form of a fine mist.

agranulocytes: a term referring to lymphocytes, monocytes, and megakaryocytes.

***AIDS:** acquired immune deficiency syndrome; a viral disease caused by the human immunodeficiency virus (HIV), which damages the immune system leaving the patient susceptible to other infections. It is contracted through infected blood and other body fluids and sexual contact.

-algia: pain.

***aliquot:** a portion of a sample used for testing.

***Allen Test:** a test performed to verify blood flow to the hand from the radial and ulnar arteries before performing arterial blood gas testing.

***anaerobic:** able to live without oxygen.

***analytical balance:** a very sensitive scale used in chemical analyses.

***anchoring:** holding a vein in position before performing a venipuncture.

***anemia:** a reduction in the number of circulating erythrocytes (red blood cells), the amount of hemoglobin, or the volume of packed red blood cells in a given volume of blood.

angi/o: vessel, either blood or lymph.

aniso-: unequal

ante-: before; preceding.

***antecubital space:** the area of the arm located in the vicinity of the bend of the elbow where the major veins for venipuncture are located.

anti-: against.

***anticoagulant:** a substance that prevents blood from clotting.

***antigen/antibody reactions:** reactions where a foreign substance (antigen) introduced into the body is attacked by a protein substance (antibody) produced by the body in response to the invader.

antiseptic: an agent capable of inhibiting the growth of microorganisms. Used when referring to living tissue.

aorta: the main artery in the body.

arteri/o: artery.

***arterial blood gas:** any of the gases that normally occur in the blood, such as oxygen and carbon dioxide, when analyzed from the artery rather than from a vein.

arterial blood gas test: a blood test used to determine acidity or alkalinity as well as the oxygen and carbon dioxide levels in the arterial blood.

arteries: blood vessels that carry oxygenated blood from the heart to the tissues.

arterioles: a tiny artery that joins directly to a capillary.
*artery: a blood vessel that transports highly oxygenated blood away from the heart to the tissues.
arthr/o: joint.
*articulation: speaking in a clear, precise manner.
*ASAP: as soon as possible.
asepsis: a condition in which no pathogens, infection, or any form of life is present.
aseptic technique: the practices and procedures designed to ensure a clean environment by removing or destroying pathogens.
aspiration: removal or drawing in by suction.
*assault: the threat of an immediate harmful or offensive contact, without actual commission of the act.
*atria: the upper left and right chambers of the heart; also known as the receiving chambers.
atrium: either the upper right or left chamber of the heart, also known as a receiving chamber.
auto-: self.
*autopsy: an examination after death of organs and tissues of the body to determine a cause of death or pathological condition.
*avoider: one who evades, shuns, or bypasses.
*backup: the duplication of files to protect information; often done on a computer once or twice a day.
baso-: blue.
basophil: the least prevalent white blood cell; may play a role in acute allergic reactions.
*battery: the unlawful touching of an individual without consent.
*beaker: a wide-mouthed, straight-sided piece of glassware with a pouring spout in the rim; glassware not critically calibrated.
*bevel: the point of a needle that has been cut on a slant for ease of entry.
bi/o: life.
*bilirubin: a product produced from the breakdown of red blood cells; excessive blood levels may indicate liver disease.
-blast: germ; primitive.
*bleeding time test: a procedure designed to evaluate how long it takes a patient to stop bleeding from a standardized tiny incision.
*blood bank: immunohematology; a clinical laboratory department that processes blood products for transfusion.
*bloodborne pathogens: the disease-causing microorganisms that are present in human blood. Examples include the human immunodeficiency virus (HIV) and the hepatitis B virus (HBV).
*blood culture: a liquid broth with a blood sample added to test for possible infection in the blood.
boot: to start up a computer.
brachi/o: arm.
brachial: refers to the large artery in the arm on the anterior inner aspect of the elbow.
*brachial artery: the large artery in the arm on the anterior inner aspect of the elbow.
bronch/o, bronchi/o: bronchial tubes (air tubes in the lungs).
*buffy coat: in a coagulated blood sample, the layer of white blood cells and platelets that settles between the plasma and the red blood cell layer.
*burden of proof: the obligation to prove the facts of a dispute by evidence presented.
*butterfly infusion set: a needle and tubing connected with a plastic wing-shaped holder; used for fragile veins when a small volume of blood is sufficient.
*calibration: a determination of the accuracy of an instrument by comparing a measurement with a known standard.
*canine: of or pertaining to dogs.
*cannula: a tube or sheath.
*capillaries: tiny blood vessels in the circulatory system that link arteries and veins.
*capillary action: a process by which blood is drawn up by contact only into a small tube.
capillary beds: areas containing capillaries; sites of capillary punctures.
*capillary tubes: tubes used to collect blood obtained during a skin puncture.
cardi/o: heart.
*cardiopulmonary resuscitation: CPR; the basic lifesaving procedure of artificial ventilation and chest compressions that is done in the event of a cardiac arrest.
*carrier: a human or animal who is infected with a pathogen, and who can spread the disease to others, but who does not show any outward signs or symptoms of disease.

***cathode ray tube:** CRT; a visual display unit with a screen that is connected to a computer.

***caustic materials:** materials destructive to living tissue.

CBC: complete blood count; a blood test that determines the number of erythrocytes, leukocytes, and platelets that are present in the patient's blood, as well as the hemoglobin and hematocrit, among other determinations.

CCU: an abbreviation for critical care unit.

CDC: Centers for Disease Control and Prevention; the government agency responsible for protecting public health through the prevention and control of disease.

***Celsius:** a temperature scale used in medicine, that uses 100° as the boiling point of water and 0° as the freezing point of water.

***Centers for Disease Control and Prevention:** CDC; the government agency responsible for protecting public health through the prevention and control of disease.

-centesis: puncture to remove fluid.

centi-: in the metric system, a prefix referring to $^1/_{100}$ (.01).

***central processing:** also known as specimen processing, the area of the clinical laboratory where specimens are processed for testing in various departments of the clinical laboratory as well as for preparing specimens for transport to other facilities.

***central processing unit:** CPU; the central processing unit or the brains of the system; the CPU's memory is made up of bits.

centrifugal force: the force that moves an object outward from the center of rotation.

***centrifugation:** the application of centrifugal force to spin and separate substances of different densities.

***centrifuge:** a device used to separate substances of different densities through spinning.

centrifuge tube: tubes generally made of plastic or glass that are designed to withstand the stress encountered during centrifugation.

cephal/o: head.

***cephalic vein:** a superficial vein of the arm and forearm that winds anteriorly up the arm; a common venipuncture site in the antecubital area (in front of the elbow at the bend of the elbow).

***cerebrospinal fluid:** CSF; the clear, watery fluid that flows through the brain and spinal column, protecting the brain and spinal cord.

***certification:** a process resulting in completion of defined academic and training requirements and attainment of a satisfactory score on a national examination.

***CHAMPVA:** the Civilian Health and Medical Program of the Veterans Administration; a governmental healthcare insurance program for surviving spouses and dependent children of persons who died or are permanently disabled as a result of military service.

chief laboratory technologist: an employee in the clinical laboratory who is in charge of all laboratory testing procedures.

***chemistry autoanalyzer:** a general term for highly automated, computerized equipment used to run tests in the chemistry department.

***chemotherapy:** the use of drugs or chemicals to treat or control diseases such as cancer.

chol/e-, chol/o: bile; gall.

chrom/o: color.

-cid; -cide: kill or destroy.

***circulatory system:** the network of vessels that carries blood to all parts of the body.

***clean-catch urine specimen:** a method of obtaining a urine specimen so that it is free of contaminating matter from external genital areas.

***clinical chemistry:** a department of the clinical laboratory in which quantitative analyses of blood and other fluids are performed, including many blood chemistries and drug analyses.

clinical laboratory: a department within a healthcare facility where blood and other body fluids and tissues are analyzed in a precise, accurate and timely manner.

clinical laboratory aide: an unskilled clinical laboratory employee; often involved in cleaning laboratory glassware, restocking supplies, and performing general cleanup.

clinical laboratory assistant/phlebotomist: a clinical laboratory employee whose duties include obtaining blood specimens, requisitioning laboratory tests in the computer, transporting specimens, preparing specimens for testing, and performing testing in different areas of the clinical laboratory.

clinical laboratory clerical worker: a clinical laboratory employee whose duties include continually interfacing with the laboratory computer system, entering tests into the computer and retrieving results for physicians, operating the telephone system of the laboratory, distributing reports, filing, and many other clerical duties.

CLIA '88: Clinical Laboratory Improvement Act of 1988; an act, signed into federal law in 1988, which mandates that all laboratories be regulated using the same standards regardless of location, type, or size.

*Clinical Laboratory Improvement Act of 1988: CLIA '88; an act, signed into federal law in 1988, which mandates that all laboratories be regulated using the same standards regardless of location, type, or size.

*clinical laboratory manager: a professional with a business or management education who is responsible for business operations in the clinical laboratory.

clinical laboratory technician: a clinical laboratory position requiring two years of training. A person in this position performs testing in the laboratory under the direction of a clinical laboratory technologist.

*clinical laboratory technologist: a clinical laboratory professional often employed as a supervisor of one of the clinical laboratory departments; responsible for results produced during laboratory testing.

CO_2: the chemical symbol for carbon dioxide.

*coagulation: the process of blood clotting.

*COBRA: Continuation of Benefits Reconciliation Act; provides healthcare continuation coverage to employees when employment ends, or to employee spouses who become divorced or separated.

colorectal cancer: a cancerous condition affecting the colon and the rectum.

*collaborator: one who assists, acting as a partner.

*combining form: a root word plus a combining vowel.

*combining vowel: a vowel that is placed between two word elements to join the two word parts.

compact disks: abbreviated CD; a high volume data storage device.

*complete blood count: CBC; a blood test that determines the number of erythrocytes, leukocytes, and platelets that are present in the patient's blood, as well as the hemoglobin and hematocrit, among other determinations.

*compound microscope: a microscope that utilizes two lens systems; the most commonly used microscope in the clinical laboratory.

*compromiser: one who adapts, adjusts, and negotiates.

*confidentiality: privacy; refers to the limiting of access to patient information to authorized personnel only.

Continuation of Benefits Reconciliation Act: COBRA; provides healthcare continuation coverage to employees when employment ends, or to employee spouses who become divorced or separated.

*continuing education: courses, workshops, and seminars offered to continually upgrade professional skills and knowledge.

contra-: opposite; opposed; against.

*controller: one who rules and manages.

*controls: comparisons of known values that are run with patient tests to check equipment, reagents, and technique.

co-payment: a type of cost sharing where the insured pays a specified amount per unit of service and the insurer pays the rest of the cost.

*cover letter: a letter that accompanies a resumé to explain or introduce its contents.

CPR: the abbreviation for cardiopulmonary resuscitation; the basic lifesaving procedure of artificial ventilation and chest compression that is done in the event of a cardiac arrest.

CPU: central processing unit; the brains of the computer system.

CRT: cathode ray tube; a visual display unit with a screen that is connected to a computer.

*critical measurements: measures that must be made in an exacting manner.

*cross-training: the gaining of skills of other job descriptions in addition to one's own position.

CSF: cerebrospinal fluid; the clear, watery fluid that flows through the brain and spinal column, protecting the brain and spinal cord.

culture and sensitivity: a laboratory test for bacterial growth that involves instilling microorganisms in special media, monitoring them for the growth of pathogens, and then determining how susceptible the patient's bacterial infection is to certain antibiotics or antibacterial drugs.

cursor: a marker on the screen showing where the next letter, number, or symbol will be placed; can be a blinking underline, rectangle, or square.

*customer service: efforts made to provide the customer (patient) with the best service available in the facility.

cutane/o: skin.

cyan/o: blue.

*cyanotic: affected by cyanosis; the bluish discoloration of the skin and mucous membranes due to a decrease in oxygen.

cyst/o: fluid-filled sac; urinary bladder; bag.

cyt/o, -cyte: cell.

cytologist: a person trained to examine body fluids and other tissue specimens in order to detect and diagnose cell changes that might indicate cancer.

*cytology: the science that deals with the formation, structure, and function of cells.

database: a software program that manipulates data, including functions such as editing, and comparisions.

deca-: in the metric system, a prefix denoting 10.

deci-: in the metric system, a prefix denoting $^1/_{10}$ (0.1).

decontaminated: having rendered an object, person, or area free of a contaminated substance.

*deductible: the amount of medical expenses that must be met before an insurance policy begins to pay.

Department of Commerce: a federal government department that deals with the exchange of both foreign and domestic goods.

derm/o, -derma, dermat/o: skin.

di-: two; twice; double.

*diabetes mellitus: a chronic disorder caused by the failure of the pancreas to produce enough insulin or the failure of cells to accept insulin, causing an increase in blood sugar; commonly referred to as diabetes.

*diagnosis related groups: DRGs; a system of disease classification used to determine reimbursement rates.

*differential cell count: the counting of 100 white blood cells to obtain the percentage of each type of white blood cells in a blood sample; also includes evaluation of platelet and red blood cell morphology.

*diluent: an agent that dilutes a substance or solution to which it is added.

dilution: to make a liquid thinner or weaker by the addition of water or other appropriate liquid.

dipl/o: two; twice; double.

dis-: to cut apart.

disk: a magnetic storage device made of rigid material (hard disk) or flexible plastic (floppy disk).

disk drive: a device used to get information on to and off of a disk.

DOS: disk operating system; a program that tells the computer how to use the disk drive.

downtime: a period of lost work time when the computer is not operating or is malfunctioning.

DRG: diagnosis related group; a system of disease classification used to determine reimbursement rates.

*duty of care: a legal term referring to the healthcare worker's duty to treat the patient according to common or average standards of practice expected in the community.

dys-: painful; difficult; bad; disordered.

e-: out; outside.

-ectomy: surgical removal; excision.

*edema: swelling due to fluid in the tissues; fluid retention.

edematous: a condition in which body tissues contain excessive amounts of tissue fluid.

*electronic cell counter: an automated system used to count and access formed elements of the blood.

electronic mail: e-mail; transmission of letters, messages, results, memos, and so on from one computer to another by the use of telephone lines.

*emancipated minor: a person under the age of 18 who is financially responsible for himself/herself and free of parental care.

-emia: blood.

*empathy: to understand and relate to the emotional state of another; to show concern.

*employee evaluation: an assessment of an employee's job performance by an employer.

*employment agency: a business that connects job seekers with potential employers.

encephal/o: brain.

endo-, end/o-: inside; interior; within.

*English System: a system of measurement not accurate enough to be used for science; used for most measurements in the United States and Great Britain.

epi-: upon; over; upper.

erythr/o: red.

*erythrocyte: a red blood cell.

eosinophil: a white blood cell active in allergic reactions and parasitic infections.

*ethics: principles of conduct that establish standards and morals that govern decisions and behavior.

euthanized: having ended the life of an animal through artificial means.

*evacuated tubes: premeasured vacuum tubes that receive the patient's blood during venipuncture.

ex/o, ex-: out; outside.

*facsimile (fax) machine: a machine that sends documents from one location to another by telephone lines.

*Fahrenheit: a temperature scale used in medicine that uses 212° as the boiling point of water and 32° as the freezing point of water.

false imprisonment: restraining a person against his or her will, either physically or with verbal threats.

fasting: abstaining from food and drink (except water).

febr/o: fever.

*feedback: a receiver's way of assuring that the message that was understood is the same as the message that was sent.

*feline: of or pertaining to a cat.

*femoral artery: the largest artery used to obtain blood; access in the groin area near the femur.

*femoral vein: a large vein located in the groin area.

*fever of unknown origin: FUO; an illness of at least three weeks duration with a recurrent fever and no diagnosis.

first morning specimen: a specimen collected at the beginning of the day; first voiding after a patient arises.

*flask: common clinical laboratory glassware that comes in a variety of sizes, usually with rounded sides, a flat bottom, and a long cylindrical neck.

*floor book: a guide, often at a nurses' station, that lists the correct vacuum tube, amount of blood, and blood specimen considerations for each test.

*floppy disk: a flexible magnetic storage device for computer programs and information; usually $3^{1}/_{2}$ inches.

flora: plant life occurring in or adapted to living in a specific environment, such as the intestine, vagina, skin, etc.

font: an assortment of print characters of a given size or style.

*forensic: pertaining to the law.

FUO: fever of unknown origin; an illness of at least three weeks duration with a recurrent fever and no diagnosis.

gaster-, gastr/o: stomach.

*gastric secretions: fluid collected from the stomach.

*gauge: a standard for measuring the diameter of the lumen of a needle.

gastrointestinal: of or relating to the stomach and the intestine.

gastrointestinal lesions: an injury or wound in the stomach or intestine.

gen/o, -genic: origin or produced by or in.

*general containers: containers such as beakers, graduated cylinders, and certain flasks designed to hold and measure inexact volumes.

*glucose tolerance test: GTT; a test for imbalance in glucose metabolism in which a patient follows a special diet and has blood drawn in timed intervals after ingesting a glucose drink. Urine also is tested at timed intervals as part of the test.

glyc/o: sugar; glucose.

graduated cyclinders: cylindrical pieces of glassware with several calibrated markings; available in sizes from 5 ml to many liters.

-gram: record.

*gram: the basic unit of weight in the metric system.

-graph: instrument used for recording.

*Gram stain: the most common stain performed in the microbiology department of the clinical laboratory; a stain used to observe the gross morphological features of specimens under a microscope.

granulocytes: leukocytes that contain granules in their cytoplasm.

Greenwich system: time expressed on a 12 hour clock, with the time before noon as a.m., and the time after noon as p.m.

growth media: solid or liquid substances containing nutrients on which microorangisms are placed for isolations and study.

GTT: glucose tolerance test; a test for imbalance in glucose metabolism in which a patient follows a special diet and has blood drawn in timed intervals after ingesting a glucose drink. Urine also is tested at timed intervals as part of the test.

gyne-, gynec/o: woman or female.

*hard copy: the readable paper copy or printout from a computer.

*hard disk: a magnetic storage device for information, usually located inside of the computer.

*hardware: the electronic, magnetic, and mechanical equipment of a computer (keyboard, monitor, and so on).

*HCG: human chorionic gonadotropin; a hormone found in the blood and urine of a pregnant human female.

*health maintenance organization: HMO; a type of prepaid group healthcare program that provides health maintenance and treatment services to its members.

hecto-: in the metric system, a prefix denoting 100.

hema-, hemo-, hemat/o: blood.

hematologist: a physician who specializes in the study of the blood and in the diagnosis and treatment of disorders of blood and blood-forming tissues.

*hematology: the clinical laboratory department concerned with the qualitative and quantitative evaluation of the formed elements of the blood and bone marrow.

*hematoma: a blood-filled swollen area; a goose egg caused by bleeding under the tissues.

hemi-: half.

*hemoconcentration: an increase in the concentration of formed blood elements caused by lack of fluid in the blood; often caused by a tourniquet too tightly applied to the arm or left on too long.

*hemoglobin: a complex protein that gives erythrocytes their red color; a molecule that transports oxygen throughout the body.

*hemorrhage: the severe, abnormal internal or external discharge of blood.

*heparin: a natural blood thinner produced by the liver; also used as a medication for patients who are prone to abnormal blood clotting.

hepat/o: liver.

*hepatitis: inflammation of the liver.

hepatitis A: inflammation of the liver that is caused by the hepatitis A virus and spread by the oral-fecal route either from poor handwashing or contaminated food or water.

hepatitis B: inflammation of the liver that is caused by the hepatitis B virus and spread through contact with infected blood or other body fluids; the most common form contracted by healthcare workers.

hepatitis C: inflammation of the liver caused by the hepatitis C virus and spread through contact with infected blood or body fluids.

hist/o: tissue.

*histology: the study of the microscopic structure of tissue.

HMO: health maintenance organization; a type of prepaid group healthcare program that provides health maintenance and treatment services to its members.

horizontal: parallel to ground level.

hub: a clear plastic section of a needle.

*human chorionic gonadotropin: HCG; a hormone found in the blood and urine of a pregnant human female.

hyper-: excessive; above; increased.

hypo-: below; deficient; under.

hyster/o: uterus; womb.

*icteric: referring to jaundice; yellow discolorization of skin and eyeballs caused by excess bilirubin in the blood.

*immune globulin: a preparation injected into an individual to boost the immune system; often given to employees who have just stuck themselves with a contaminated needle.

immunohematology: blood bank; a clinical laboratory department that processes blood products for transfusion.

*incident report: a report made by a healthcare worker when an event occurs that is not consistent with the routine operation of the healthcare facility.

infection: the invasion of the body or a part of the body by a pathogen.

*infection control: efforts taken to control infectious agents in a healthcare facility.

Infection Control Department: the department in a hospital responsible for developing policies and procedures concerned with reducing the risk of transferring communicable diseases to both the staff and patients.

*infection cycle: a pattern that describes the origin and transmission of a disease or illness.

inoculated: having injected a specimen into a medium that promotes the growth of microorganisms.

*inpatient: a patient who is admitted into a healthcare facility and receives treatment within the facility itself.

input: data put into the computer via the keyboard or floppy disk.

inter-: between.

interface: the hardware and software that allow computers to interact.

*interstitial fluid: the fluid outside the cell (extracellular fluid), excluding the fluid within the blood and lymph vessels.

invasion of privacy: public discussion of private information.

intra-: within.

iso-: equal, same

-itis: inflammation.

*jaundice: yellow discolorization of skin and eyeballs caused by excess bilirubin in the blood.

JCAHO: Joint Committee for Accreditation of Healthcare Organizations; a voluntary nongovernmental agency charged with establishing standards for the operation of hospitals and other health-related facilities and services.

*Joint Committee for Accreditation of Healthcare Organizations: JCAHO; a voluntary nongovernmental agency charged with establishing standards for the operation of hospitals and other health-related facilities and services.

*jugular vein: the major vein that runs on either side of the trachea; a major venipuncture site in animals.

K: computer shorthand for 1,024 bytes; a term used to measure the memory capacity of the computer.

keyboard: an input device like a typewriter keyboard that converts keystrokes into electrical signals displayed on the screen as letters and symbols.

kilo-: in the metric system, a prefix referring to 1,000.

*laboratory requisition form: a form filled out by physicians or nurses to order clinical laboratory tests.

lancet: a sterile, disposable sharp-pointed instrument used to pierce the skin to obtain droplets of blood used for testing.

lapar/o: abdomen

*lateral saphenous vein: a superficial vessel that obliquely crosses the lateral surface of the distal tibia; a common venipuncture site for dogs.

leuk/o: white.

*leukocytes: white blood cells that are responsible for fighting infection.

leukocytosis: an increase in leukocytes normally found in the circulating blood.

leukopenia: a decrease in leukocytes normally found in the circulating blood.

*libel: false and malicious writing about another constituting a defamation of character.

lip/o: fat.

*liter: the basic unit of volume in the metric system; a metric fluid measurement that is equivalent to 1,000 milliliters, or approximately one quart.

lith/o: stone or calculus.

*litigation: a lawsuit.

-logist: specialist; one who studies.

*Luer adapter: a device for connecting a syringe to the needle and when locked into place gives a secure fit.

*lumbar puncture: a diagnostic test in which a specimen of cerebrospinal fluid is removed and analyzed for diseases such as meningitis; a spinal tap.

lymphocyte: a type of leukocyte found in blood, lymph, and lymphatic tissue that helps fight infection.

macro-: large; long.

magnetic tapes: digital data storage media for the computer.

*mainframe: the largest of computers, capable of performing multiple tasks at rapid speeds; usually found in large facilities.

mal-: abnormal; bad; disordered.

*malpractice: professional misconduct or lack of professional skill that results in injury to the patient; negligence by a professional, such as a physician or nurse.

manual differential cell count: counting by hand 100 leukocytes, using a microscope and a stained peripheral blood smear.

mass: the physical measurement of how much an object weighs, regardless of the gravity exerted on the object.

mast/o-: breast.

*material safety data sheet: MSDS; an official required document that identifies all the chemicals that are used in a specific department and that details important information regarding those chemicals.

meatus: the anatomical opening where urine is expelled from the body.

*medial saphenous vein: a superficial vein that travels along the medial surface of the ankle (tibiotarsal joint) and the distal tibia; a common venipuncture site for cats.

median cubital: pertaining to the middle of the forearm.

*Medicaid: a program funded by the state and federal government for providing medical care to the poor and disabled.

*medical law: laws that govern the legal conduct of the members of the medical profession; includes local, state, and federal laws.

*Medicare: a federally-funded program enacted in 1965 that provides healthcare to people over the age of 65 as well as to the disabled, regardless of financial status.

mega-, megal/o, -megaly: enlarged.

megakaryocytes: large cells that break apart in the bone marrow to form platelets.

memory: data that is held in storage.

mening/o: membrane; meninges.

***meningitis:** inflammation of the membranes covering the spinal cord and brain; marked by severe headache, vomiting, fever, and a stiff neck, and usually caused by infection.

***meniscus:** the curvature of a liquid's upper surface when the liquid is placed in a container.

menu: a list of available computer functions for selection by the operator; usually appears when the computer is turned on.

meta-: after, next.

-meter: instrument that measures.

***meter:** the basic unit of linear measurement in the metric system.

***metric system:** a decimal system of weights and measures based on the basic units of meters, grams, and liters.

micro-, micr/o: small.

***microbiology:** a department in the clinical laboratory that grows and identifies organisms that can cause infection, disease, or both in humans.

microcapillary tube: a small tube used to collect capillary blood.

***microcomputer:** a self-contained computer system that uses a microprocessor as the CPU; often called a PC (personal computer).

microneedle: a tiny needle.

***midstream urine specimen:** a urine sample collected in the middle of the urine flow.

military time: time measured on a 24-hour clock and expressed in hundreds, such as 0800; used in healthcare facilities.

milli-: in the metric system, a prefix denoting $1/1000$ (0.001).

***minicomputer:** a computer system often used in a clinical laboratory setting; larger than a microcomputer and smaller than a mainframe computer.

modem: a peripheral device that allows the computer to communicate with other computers or terminals over the telephone lines.

monitor: a visual display unit with a screen called a cathode ray tube (CRT).

mon/o, mono-: one; single.

monocytes: the largest white blood cells.

morbidly obese: a condition in which an individual is 100 lbs or more over the desired weight.

mouse: a handheld computer input device, usually separate from the keyboard, used to control cursor position.

MSDS: material safety data sheet; an official required document that identifies all the chemicals that are used in a specific department and that details important information regarding those chemicals.

multiple-sample needle: a needle used for venipuncture that has both ends beveled; one end pierces the patient's skin, and the other end pierces a vacuum tube.

myel/o: spinal cord; bone marrow.

NAACLS: National Accrediting Agency for Clinical Laboratory Sciences; an organization responsible for evaluating the quality of laboratory educational programs.

***nasopharyngeal:** of or relating to the nose and throat.

***National Accrediting Agency for Clinical Laboratory Sciences:** NAACLS; an organization responsible for evaluating the quality of laboratory educational programs.

National Committee for Clinical Laboratory Standards: NCCLS; a national organization that develops standards for the accurate performance of laboratory procedures based on voluntary consensus.

***NCCLS:** National Committee for Clinical Laboratory Standards; a national organization that develops standards for the accurate performance of laboratory procedures based on voluntary consensus.

***negligence:** the failure to give reasonable care or to do what another prudent person with similar experience, knowledge and background would have done under the same or similar circumstances.

necr/o: pertaining to death.

neo-: new.

neph-, nephr/o: kidney.

neur/o: nerves or nervous system.

neutr/o: neutral.

neutrophils: the most prominent white blood cells, with a three or four-lobed nucleus.

***nonverbal communication:** a form of communication that involves body language, tactile stimulation (touch), and facial expressions.

***nosocomial infection:** an infection that is acquired during a stay at a hospital.

*occult blood testing: an examination for blood, especially in the stool, that is present in such minute quantities that it cannot be visually detected.

*occupational exposure: exposure to infectious materials that can be reasonably anticipated to occur during the course of one's work; exposure can be to the eye, skin, mucous membranes, or through needle sticks or breaks in the skin.

*Occupational Safety and Health Administration: OSHA; a government agency that develops safety standards and establishes maximum levels of exposure to many biohazardous materials.

-oma: tumor.

onc/o: tumor.

*oncology: the area of medicine concerned with the diagnosis and treatment of tumors.

orth/o: straight.

OSHA: Occupational Safety and Health Administration; a government agency that develops safety standards and establishes maximum levels of exposure to many biohazardous materials.

-osis: abnormal condition.

oste/o: bone.

*osteochondritis: inflammation of the bone and cartilage.

*osteomyelitis: severe inflammation of bone and bone marrow, resulting from a bacterial infection.

*outpatient: a patient who receives treatment from a facility without being admitted into the hospital.

output: what the computer produces after information is processed and printed out.

*ova and parasite testing: a microbiology test performed on stool to determine whether a patient has parasite eggs and/or parasites themselves in the stool.

*oxygenated blood: blood that contains a sufficient level of oxygen necessary for proper functioning of the body systems.

panels: a method of organizing blood tests into groupings; examples include liver function panels, kidney function panels, and so on; also known as profiles.

*Pap smear: the scraping and examination of cells from the body, especially the cervix and the vaginal walls; used in the detection of cancer; Papanicolaou test.

para-: beside; beyond; apart from; near; abnormal; irregular; opposite; adjacent to.

path/o, -pathy: disease.

*pathogenic: disease-producing.

*pathologist: a physician with a specialty in pathology (the study of disease); oversees laboratory operations and aids other physicians in the diagnosis and treatment of disease.

*Patient's Bill of Rights: a document that identifies the basic rights of all patients.

*peak level: a drug level in the blood collected 15 to 20 minutes after the dosage has been administered or when the highest serum concentration of the drug is expected.

ped/o: child (Gr.); foot (Lat.)

-penia: lack of; deficiency.

*percentage solutions: the percentage strength of some clinical laboratory solutions expressed in parts per 100.

peri-: surrounding; around.

peripheral: anything plugged into the computer, including the printer, disk drive, monitor, and so on.

*pericardial fluid: fluid surrounding the heart.

*peripheral blood smear: a blood smear made from EDTA-anticoagulated blood or capillary blood that is stained for the purpose of microscopic viewing of blood elements.

peripheral circulation: blood flow to the surface of the skin, extremities, ears, nose, and face.

*peritoneal fluid: the clear fluid secreted by the tissue in the peritoneum.

*petechiae: red spots seen on skin, associated with a decrease in platelet function.

-phil: attraction.

*phenylketonuria testing: PKU testing; testing on a newborn for a recessive, inherited disease in which a body is unable to break down the amino acid phenylalanine.

phleb/o: vein.

phlebotomy: the act of taking blood from a vein.

*phlebotomist: Also known as the clinical laboratory assistant/phlebotomist; a clinical laboratory employee whose duties include obtaining blood specimens, requisitioning laboratory tests on the computer, transporting specimens, preparing specimens for testing, and performing testing in different areas of the clinical laboratory.

*pipette: a narrow glass or plastic tube with both ends open; used for transferring and measuring liquids by bringing liquids into the tube with a pipetting device.

pipette aid: a device that allows fluid to be pulled into a pipette; used instead of pipetting by mouth.

PKU testing: phenylketonuria testing; testing on a newborn for a recessive, inherited disease in which a body is unable to break down the amino acid phenylalanine.

*plasma: the fluid part of the blood that contains serum, proteins, solids, chemical substances, and gases; collected using an anti-coagulated tube.

-plasty: surgical repair.

*platelets: cells found in the blood that assist in clot formation; thrombocytes.

*pleural fluid: fluid in and around the lungs.

-pnea: breathing.

pneum/o: lung.

*pocket resumé: a list to carry with you of important details that are usually requested on job applications, such as a Social Security number, names and addresses of schools attended, and so on.

*point-of-care testing: collection of a blood sample and immediate testing at the site of patient care.

-poiesis: to make.

poly-: many.

post-: following; after.

pre-: in front of; before.

preadmission testing: PAT; a battery of tests routinely performed on patients who are being admitted to the hospital; often includes a complete blood count and a urinalysis.

*prefix: a word element placed in front of a root to modify its meaning.

printer: a device that produces a hard copy; types include laser, dot matrix, and letter quality printers.

*privileged information: confidential data; all data concerning a patient that is disclosed within the healthcare facility.

program: a set of instructions written in computer language, designed to tell the computer how to complete operations.

*prothrombin time: PT; a common blood test used to assess a part of the coagulation system; commonly used to monitor oral anticoagulant therapy such as coumadin therapy.

*proxemics: the study of an individual's concept and use of space.

pseud/o: false.

PT: prothrombin time; a common blood test used to assess a part of the coagulation system; commonly used to monitor oral anticoagulant therapy such as coumadin therapy.

pulm/o, pulmon/o: lung.

pulmonary circulation: the passage of blood from the heart to the lungs for reoxygenation and its return to the heart.

.py/o: pus.

QA: quality assurance; a process of policies, principles, and procedures that provides accurate, reproducible, and reliable test results.

QC: quality control; also called quality assurance; a program throughout the healthcare facility that contains specific policies and procedures that help ensure patient safety and accurate testing results; the program includes maintaining procedure manuals, monitoring equipment, maintaining records, and hospital inspections.

*QNS: an abbreviation for *quantity not sufficient*; in the clinical laboratory, a term often used when a blood sample is insufficient in quantity for testing.

*quality assurance: QA; a process of policies, principles, and procedures that provides accurate, reproducible, and reliable test results.

*quality control: QC; also called quality assurance; a program throughout the healthcare facility that contains specific policies and procedures that help ensure patient safety and accurate testing results; the program includes maintaining procedure manuals, monitoring equipment, maintaining records, and hospital inspections.

*radial artery: the artery located near the radius in the wrist; one of the places suitable for taking a pulse.

RAM: random access memory; temporary or programmable memory that stops when the machine is turned off.

*random urine specimen: a urine specimen collected at any time of the day or night.

rapport: a satisfactory relationship with others.

*ratio: a relationship between two substances in degree or number.

*reagent: a substance used in laboratory testing procedures to detect and measure other substances.

*reasonable care: care that a healthcare worker is expected to provide to patients.

*red blood cells: also known as erythrocytes; cells primarily involved in the transportation of oxygen to the cells of the body.

removable disks: information storage devices that can be removed from a computer.

ren/o: kidney.

reproducibility: the ability to obtain the same or nearly the same results after testing a specimen several times.

*resistance: the ability to fight off a particular force, such as an infection.

*resumé: a brief, written account of personal and professional qualifications and experience that is prepared by an applicant for a position.

resuscitate: to revive or bring back to life.

-rhage, -rhagia: bursting forth; excessive flow of blood.

ROM: read only memory; permanent memory in a computer determined by the computer manufacturer.

*safety hood: a device that separates a laboratory employee from a specimen or potentially toxic materials by a glass in front of the face. Fumes and aerosols are drawn through the top of the hood and away from the employee.

*satellite blood drawing station: an area separate from the clinical laboratory where specimens are collected and transported to the main clinical laboratory for testing.

scler/o: hardening; sclera (white of the eye).

sclerosed veins: veins that are hardened, often due to excessive growth of fibrous tissue.

-scope: instrument used to examine or look into a part.

*scope of practice: a legal description of what a specific health professional may and may not do.

scrolling: moving the cursor up, down, left or right through information on the computer display.

security code: a code you must enter before accessing a computer system; especially important in a health-care facility where much information is privileged.

*semen: the thick, white secretion discharged by the male sex organs that carries sperm.

seminal fluid: semen.

semi-: half.

sept/o: poison.

*septicemia: the presence in the bloodstream of infectious microorganisms or their toxins.

*serology: often a subdepartment of the blood bank; concerned with tests using antigen/antibody reactions.

*serum: the liquid portion of the blood after blood coagulation.

*serum separator tubes: vacuum tubes that can contain thixotropic gel that forms a physical barrier of separation, glass particles that accelerate clotting, and a filter that separates the cellular from the liquid components of blood.

*sharps: a general term given to all items in the operating room that are sharp; includes scalpel blades, needles, and glass items.

*skin puncture: also known as a capillary puncture; collecting blood after puncturing the skin with a lancet or similar skin puncture device.

*slander: a spoken attack on a person's reputation.

sodium fluoride: an agent used in the clinical laboratory as a preservative for drawing glucose blood levels.

*software: computer programs necessary to direct the hardware of a computer system.

specimen: a sample of something tested to determine the nature of characteristics of the whole, such as blood, sputum, stool and other bodily substances, that is submitted to the clinical laboratory for testing.

*specimen processing: also known as the *central processing area*; the area of the clinical laboratory where specimens are processed for testing in various departments of the clinical laboratory as well as specimens for transport to other facilities.

spinal tap: also known as a spinal or lumbar puncture; a needle puncture of the spinal cavity at the lumbar level to extract spinal fluid for diagnostic purposes.

spreadsheet: a computer program that has mathematical processing capabilities.

*sputum: mucous coughed up from the lung.

*Standard Precautions: guidelines developed by The Centers for Disease Control and Prevention for protecting healthcare workers from exposure to bloodborne pathogens in body secretions.

*standards: substances having a known value used in quality control testing.

-stasis: stopping

sten-, steno-: contracted; narrow.

stomat/o: mouth.

-stomy: surgical creation of an opening.

*stool: feces.

streptococcus: a spherical bacterium that appears in chain-like formations; can cause pathologic conditions in human beings.

sub-: under; below.

*suffix: a word element placed at the end of a root to modify its meaning.

super-: over; above.

supra-: over; above.

*syncope: fainting; sudden, brief, and temporary loss of consciousness; passing out.

*synovial fluid: the clear fluid surrounding a joint.

*syringe: a device used to inject fluids or medications into the body or withdraw them from the body.

systemic circulation: circulation throughout the body except to the lungs.

tachy-: fast; rapid; swift.

*TC: initials meaning *to contain*; glassware calibrated to contain the measurement specified.

*TD: initials meaning *to deliver*; glassware that has been calibrated to deliver a specific volume of liquid into another vessel.

TDM: therapeutic drug monitoring; collection and testing of blood to evaluate and manage medication therapy effectively and safely.

terminal: a device used to communicate with a computer, usually a keyboard and a monitor; a medical office may have several terminals and one computer, which is located elsewhere in the office or building.

test tube: a small plastic or glass tube that is available in a variety of sizes; the container used most commonly in the clinical laboratory.

*therapeutic drug monitoring: TDM; collection and testing of blood to evaluate and manage medication therapy effectively and safely.

therm/o: heat.

thorac/o: chest.

thromb/o: clot.

thrombocytes: blood platelets.

thrombocytopenia: an abnormal decrease of platelets in the circulating blood.

thrombocytosis: an abnormal increase in the number of platelets in the circulating blood.

*thrombi: blood clots.

*thrombosed: clotted with blood.

thrombotic: related to the formation, development, or existence of a blood clot within the vascular system.

-tomy: cutting into; incision.

*Total Quality Management: TQM; an overall institutional process to assess quality and constantly improve patient care.

*tourniquet: a device, often a rubber band at least $^{1}/_{2}$ inch wide, that reduces the flow of blood in the veins and allows the veins to become more prominent.

tox/o, toxi-: poison.

*toxicology: specimens evaluated for the presence of drugs.

TQM: Total Quality Management; an overall institutional process to assess quality and constantly improve patient care.

trans-: across; through.

Transmission-based Precautions: guidelines developed by The Centers for Disease Control and Prevention to help prevent transmission of specific infectious and communicable diseases of patients either suspected of having, or confirmed to have, certain pathogens.

*TRICARE: formerly known as CHAMPUS; a government healthcare insurance program that covers dependents of active-duty and retired military personnel.

*trough level: a drug level in the blood collected when the lowest serum concentration is expected, which is usually immediately before the administration of the next dosage.

*turbidity: the appearance of cloudiness in a normally clear liquid. In the laboratory, often due to the growth of microorganisms in the specimen.

*2-hour post prandial: a blood test drawn 2 hours after a meal.

*24-hour urine specimen: urine collected in a container over a period of 24 hours.

*ulnar artery: an artery located in the wrist opposite the radial artery; not used for arterial puncture.

-uria: present in urine.

*urinalysis: the examination of urine to observe the physical, chemical, and microscopic characteristics to assess the possibility of infection, disease, or damage to the urinary tract.

*urinary tract infection: UTI; a cluster of symptoms characterized by dysuria, frequent urination, urgency, and white blood cells in the urine.

*urine culture and sensitivity: a test where a urine specimen is placed on special growth media to grow an organism for identification and also for testing with antibiotics to ascertain the best antibiotic to use to kill the infectious organism.

uro-: presence in urine.

*vacuum tube system: a system used for blood collection; contains a disposable needle, an adapter (holder), and various types of blood collection tubes.

VAD: vascular access device; a device used to automatically remove blood from a patient without having to stick the patient with a needle.

vas/o: duct; vessel; vas deferens.

*vascular access device: VAD; a device used to automatically remove blood from a patient without having to stick the patient with a needle.

*vein: a blood vessel that carries low-oxygenated blood to the heart.

ven/o: vein.

venous: of or relating to a vein.

venules: microscopic veins that attach directly to capillaries.

*ventricles: the pumping chambers of the heart, located inferior to the atria.

*verbal communication: communication by the spoken word.

vertical: perpendicular to the horizon.

*void: to urinate.

volume: the space occupied by a substance, usually a gas or a liquid.

volume-to-volume percentage: a calculation used when determining how much of two liquids are to be mixed together.

*volumetric glassware: carefully manufactured glassware to contain, transfer, or deliver exact amounts of substances.

volumetric pipettes: pipettes that are carefully calibrated to measure exact amounts of liquids.

weight: the physical measure of an object depending on the physical force of gravity.

weight-to-volume percentage: a calculation used when determining how much of a solid to dissolve in a liquid.

*white blood cells: also known as *leukocytes*; blood cells responsible for fighting infection.

word processing: a computer application that allows the user to input, format and edit documents before printing them out.

*word root: the body or main part of the word, referring to the primary meaning of a word as a whole.

*Workers' Compensation: a program established by law in each state providing income and healthcare insurance to persons who become ill or injured in the course of their employment.

* denotes Key Term.

Common Medical Abbreviations

ABO: blood group system.
AIDS: acquired immune deficiency syndrome.
aka: also known as.
alk phos: alkaline phosphatase.
ALL: acute lymphocytic leukemia.
ALT: alanine transaminase.
AML: acute myelocytic leukemia.
ASAP: as soon as possible.
ASCP: American Society of Clinical Pathologists.
AST: asparate aminotransferase.
BID or **bid:** twice daily.
bl: blood.
BP: blood pressure.
BUN: blood urea nitrogen.
c̄: with.
Ca: calcium.
CA: cancer.
CAD: coronary artery disease.
CBC: complete blood count.
cc: cubic centimeter.
CCU: Coronary Care Unit.
cm: centimeter.
CML: chronic myelogenous leukemia.
CNS: central nervous system.
CO: carbon monoxide.
CO_2: carbon dioxide.
COPD: chronic obstructive pulmonary disease.
CPR: cardiopulmonary resuscitation.
CSF: cerebrospinal fluid.
CVA: cerebrovascular accident.
diff: differential white blood cell count.
dil: dilute.
DOB: date of birth.
DRG: diagnosis related group.
Dx: diagnosis.
EBV: Epstein-Barr virus.
ECG or **EKG:** electrocardiogram.
EEG: electroencephalogram.
EENT: eye, ear, nose, and throat.
eos: eosinophils.
ER: emergency room.
ESR: erythrocyte sedimentation rate.
FBS: fasting blood sugar.
Fe: iron.
FUO: fever of undetermined origin.
g, Gm, or **gm:** gram.

GI: gastrointestinal.
GTT: glucose tolerance test.
Gtt, gtt: drops.
GYN or **gyn:** gynecology.
h: hour.
hb or **hgb:** hemoglobin.
HBV: hepatitis B virus.
HCG: human chorionic gonadotropin.
HCl: hydrochloric acid.
Hct: hematocrit.
HDL: high-density lipoprotein.
HIV: human immunodeficiency virus.
ICU: Intensive Care Unit.
IM: intramuscular.
IV: intravenous.
IVP: intravenous pyelogram.
K: potassium.
Kg: kilogram.
L or **l:** liter; left.
LD or **LDH:** lactic dehydrogenase.
LDL: low-density lipoprotein.
LE: lupus erythematosis.
MCH: mean corpuscular hemoglobin.
MCHC: mean corpuscular hemoglobin concentration.
MCV: mean corpuscular volume.
mEq: milliequivalents.
mg: milligram.
Mg: magnesium.
MI: myocardial infarction.
ml: milliliter.
mm: millimeter.
mono: monocyte.
Na: sodium.
neg: negative.
NG: nasogastric.
nm: nanometer.
NPO: nothing by mouth.
O_2: oxygen.
OB or **Obs:** obstetrics.
OR: operating room.
path: pathology.
peds: pediatrics.
pH: hydrogen ion concentration (potential of hydrogen); the expression of degree of acidity or alkalinity of a substance.

PKU: phenylketonuria.
PMNs: polymorphonuclear leukocytes.
pos: positive.
post-op: after the surgery.
PP: postprandial (after meals).
PT: prothrombin time/protime or physical therapy.
PTT: partial thromboplastin time.
pt: patient.
QNS: quantity not sufficient.
RBC: red blood cell/count.
RIA: radioimmunoassay.
R/O: rule out.
RT: respiratory therapy.
s̄: without.
sed rate: erythrocyte sedimentation rate (ESR).
segs: segmented white blood cells.
SLE: systemic lupus erythematosis.
SpGr or **sp gr:** specific gravity.

staph: staphylococcus.
STAT: immediately, at once.
STD: sexually transmitted disease.
strep: streptococcus.
TB: tuberculosis.
T-cells: lymphocytes from the thymus.
T & C: type and cross-match.
TIBC: total iron binding capacity.
trig: triglycerides.
TSH: thyroid-stimulating hormone.
TURP: transurethral resection of the prostate.
UA: urinalysis.
URI: upper respiratory infection.
UTI: urinary tract infection.
UV: ultraviolet.
VD: venereal disease.
WBC: white blood cell/count.

Frequently Ordered Clinical Laboratory Tests

PROCEDURE	SPECIMEN TYPE	NORMAL RANGE
Hematology Testing		
Complete Blood Count	EDTA, > ½ full	
WBC		$4.4\text{-}10.04 \times 10^3$ µL
RBC		Females: $4.0\text{-}5.3 \times 10^6$ µL
		Males: $4.5\text{-}5.9 \times 10^6$ µL
Hemoglobin (Hgb)		Females: $11.8\text{-}15.8 \times 10^6$ µL
		Males: $13.4\text{-}17.8 \times 10^6$ µL
Hematocrit (HCT)		Females: 36-50%
		Males: 42-54%
MCV		Females: 86-100 fL
		Males: 84-100 fL
MCH		27.2 -32.2 pg
MCHC		31.3-34.7 g/dL
Platelets		6.5 - 9.3 fL
Differential (Diff)		100%
Neutrophils (Segs)		40-74%
Lymphocytes (Lymphs)		18-44%
Monocytes (Monos)		3-9%
Eosinophils (Eos)		0-5%
Basophils (Basos)		0-2%
Reticulocyte Count	EDTA, > ½ full or capillary puncture	0.5 - 1.5% Adults At birth: 2.5 to 6.5%
Sickle Cell Prep	EDTA, > ½ full	Negative
Sedimentation Rate (Westergren)	EDTA, > ½ full	Females < 50: 0-25 mm/h Females > 50: 0-30 mm/h Males < 50: 0-15 mm/h Males > 50: 0-20 mm/h

PROCEDURE	SPECIMEN TYPE	NORMAL RANGE
Coagulation Testing		
APTT (Activated partial thromboplastin)	Citrate, 4.5 ml/ full	22-35 seconds
Bleeding Time - Ivy (Simplate®, Surgicutt®)	Forearm	1.6 - 8 minutes
Clot Retraction	Red clot tube	1.6-8.0 minutes
FDP/FSP (Fibrin degradation products/Fibrinogen split products or D-Dimer)	Special blue tube with yellow label 2.0 ml citrate, full	Negative <10 µg/ml
Fibrinogen	Citrate, full	200-400 mg/dL
Prothrombin Time (Protime, PT)	Citrate, full	10.9-12.9 seconds
Thrombin Time	Citrate, full	Clot forms within 10 seconds; solid gel clot at 60 seconds
Urine Testing		
Urinalysis, Routine	Random urine, at least 10 ml	
Color		Yellow, straw, dark yellow
Appearance		Clear, hazy
Specific gravity		1.003-1.030
pH		5-6 in 1st AM specimen
Glucose		Negative
Ketone		Negative
Bilirubin		Negative
Protein		< 25 mg/dl
Blood		Negative
Urobilinogen		0.2 - 1.0 Ehrlich units/dl
Nitrite		Negative
Leucocyte Esterase		Negative

PROCEDURE	SPECIMEN TYPE	NORMAL RANGE
Chemistry Testing		
Alcohol, blood	EDTA, 0.5 ml or SST	Legal Limit: 0.08 G% (varies among states)
Alkaline phosphatase (alk phos; ALP)	SST, 1.0 ml serum Iced	30-115µ/L
Ammonia (NH_3)	Heparin, 0.5 ml	0-90 µg/dL or 0-50 µmol/L
Amylase	SST, 0.3 ml	20-110 µ/L
Bilirubin, Total	SST, 1.0 ml	0.2-1.2 mg/dL Newborn: 2.0-6.0 mg/dL 48 hrs: 6.0 - 7.0 mg/dL 3-5 days: 4.0-12.0 mg/dL
Bilirubin, Direct and Indirect	SST, 1.0 ml	Direct: 0 - 0.4 mg/dL Indirect: 0.2-1.2 mg/dL
Blood Urea Nitrogen (BUN)	SST, 1.0 ml	7-26 mg/dL
Calcium	SST, 1.0 ml	8.5-10.5 mg/dL
Biocarbonate (CO_2; carbon dioxide)	SST, 1.0 ml	24-30 mEq/L
Chloride, serum	SST, 1.0 ml	101-111 mEq/L
Cholesterol	SST, 1.0 m	Desirable: under 200 mg/dL
Creatine Phosphokinase (CPK, CK)	SST, 0.3 ml	0-225 U/L
Creatinine, serum	SST, 0.3 ml	0.7-1.5 mg/dL
Gamma GT (GGT, GTP)	SST, 0.3 ml	Females: 5-45 U/L Males: 9-85 U/L
Glucose, serum (blood sugar; FBS)	SST, 1.0 ml sodium fluoride (gray tube)	Fasting: 85-125 mg/dL >50 yr 70-115 mg/dL <50 yr
Glucose, serum/ 2-hour pp	sodium fluoride (gray tube)	<130 mg/dL

Lactic dehydrogenase (LDH, LD)	SST, 1.0	60-200 U/L
Potassium, serum (K)	SST, 1.0 ml	3.5-5.0 mEq/L
Protein, total serum	SST, 1.0 ml	6.0-8.5 g/dL
SGOT (AST) (serum glutamic oxaloacetic transaminase)	SST, 1.0 ml	0-41 U/L
SGPT (ALT) (glutamic pyruvate transaminase)	SST, 1.0 ml	0-45 U/L
Sodium, serum (Na)	SST, 1.0 ml	136-145 mEq/L
Therapeutic Drug Monitoring (TDM)	SST, 1.0	
Dilantin/Phenytoin		Therapeutic: 10-20 µg/L Toxic: 30 µg/L
Gentamicin/Garamycin		Therapeutic: Trough - < 2.0 µg/L Peak: 5-10 µg/L
Lithium (Li)		Therapeutic: 0.4-1.0 mEq/L
Theophylline/Theo-Dur/Aminophylline		Therapeutic: 10-20 µg/L
Triglycerides	SST, 1.0 ml	30-175 mg/dL
Uric Acid	SST, 1.0 ml	Females: 2.2-7.7 mg/dL Males: 3.9-9.0 mg/dL

Microbiology Testing

Blood Culture	Aerobic/anaerobic bottles; 5-10 ml of blood for each	No growth
KOH Prep	Skin scraping or hair from infected area	Negative
Occult Blood, Stool (Guaiac Test)	Fresh feces only	Negative

Streptococcus A (Rapid Antigen Detection; Rapid Strep A Test)	Throat swab	Negative
Susceptibility Testing (MIC; sensitivity testing)	Any specimen to be tested	No growth

Blood Bank (Immunohematology) Testing

ABO, Rh Blood Type (Type and Rh)	Clot tube, 1-10 ml	
Antibody Identification Panel	Clot tube, 1-10 ml and 1-5 ml EDTA	
Crossmatch, whole blood	Clot tube, 10 ml	
Direct Coombs	EDTA	Negative
Indirect Coombs Antibody Screen	Clot tube	Negative

Immunology/Serology Testing

ANA (antinuclear antibody)	SST, 1.0 ml	< than 1:40
ASO (antistreptolysin O)	SST, 1.0 ml	0-124.9 IU/ml
Cold Agglutinin	SST, 1.0 ml	< 1:40
Heterophile/Mononucleus Screen (Infectious Mono Test)	SST, 1.0 ml	Negative
HIV AIDS Screen (HTLV-III)	SST, 1.5 ml	Negative
RPR	SST, 1.5 ml	Negative
Serum Pregnancy	SSGT, 0.5 ml	Negative

Metric Conversions
for the Clinical Laboratory

MASS

1 ounce (oz) = 28.35 grams (g)

1 pound (lb) = 453.6 grams (g)

2.205 pounds (lb) = 1 kilogram (kg)

LENGTH

1 inch (in) = 2.54 centimeters (cm)

1 foot (ft) = 30.48 centimeters (cm)

39.37 inches (in) = 1 meter (m)

1 mile (mi) = 1.61 kilometers (km)

VOLUME

1 fluid ounce (fl oz) = 29.57 milliliters (mL)

1.057 quarts (qt) = 1 liter (liter or L)

1 gallon (gal) = 3.78 liters (liter or L)

Formulas and Calculations
Frequently Used in the Clinical Laboratory

Area   square meter (sq m or m^2)

Centrifugal   A measure of the force of centrifugation acting on blood
Force   components and allowing them to separate. Often used
                            in calibration of centrifuges.

                            rcf = 1.118 X 10^{-5} X r X n^2
                            r = rotating radius (centimeters)
                            n = speed of rotation (revolutions per minute)

Density   kilogram/liter (kg/L)

Dilutions   Final concentration = Original concentration X dilution 1
                            X dilution 2, and so on

Hematology math   Mean cellular volume (MCV) = average volume of red
                            blood cells (RBCs); expressed in cubic microns (μm^3) or
                            femtoliters (fL)

                            $$MCV = \frac{Hct \times 10}{RBC\ count\ (in\ millions)}$$

                            Hct = hematocrit value

                            Mean cellular hemoglobin (MCH) = average weight of
                            hemoglobin in RBC; expressed in picograms (pg)

                            $$MCH = \frac{Hgb\ (g) \times 10}{RBC\ count\ (in\ millions)}$$

                            Hgb = hemoglobin value

                            Mean cellular hemoglobin concentration (MCHC) =
                            hemoglobin concentration of average RBC

                            $$MCHC = \frac{Hgb\ (g) \times 100}{Hct}$$

                            Red blood cell distribution width (RDW) = expression of
                            variation of RBC size, dispersion of RBC volumes about the
                            mean

                            $$RDW = \frac{SD\ (standard\ deviation)\ of\ RBC\ size}{MCV}$$

Mass   kilogram/liter (kg/L)

Proportion $\dfrac{C}{A + b} = V$

Quality Control   variance (s^2) $s^2 = \dfrac{(x - x)^2}{n-1}$
Calculations

                             standard deviation (SD) $SD = \sqrt{2}$

                             % Coefficient of variation $\%CV = \dfrac{s}{X} \times 100$

Solutions   Specific gravity (sp gr) :

                             sp gr + $\dfrac{\text{weight of a solid or liquid}}{\text{weight of equal volume of } H_2 0 \text{ at } 4°C}$

Substrate   mole/liter (mol/L)

Temperature   Celsius (Centigrade): $°C = K - 273$
                                                     $°C = \dfrac{5}{9} (F- 32)$

                             Kelvin: $°K = °C + 273$
                                       $°K = \dfrac{5}{9} (°F) + 255$

                             Fahrenheit: $°F = \dfrac{9}{5} C + 32$

Vacuum Tube Selection Guide

LAB DEPARTMENT	SPEC. TYPE	STOPPER	ADDITIVE
BLOOD BANK	Clotted blood	Red	None
CHEMISTRY	Serum	Red/yellow marbled (serum separator tube)	Glass particles (activate lot)
	Serum	Red/gray (serum separator)	Thixotropic gel
	Serum	Navy Blue	None
	Plasma	Navy Blue	Sodium heparin
	Plasma for sugar testing	Gray	Sodium fluoride
	Plasma	Green	Lithium heparin
	Plasma	Green	Sodium heparin
COAGULATION	Plasma	Light blue	Sodium citrate
HEMATOLOGY	Whole blood	Purple	EDTA (anticoag.)
IMMUNOLOGY	Serum	Red (serum separator)	None
MICROBIOLOGY	Whole blood	Yellow Ivory	Sodium polyanethole sulfonate (SPS)

Normal Laboratory Values for Selected Animal Blood Tests

The values listed in this chart are an average of laboratory values found using a variety of laboratory methods. Values are given for adult animals. There can be variation among breeds of these animals.

TEST	DOG	CAT	RAT	MOUSE	GUINEA PIG	RABBIT
WBC (10^3/ mL)	6,000–17,000	5,500–19,500	8–10,000	8,000–10,000	5,000–12,000	8,000–10,000
RBC (10^6/mL)	5,5–8.5	5.5–10.0	7.2–9.6	9.3–10.5	4.5–7.0	3.2–7.5
HGB (gm/dL)	12–18	8–14	14.5–15	12–14.9	11–15	10–15
HCT (%)	37–55%	24–45%	40–50%	35–50%	35–50%	35–45%
DIFF (out of 100)						
Segs	60–77	35–75	30	26	42	30–50
Lymphs	12–30	20–55	65–77	55–80	45–81	30–50
Monos	3–10	1–4	4	5	8	9
Eos	2–10	2–12	1	3	5	1
Basos	Rare	Rare	0	0	2	0
SODIUM (mEq/L)	144–154	146–161	144	114–154	120–155	100–145
POTASSIUM (mEq/L)	3.8–5.8	3.7–4.9	5.9	3.0–9.6	6.5–8.2	3.0–7.0
GLUCOSE (mg/dL)	50–120	70–150	50–115	108–192	60–125	50–140
BUN (mg/dL)	10–22	5–30	10–20	8–30	8–20	5–30
ALK PHOS (IU/L)	20–30	10–80	4.1–8.6	2.4–4.0	1.5–8.1	2.1–3.2
BILIRUBIN (mg/dL)	0–0.6	0–0.8	0.42	0.18–0.54	.24–.30	0.15–0.20

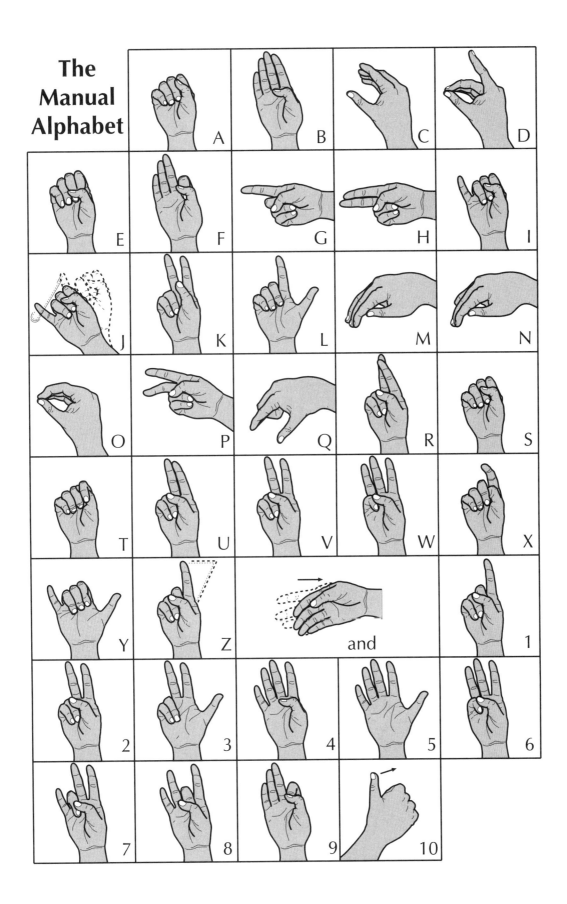

Bibliography

Chabner, Davi-Ellen, *The Language of Medicine, 5th Edition*. Philadelphia, PA: W.B. Saunders Company, 1996.

Crouch, James E., PhD. *Text-Atlas of Cat Anatomy*. Philadelphia: Lea & Febiger, 1961.

Davis, Bonnie K. *Phlebotomy: A Client-Based Approach*. Albany, New York: Delmar Publishers, 1997.

Flynn, John C., Jr. *Procedures in Phlebotomy*. Philadelphia, PA: W.B. Saunders Company, 1994.

Fordney, Marilyn T., Follis, Joan J. *Administrative Medical Assisting, 3rd edition*. Albany, New York: Delmar Publishers, Inc., 1993.

Fremgen, Bonnie F. *Medical Terminology: An Anatomy and Physiology Systems Approach*. New Jersey: Prentice Hall, 1997.

Garber, Debra L. *Introduction to Clinical Allied Healthcare, Second Edition*. Orange, California: Career Publishing, Inc., 1996.

Garza, Diane, and Becan-McBride, Kathleen. *Phlebotomy Handbook, 4th edition*. Stamford, Connecticut: Appleton & Lange, 1996.

Glanze, Walter, ed. *The Mosby Medical Encyclopedia, Revised Edition*. St. Louis: The C.V. Mosby Company, 1992.

Iverson, Cheryl; Dan, MD, Bruce B.; Glitman, Paula; King, MD, Lester S.; Knoll, PhD, Elizabeth; Meyer, MD, Harriet S.; Raithel, Kathryn Simmons; Riesenberg, MD, Don; Young, Roxanne K; *American Medical Association Manual of Style, 8th Edition*. Chicago: American Medical Association, 1989.

Katz, N.H., and Lawyer, J.W. *Communication and Conflict Resolution Skills*. Dubuque: Jendall/Hunt Publishing, 1985.

Keir, Lucille, Wise, Barbara A., Krebs, Connie. *Medical Assisting: Administrative and Clinical Competencies, 3rd edition*. Albany, New York: Delmar Publishers, Inc., 1993.

Kovanda, Beverly M., ed. *Phlebotomy Collection Procedures for the Health Care Provider*. Albany, New York, 1998.

Marshall, Jacquelyn R. *Being a Medical Clerical Worker, 2nd Edition*. Upper Saddle River, New Jersey: Brady , 1998.

Marshall, Jacquelyn R. *Fundamental Skills for the Clinical Laboratory Professional.* Albany, New York: Delmar Publishers, 1993.

Marshall, Jacquelyn R. *Medical Laboratory Assistant.* Englewood Cliffs, New Jersey: Brady, 1990.

Martini, Frederic H. *Fundamentals of Anatomy and Physiology/Applications Manual.* New Jersey: Prentice Hall, 1997.

McBrien, Marianne. *The Emergency Room Technician.* Orange, California: Career Publishing, Inc., 1995.

McCall, Ruth E., and Tankersley, Cathee M. *Phlebotomy Essentials.* Philadelphia: J.B. Lippincott Company, 1993.

Evans, H., PhD and Christensen, George, DVM. *Miller's Anatomy of the Dog.* Philadelphia: W.B. Saunders Company, 1993.

National Committee for Clinical Laboratory Standards. H18A: *Procedures for the Handling and Processing of Blood Specimens.* Villanova, PA, 1991.

National Committee for Clinical Laboratory Standards. *117P: Protection of Laboratory Workers from Instrument Biohazards: Proposed Guidelines.* Villanova, PA, September, 1991.

National Committee for Clinical Laboratory Standards. *H3-A4: Procedures for the Collection of Diagnostic Blood Specimens by Venipuncture, 4th edition, Approved Standard.* Villanova, PA, 1997.

National Committee for Clinical Laboratory Standards. *M29-A: Protection of Laboratory Workers from Infectious Disease Transmitted by Blood, Body Fluids, and Tissue, Approved Standard.* Villanova, PA, 1997.

O'Toole, Marie T., ed. *Miller-Keane Encyclopedia and Dictionary of Medicine, Nursing, and Allied Health, Sixth Edition.* Philadelphia: W.B. Saunders, 1997.

Suckow, Mark A., DVM, and Douglas, Fred A., BS, LATG. *The Laboratory Rabbit.* New York: CRC Press, 1997.

Thomas, Clayton L., MD, MPH. *Taber's Cyclopedic Medical Dictionary, 18th Edition.* Philadelphia: F.A. Davis Company, 1997.

Virgilio, Mary. *The Operating Room Aide.* Orange, California: Career Publishing, Inc., 1997.

Index

Clinical Allied Healthcare Series

*Created by healthcare professionals and experienced educators, this Series brings students the knowledge and training essential for careers in hospitals, medical centers, and physicians' offices. **Career's Clinical Allied Healthcare Series** encourages students to master concepts and skills in its intelligent, reader-friendly text, informative illustrations and graphs, critical thinking exercises, and student enrichment activities. This Series offers administrators the coursework texts that fill classrooms—and students and instructors a text series that is the most versatile and comprehensive in its field.*

Introduction to Clinical Allied Healthcare, 2nd Edition (Core Text)

Introduction to Healthcare Facilities • The Acute Care Hospital • Hospital Employees and Medical Staff • The Allied Health Worker, the Law, and Professional Ethics • Understanding the Patient as a Person • Communication Skills • The Safe Workplace • Disasters: Preparedness, Hazards, & Prevention • Infection Control • Fundamental Skills • Fundamental Patient Care Equipment • Introduction to Medical Terminology • Introduction to the Human Body • Support, Movement, & Protection: The Skeletal, Muscular, and Integumentary Systems • Transporting and Transmitting: The Circulatory, Lymphatic, and Nervous Systems • Excretion: The Respiratory, Digestive, and Urinary Systems • The Specialties: The Sensory and Reproductive Systems • Basic First Aid • Healthful Living • Career Planning

ISBN 0-89262-551-1 .... **CALL FOR QUOTE**
Workbook **ISBN 0-89262-550-3** .... **CALL**
Instructor's Guide **ISBN 0-89262-552-X**

The Emergency Department Technician

Health Careers in Emergency Care • Introduction to Emergency Medical Services • The Working Environment • Asepsis • Admitting Procedures • Patient Evaluation • Safety In the Emergency Department • Basic Life Support • Emergencies of the Eye, Ear, Nose, and Throat • Medical Emergencies • Abdominal Emergencies • Emergencies of the Reproductive System • Wound Care • Traumatic Emergencies • Bone and Joint Injuries • Moving and Positioning Patients • Environmental Emergencies • Poisoning and Overdose • Emotional and Behavioral Emergencies • Caring for Children • Care of the Elderly

ISBN 0-89262-432-9 .... **CALL FOR QUOTE**
Instructor's Guide **ISBN 0-89262-440-X**

The Clinical Laboratory Assistant/Phlebotomist

Introduction to the Career of Clinical Laboratory Assistant/Phlebotomist • Departments in the Clinical Laboratory • Medical Terminology for the Clinical Laboratory Assistant/Phlebotomist • Ethical and Legal Considerations for the Clinical Laboratory Assistant/Phlebotomist • Infection Control Practices in the Clinical Laboratory • General Safety Issues in the Healthcare Environment • An Introduction to Blood Drawing: The Circulatory System • Preparing for Blood Collection • Performing the Venipuncture • Performing the Skin Puncture • Special Blood Collection Procedures • Hazards and Complications of Blood Drawing • Obtaining Blood Samples from Animals • Urine Specimen Collection • Collection of Other Non-Blood Specimens • Quality Assurance and the Clinical Laboratory Assistant/Phlebotomist • Transporting, Processing, and Distributing Clinical Specimens • Operating Laboratory Equipment • Measurements and Calculations • Reception and Telephone Technique • The Computer System and Other Office Machines • Health Insurance • Customer Service Skills • Conflict Management in the Clinical Laboratory • Obtaining the Right Job for You • The Excellent Clinical Laboratory Employee • Certification, Regulations, and Continuing Education Requirements

ISBN 0-89262-434-5 .... **CALL FOR QUOTE**
Instructor's Guide **ISBN 0-89262-442-6**

The Operating Room Aide

Introduction to the Operating Room • Medical Terminology for the Operating Room • Principles of Microbiology & Infection Control • Medical and Surgical Asepsis • Operating Room Design and Surgical Equipment • Safety & Patient Care in the Operating Room • Procedures in the Operating Room • Emergencies in the Operating Room • The Operating Room Aide in the Instrument Room

ISBN 0-89262-433-7 .... **CALL FOR QUOTE**
Instructor's Guide **ISBN 0-89262-441-8**

The Mental Health Worker: Psychiatric Aide

Mental Health Care: Past and Present • Normal Growth and Development • Anxiety • Trust and Communication • Safety in the Workplace • General Patient Care • Chemical Dependency • Common Psychiatric Disorders • Developmental Disorders Affecting Children and Adults • Alzheimer's Disease and Other Dementias • Mental Retardation and Other Developmental Anomalies • Assaultive and Other Unsafe Behaviors • Documenting Patient Status • Patients' Rights

ISBN 0-89262-437-X .... **CALL FOR QUOTE**
Instructor's Guide **ISBN 0-89262-445-0**

The Pharmacy Aide

Introduction to the Role of the Pharmacy Aide • The Pharmacy Team The Role and Responsibilities of the Pharmacy Aide • Pharmacology Basics • The Prescription • Inventory Control in the Pharmacy • Staying Healthy as a Pharmacy Aide

ISBN 0-89262-438-8 .... **TBA**
Instructor's Guide **ISBN 0-89262-446-9**

Essentials of Athletic Training and Physical Rehabilitation

Introduction • Athletic Training • Personal Fitness Training • Physical Therapy • Basic Nutrition & Weight Control • Basic Skills • The First Aid Kits • Emergency Preparedness & Assessment • Basic Life Support • The Tissues The Head and Spine • The Shoulders and Upper Extremities • The Chest and Abdomen • The Groin and Lower Extremities • Environmental and Medical Emergencies • Assessment of Physical Fitness • Developing an Individual Training Program • Weight Training • Therapeutic Modalities • Physical Rehabilitation • The Law and Ethics • Resumé and Interview

ISBN 0-89262-436-1 .... **TBA**
Instructor's Guide **ISBN 0-89262-444-2**

The Electrocardiograph Technician

The ECG Technician • Fundamental Concepts • Cardiac Anatomy & Physiology • ECG Basics—The Heartbeat as a Waveform • The 12 Lead ECG • Recognizing Arrhythmias • Bedside Monitoring & Troubleshooting

ISBN 0-89262-435-3 .... **TBA**
Instructor's Guide **ISBN 0-89262-443-4**

The Pharmacy Technician

Content to be determined.
ISBN 0-89262-455-8 .... **TBA**
Instructor's Guide **ISBN 0-89262-446-9**

Phone *Toll Free* — From the U.S./Alaska, Hawaii, Canada & Puerto Rico **1-800-854-4014 (FAX 1-714-532-0180)**

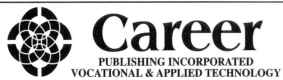

Career
PUBLISHING INCORPORATED
VOCATIONAL & APPLIED TECHNOLOGY

910 N. Main Street • Orange, CA 92867-5403
P.O. Box 5486 • Orange, CA 92863-5486

Call our Order Dept. at our
National Toll Free Number

1-800-854-4014

includes Alaska, Hawaii,
Puerto Rico, and Canada

FAX ORDERS
1-(714)-532-0180
24 HOURS

ORDER FORM

Clinical Allied Healthcare Series

PLEASE SEND THE FOLLOWING

QTY.	CODE	TITLE	NET PRICE	TOTAL
	0-89262-551-1	**Intro. to Clinical Allied Healthcare, 2nd Edition** (*Core Text*)	CALL FOR QUOTE	$
	0-89262-550-3	**Introduction to Clinical Allied Healthcare** *Workbook*		$
	0-89262-552-X	**Intro. to Clinical Allied Healthcare, 2nd Ed.** *Instructor's Guide*		$
	0-89262-432-9	**The Emergency Department Technician**		$
	0-89262-440-X	**The Emergency Department Technician** *Instructor's Guide*		$
	0-89262-433-7	**The Operating Room Aide**		$
	0-89262-441-8	**The Operating Room Aide** *Instructor's Guide*		$
	0-89262-437-X	**The Mental Health Worker: Psychiatric Aide**		$
	0-89262-445-0	**The Mental Health Worker: Psychiatric Aide** *Instructor's Guide*		$
	0-89262-434-5	**The Clinical Laboratory Assistant/Phlebotomist**		$
	0-89262-442-6	**The Clinical Lab. Assistant/Phlebotomist** *Instructor's Guide*		$
	0-89262-438-8	**The Pharmacy Aide**	TBA	$
	0-89262-446-9	**The Pharmacy Aide** *Instructor's Guide*	TBA	$
	0-89262-436-1	**Essentials of Athletic Training and Physical Rehabilitation**	TBA	$
	0-89262-444-2	**Essentials of Athletic Train./Phys. Rehab.** *Instructor's Guide*	TBA	$
	0-89262-435-3	**The Electrocardiograph Technician (EKG)**	TBA	$
	0-89262-443-4	**The Electrocardiograph Technician (EKG)** *Instructor's Guide*	TBA	$
	0-89262-455-8	**The Pharmacy Technician**	TBA	$
	0-89262-446-9	**The Pharmacy Technician** *Instructor's Guide*	TBA	$

Payable in U.S. Funds — F.O.B. Orange CA

Shipping, Handling, & Insurance
A single charge to cover shipping, handling, and insurance will be added as a percentage of the total order as follows:

Orders less than $100.00 .... 13%
Orders $100.00 to $499.99 .... 11%
Orders $500.00 to $999.99 .... 9%
Orders of $1,000.00 and over 7%
There will be a minimum charge of $6.00 per order. These costs may be higher for shipments outside the continental United States.

Subtotal $ _____

*Calif. Orders Add Tax _____

TOTAL AMOUNT $ _____

Shipping, Handling, & Insurance Charges _____

GRAND TOTAL $ _____

*California Sales Tax will be added as applicable without Resale Number on file.
PRICES (INCLUDING SHIPPING) AND PUBLICATION DATES SUBJECT TO CHANGE WITHOUT NOTICE.

School/Company/Individual _____ Date _____

Street _____ Phone (___) _____

City _____ State _____ Country _____ Zip _____

Authorized By _____ Title _____

☐ MasterCard ☐ VISA ☐ AMERICAN EXPRESS   Card # _____ Exp. _____
MasterCard   Visa   American Express   16 Digits   Mo/Yr
Signature _____ Exact Name on Card _____

Send me ☐ Order Forms ☐ Catalog ☐ Check enclosed   Purchase Order Number (PO) _____

Printed in the U.S.A.